Clinical Concepts of Infectious Diseases

Clinical Concepts of Infectious Diseases

AUTHORED AND EDITED BY

LEIGHTON E. CLUFF, M.D.

Professor of Medicine;
Chairman, Department of Medicine,
University of Florida College of Medicine,
Gainesville

JOSEPH E. JOHNSON, III, M.D.

Professor of Medicine;
Head, Division of Infectious Diseases
and Clinical Immunology, Department of Medicine,
University of Florida College of Medicine,
Gainesville

The Williams & Wilkins Company BALTIMORE

SANS TACHE

Made in the United States of America

Library of Congress Catalog Card Number 72-187529
SBN 683-01657-1

Composed and printed at the
Waverly Press, Inc.
Mt. Royal and Guilford Aves.
Baltimore, Md. 21202, U.S.A.

PREFACE

Textbooks of Medicine invariably include chapters or sections on infectious diseases and immunology. In some, this may consume 20 percent or more of the text. Usually, comprehensive coverage is attempted, including presentations on almost all microbial diseases, whether esoteric or common, clinically important or unimportant in the United States. Therefore, a proportion of the material covered has limited relevance to training or practice of students, housestaff, and practicing physicians. They serve as essential reference sources but are not prepared for reading and perspective.

Involvement with preclinical education, student clerkships, housestaff, and postdoctoral clinical and research fellowship training over several years convinced us that a collection of selected essays emphasizing concepts of infectious diseases could serve a useful purpose. Therefore, we have arbitrarily chosen to cover aspects of host resistance which have clear clinical implications. We have selected a few clinical problems with broad ramifications, particularly important but not restricted to hospital practice. The principles of prevention of infectious diseases are presented to emphasize an approach to clinical management. Each section is preceded by an introduction to set the stage for the reader.

Our hope is that those reading this book will attain a perspective of the approaches important for thinking about problems in infectious diseases and caring for patients.

To serve as an entry to consideration of infectious diseases not covered fully in the text, we have elected to provide a selected list of references directing the interested reader to some of the important sources of information. The table preceding this section can serve to refresh the reader's memory or orient his thinking about other infectious diseases. Conceivably, in the future, it might be desirable to include sections on infectious diseases not covered in this text or to replace present ones with others.

For example, poliomyelitis would certainly have been included two decades ago, but can now be treated primarily as a preventable and less clinically important infectious disease.

One thing is certain. Infections are and probably always will be a cause of human disease. The microorganisms and their respective diseases, however, may vary from time to time in clinical and theoretical importance.

The contributing authors of this book, for the most part, are past and present associates of the editors. Their efforts are gratefully appreciated. Hopefully, they along with others active in medical education and training will find this book useful in their own teaching programs.

In particular, we wish to extend our gratitude to Mrs. Mary Bob Ellspermann. Without her loyal, efficient and helpful assistance this book would not have materialized.

Leighton E. Cluff, M.D.
Joseph E. Johnson, III, M.D.

CONTRIBUTORS

Allen, James C., Professor of Medicine, State University of New York at Buffalo, Buffalo, New York. (*Chapter 4*)

Ayoub, Elia M., Professor of Pediatrics, University of Florida College of Medicine, Gainesville, Florida. (*Chapter 2, 20*)

Block, A. Jay, Assistant Professor of Medicine, University of Florida College of Medicine, Veterans Administration Hospital, Gainesville, Florida. (*Chapter 16*)

Caldwell, Jacques R., Assistant Professor of Medicine, University of Florida College of Medicine, Gainesville, Florida. (*Chapters 6, 30*)

Cluff, Leighton E., Professor of Medicine, University of Florida College of Medicine, Gainesville, Florida. (*Chapters 7, 9, 11, 12, 13, 15, 19, 25, 33*)

Deal, William B., Assistant Professor of Medicine, University of Florida College of Medicine, Gainesville, Florida. (*Chapter 11*)

Fekety, F. Robert, Jr., Professor of Medicine, University of Michigan School of Medicine, Ann Arbor, Michigan. (*Chapter 8*)

Greer, Melvin, Professor of Medicine (Neurology), University of Florida College of Medicine, Gainesville, Florida. (*Chapter 22*)

Johnson, Joseph E., III, Professor of Medicine, University of Florida College of Medicine, Gainesville, Florida. (*Chapters 1, 14, 18, 24, 26, 33*)

Kaufman, Herbert E., Professor of Ophthalmology, University of Florida College of Medicine, Gainesville, Florida. (*Chapter 28*)

Keene, Willis R., Professor of Medicine, University of Florida College of Medicine, Gainesville, Florida and University Hospital, Jacksonville, Florida. (*Chapter 10*)

McGuigan, James E., Professor of Medicine, University of Florida College of Medicine, Gainesville, Florida. (*Chapter 23*)

Noyes, Ward D., Professor of Medicine, University of Florida College of Medicine, Gainesville, Florida. (*Chapter 10*)

Philp, James R., Senior Lecturer, St. Mary's Hospital Medical School, Wright-Fleming Institute, London, England. (*Chapter 29*)

Reynolds, Richard C., Professor of Medicine and of Community Medicine, University of Florida College of Medicine, Gainesville, Florida. (*Chapter 17*)

Robson, Hugh G., Assistant Professor of Medicine, McGill University School of Medicine, Montreal, Canada. (*Chapter 9*)

Sanders, W. Eugene, Associate Professor of Medicine, University of Florida College of Medicine, Gainesville, Florida. (*Chapters 9, 21, 27*)

Small, Parker A., Jr., Professor of Medical Microbiology and Immunology, University of Florida College of Medicine, Gainesville, Florida. (*Chapter 3*)

Streiff, Richard R., Associate Professor of Medicine, University of Florida College of Medicine, Veterans Administration Hospital, Gainesville, Florida. (*Chapter 10*)

Waldman, Robert H., Assistant Professor of Medicine, University of Florida College of Medicine, Gainesville, Florida. (*Chapters 4, 31*)

CONTENTS

Section 3.
SPECIFIC INFECTIOUS DISEASES

Section 4.
MANAGEMENT AND PREVENTION OF INFECTIOUS DISEASES

Section 5.
TABULATION AND OTHER REFERENCES OF INFECTIOUS DISEASES

SECTION ONE

MECHANISMS AND DISORDERS OF RESISTANCE TO INFECTION

Chapter 1

INTRODUCTION

Man lives in a sea of microorganisms. Intermittently seeding the air he breathes are viruses, bacteria, and spores. Growing on the surfaces of his body, in the hair follicles and cavities of the integument are still other organisms. The food and drink he ingests are virtually never sterile, as the teeming flora of his gastrointestinal tract attest. In the deeper tissues of the body, even within the cells themselves, microbial forms lie dormant....

And yet serious infection is a relatively rare event. Although minor skirmishes occur with considerable frequency, the body's defenses easily repulse or at least come to terms with the majority of microbial invaders. Although it was popular in the past to view man's posture with respect to the microbial world in terms of "nature red in tooth and claw," in actual fact for much of the time the body's ecologic relationship with this sea of microbes is one of commensalism and even occasionally a mutually beneficial symbiosis.

What then are the circumstances in which this happy state of truce collapses? What determines the events which result in tissue invasion, destruction or disease?

It is convenient to conceive of microorganisms as possessing a hierarchy of virulence. Among the flora common to the microenvironment of man are bacteria, for example, which almost never produce significant disease. It is clear that such organisms are easily susceptible to normally-present antibacterial mechanisms. *Sarcina lutea* is readily inactived by lysozyme, and *Bacillus subtilis* by beta lysin. *Staphylococcus epidermidis*, part of the "normal flora" of the skin surface, is readily ingested by the phagocyte without a requirement for specific antibodies. Still other organisms such as the pneumococcus are ordinarily dealt with quite effectively with the assistance of opsonizing antibodies which facilitate phagocytic ingestion. A third order of virulent organisms, including tubercle bacilli, listeria, and histoplasma, are capable of intracellular survival following ingestion by polymorphonuclear leukocytes. When the polymorph dies, the surviving microorganism may even withstand the intracellular assault of the immature mononuclear phagocyte and only succumb after activation produces an "angry macrophage."

Thus, some infectious diseases, especially those due to the microflora indigenous to man, ordinarily result when there is a breakdown in the normal defenses of the host. Others, said to have primary virulence, such as measles and smallpox viruses and the plague and tularemia bacilli, produce disease in virtually all human hosts on initial exposure. Immunity (i.e., resistance acquired either through previous disease or vaccination) is required for protection against these agents.

Although all host defense ultimately derives from the cells of the body, it is customary to consider two basic systems: the *humoral* and the *cellular*. Each system will be seen to have a *"natural"* or normally present component as well as an "acquired" or *immune* component. Normally-present humoral components include substances such as lysozyme, beta lysin, the "natural antibodies" and the complement system, while the cellular "first line of defense" is the phagocytic system composed of polymorphonuclear leukocytes (Chapt. 2) and of the mononuclear phagocytic system (formerly the "reticuloendothelial system"). Polymorphs are mature cells which come equipped with a full set of antibacterial enzymes and digestive factors; while the mononuclear phagocytes tend to be immature and require time and an appropriate stimulus for full activation.

The immune system also is conveniently thought of as having a humoral component—the immunoglobulins (antibodies), and a cellular component—cell-mediated immunity. Because certain of the immunoglobulins (IgA and IgE) appear to function predominantly on body surfaces (the respiratory, gastrointestinal and genital tracts), while the classic antibody systems (especially IgG and IgM) are predominantly intravascular or interstitial, it seems justifiable to separate the humoral system into circulatory (Chapt. 3) and secretory (Chapt. 4) subsystems. *Cellular immunity* (Chapt. 5) is a term which perhaps properly should be used to designate the circumstance in which cells (e.g., activated macrophages) act as the principal effector agents of immunity, showing enhanced capacity for intracellular killing of organisms such as the tubercle bacillus. *Cell-mediated immunity* is the term designated to describe the possession by certain cells (e.g., the immunologically committed lymphocytes) of surface molecular-recognition sites which react with specific antigens.

There is considerable interaction between all the components of these systems. Various complement components, for example (Chapt. 6), may function directly against certain gram-negative bacilli, they may act as chemotactic factors for polymorphs, or they may collaborate with antibodies in phagocytosis. The polymorph which may serve as the first line of defense against a pneumococcus is capable of ingesting the microorganism without the aid of specific opsonizing antibodies by the process of "surface phagocytosis," but ingestion is greatly facilitated by the collaboration of type specific anti-pneumococcal opsonins. Mononuclear phagocytes may be "activated" non-specifically to mature into "angry macrophages" or they may be stimulated by the interaction of immunologically committed lymphocytes and specific microbial antigens (Chapt. 5).

The body in its teleological wisdom fortunately seems to have available a variety of "back-up" systems such that, if one line of resistance fails, another is capable of filling the breach. This seems to hold true, for example, for the bactericidal mechanisms of the polymorph. Certain types of myeloperoxidase-deficient cells, although partially defective, nevertheless can kill many kinds of bacteria intracellularly and little difficulty is experienced by the host. It is only when more profound deficiency (probably of NADH oxidase) occurs that the cells' antibacterial mechanisms are markedly impaired and chronic granulomatous disease results (Chapt. 2). Even these cells, however, are capable of killing certain bacteria. Similarly, the host can at least partially compensate for deficiencies of a particular immunoglobulin, whose functions may be assumed by another. Defects in either the humoral or cellular systems individually may be partially compensated for by the remaining system. Catastrophic results ensue, however, when both systems are deficient.

Much of our knowledge about the biological functions of the various components of the immune defense mechanisms has been derived from observations of illnesses in which particular systems or substances are deficient or impaired. Defective polymorphs in chronic granulomatous disease result in chronic recurrent infections with staphylococci and certain gram-negative bacilli. Pneumococcal and group A streptococcal infections, however, are not increased nor are viral infections a particular problem. These observations helped direct investigations which delineated the mechanisms by which these organisms are inactivated. Studies of the consequences of deficiencies of particular immunoglobulins in the hypogammaglobulinemia syndromes or in multiple myeloma have indicated the roles played by these substances. Similarly, disorders of cell-mediated immunity have helped to clarify the biological role of this system. Common viral infections such as measles, for example, are handled without great difficulty by hypogammaglobulinemic children, pointing to a major role for cell-mediated immunity in these disorders. Modern therapeutic techniques which alter polymorph function or immune defenses at particular levels also add to understanding of biologic functions.

While the immune responses of the host are clearly beneficial in many of their aspects, nevertheless, adverse consequences of the immune response to microbial agents also account for a number of untoward reactions and disease states. Cell-mediated immunity in tuberculosis is of great assistance in resistance to this disease—in major part, it appears, through activation of macrophages—while at the same time the consequent "delayed hypersensitivity" reaction to tuberculoprotein contributes significantly to tissue destruction and many of the clinical manifestations of tuberculous disease (Chapt. 5). Immune (allergic) responses to inhaled thermophillic actinomycetes present in moldy hay result in the disease, "Farmer's lung," probably as a consequence of tissue damage from immune complexes formed in the pulmonary interstitium by precipitating antibodies and fungal antigens (Chapt. 6). Immune responses to group A streptococcal infections are clearly operative in the pathogenesis of rheumatic fever, probably through cross reactions between microbial antigens and components of heart tissue. Post-streptococcal glomerulonephritis appears to result from the deposition of immune complexes in renal tissue.

Thus the defense mechanism may at times act as a "double-edged sword." Even the helpful polymorphonuclear phagocyte can be shown to participate actively in the production of tissue damage in "immune complex" disease.

The section that follows attempts to assemble in a useful way information about key components of man's defense mechanisms against microbial infection and to illustrate the biological roles of these components by relating a variety of important disease states resulting from disorders of these systems. It is our knowledge of the mechanisms of defense which permit rational efforts to augment, reinforce or bolster the host in his continuing effort to maintain the truce with his ecological microflora. Manipulation of the immune response allows us to supplement man's defensive armamentarium by active or passive immunization, circumventing the natural requirement for suffering the disease itself. Finally, detailed understanding of the intricate mechanisms by which an immune process may turn into a "double-edged sword" points to ways in which these adverse consequences may be lessened or avoided.

Chapter 2

DISORDERS OF THE PHAGOCYTIC SYSTEM

Introduction

Of the factors that contribute to man's survival in a hostile environment, none is more overlooked than the continuous function of the *phagocytic system* in clearing the body of invading organisms. Considering that invasion of the blood stream by bacteria is a recurrent, daily event, the importance of the role of the intricate and coordinated system responsible for dealing continuously with these invaders should not be underestimated. While the organisms involved are usually part of the normal flora of the skin, respiratory and gastrointestinal tracts and might be labeled as non-pathogenic when recovered from these respective sites, their potential for being pathogenic to the host is best exemplified when there is a breakdown in the body's normal defense mechanisms.

Mechanisms of Phagocytosis

The components of the system responsible for dealing with bacterial invasion have been arbitraritly divided into humoral and cellular components. The humoral component is composed of specific antibodies in the various immunoglobulins, while the cellular component includes cells which consist of the peripheral leukocytes or wandering macrophages and the fixed macrophages of the reticuloendothelial system. One has to keep in mind that while on occasion only one component of this system might be involved in the killing of an invading organism, in most instances the various components act in concert to effect the killing and clearance of bacteria from various tissues. This can best be exemplified in the case of the group A streptococcus where the presence of the M-protein on the streptococcal cell enables the organism to resist phagocytosis by the polymorphonuclear leukocyte. However, the presence of antibody specific to the M-protein, the type-specific antibody, eliminates this resistance and greatly enhances the phagocytosis of the organism. In addition to the relevance of this phenomenon to phagocytosis by the peripheral leukocyte, recent studies have shown that specific antibodies produced late in the course of the immune response against gram-negative organisms are highly effective in the clearance of organisms by the spleen in experimental animals.

In addition to the requirement of specific antibody for the phagocytosis of certain bacteria, other less specific and more labile humoral factors, called opsonins, play a role in this process. Phagocytosis of some organisms, as with inert particles, does not always require the presence of antibody. Physical factors like the presence of an immovable surface, clumping of bacteria or the formation of fibrin clots around bacteria, all obviate the need for opsonic antibody and allow phagocytes to ingest organisms by a phenomenon described by Wood as "surface phagocytosis." This mechanism is important in effecting phagocytosis during the early stage of infection of tissue, at a time when opsonic antibody has not been produced by the affected host. Other factors that play a role in phagocytosis are the pH of the medium, osmolarity, presence of divalent cations and cationic proteins.

While the phagocytic process and the events leading to it have been the subject of study for almost a century, the mechanism by which the phagocytic cell kills and disposes of the ingested bacteria has attracted the interest of investigators only recently. The energy required for phagocytosis is derived from glycolysis. Engulfment of particles is associated with increased oxygen uptake by the leukocyte together with increased CO_2 liberation and a transient increase in lactate production. Inhibitors of glycolysis, such as iodoacetate and sodium fluoride, inhibit phagocytosis. Following ingestion, there is a shift of metabolism to the hexose monophosphate shunt. This shift is associated with a burst of leukocyte metabolic activity which results in a marked increase in hydrogen peroxide production and a fall of the pH in the area of the ingested particles. This intracellular process is mediated by a cytoplasmic, cyanide-insensitive NADH oxidase. Recent studies suggest that the H_2O_2 produced acts in concert with the leukocytic lysosomal myeloperoxidase and halide ions, iodide or chloride, to kill bacteria. Thus the addition of specific inhibitors for any of the above components in a phagocytic system would suppress the capacity of the phagocytes to either ingest or kill the ingested organism.

One of the most valuable contributions to our knowledge of leukocyte structure and function is the recent description of lysosomes and the elucidation of their role in the degradation of ingested bacteria. These structures, grossly seen as cytoplasmic granules in some cells, are bags with a membrane similar to that of the cell. Lysosomes contain a variety of hydrolytic enzymes with acid optima. Many of these acid hydrolases have the capacity of degrading macromolecular components of bacteria. The participation of these lysosomes in intraphagocytic degradation was suggested by morphological studies which showed that phagocytosis was followed by a degranulation process consisting of "popping out and disappearance" of these cytoplasmic granules. Although the exact site of the killing of the ingested bacteria has not been determined, morphological studies suggest that the intraphagocytic events that occur after bacterial ingestion follow this sequence: The ingested organism is enveloped by a vacuole to which lysosomes are attracted. The lysosomal walls fuse with the wall of the vacuole, allowing the lysosomes to discharge their content into the vacuole, now a phagosome. The acid hydrolases then act on the organisms within the phagosome and effect disintegration and digestion of their components. The rapidity with which this process occurs varies with the ingested organism and with the phagocytic cell involved. While this sequence applies to many organisms, certain bacteria such as *M. tuberculosis* and other acid fast organisms remain viable after prolonged residence within phagocytic cells. It should be emphasized that although lysosomal enzymes with the capacity of degrading some constituents of various bacteria have been described, available evidence suggests that a multitude of intraphagocytic factors work together in order to achieve killing and complete degradation of bacterial cells.

What would be the result of a breakdown in the phagocytic system? It can be assumed from the above that bacterial propagation in the host would proceed unabated, leading to overwhelming infection and a fatal outcome. The validity of such an assumption is supported by the clinical picture provided by patients who are either born with or acquire a deficiency in this system. Experimental work shows that addition of inhibitors for the various steps associated with the phagocytic process results in specific blocking of either the phagocytic or intraphagocytic killing and digestive processes. Parallel to this, nature has provided examples of specific deficiencies that have helped define the role of these factors in the phagocytic-bactericidal system. The list of these deficiency-states is growing, but they have one common manifestation: recurrent and serious bacterial infection.

Disease Associated with Disorders of the Phagocytic System

Defects in the phagocytic system can involve either the circulating phagocyte or the fixed macrophages in organs of the reticuloendothelial system. Deficiencies can occur in the humoral factors necessary for phagocytosis, in the leukocyte itself, or in both, leading to disease states associated with serious infection.

Defects in Humoral Factors Responsible for Promoting Phagocytosis

Defects in the humoral (thymic-independent) and the cell-mediated (thymic-dependent) immune mechanisms have been described in other chapters. Recurrent or persistent infections in these deficency states are related to lack of formation of serum bactericidal or opsonizing antibodies.

Another humoral deficiency state associated with secondary phagocytic dysfunction and increased susceptibility to infection is the deficiency in the *complement system.* This system of serum proteins (C_1–C_9) was initially described as active in cell lysis or bacteriolysis. Some of its components have been shown to play specific roles in the phagocytic process. Phagocytosis involves utilization of C_3 while chemotaxis, migration of normal leukocytes to the site of injury, is enhanced by $C_{5,6,7}$. Deficiency states in complement, associated with recurrent infections, have been described in a few cases. A case of a deficiency of a factor that stabilizes C_3 was reported by Alper *et al.*, while Miller and his co-workers reported the case of a familial deficiency of C_5 in an infant with recurrent infection. In these cases, phagocytosis by the patient as well as normal subjects' leukocytes was inhibited *in vitro* when the patient's plasma was used, but proceeded normally when plasma from healthy donors was substituted. In the latter case, addition of C_5 to the plasma of the mother, who was found to be similarly deficient, restored the phagocytosis enhancing capacity of the plasma.

The case of an isolated instance of defective chemotaxis has been reported by Ward and Schlegel. Chemotaxis was inhibited in the presence of the patient's serum. A younger sibling of this patient was shown to possess a similar inhibitor. In these patients, an associated deficiency in the bactericidal capacity of the patient's leukocytes was also described.

Defects in the Phagocytic Cell

Quantitative or qualitative deficiencies of the phagocytic cell lead to diminished resistance to infection. The clinical manifestations and the nature of the infectious organism can give a good clue regarding the nature of the underlying deficiency. Quantitative neutrophil defects are associated primarily with infections due to highly virulent organisms, whereas qualitative defects in the leukocytes are associated with organisms that are usually part of the normal flora of the body or environment.

Quantitative Defects. Leukopenia, a decrease in the absolute number of leukocytes, is either congenital or acquired. Reduction of the circulating leukocytes can result from either increased sequestration or destruction of the cell, usually in the spleen, or decreased production by the bone marrow. The defect can be limited to a decrease in the polymorphonuclear leukocytes, a condition called neutropenia or agranulocytosis. Infections of the skin and the respiratory tract, ulcerations in the mouth and of the rectum, all are the primary manifestations of the lack of an adequate number of circulating polymorphonuclear leukocytes, and occur when the peripheral number drops to 1,000/cu.mm. or less.

Transient neutropenia of the newborn occurs during the first two months of life and is ascribed to the presence of placentally transmitted maternal antibody to leukocytes. *Infantile agranulocytosis* is a genetically determined, autosomal recessive disease where the neutrophils are markedly reduced or absent from the peripheral blood. Recurrent severe bacterial infections with a fatal outcome characterize this disease. A milder form of neutropenia, *chronic benign neutropenia,* may be encountered. Total remission from this condition can occur during late childhood. *Cyclic neutropenia* is characterized by the occurrence of periodic episodes of neutropenia lasting about seven days. The bone marrow shows decreased numbers of neutrophil precursors. These episodes are associated with oral ulcers and high fever. Both the peripheral blood and bone marrow are normal between these episodes. Neutropenia with *abnormal cellular immunity* has been described in two patients with cartilage-hair hypoplasia. Lymphopenia was also present and the bone marrow showed failure of myeloid maturation. These patients contracted unusually severe varicella. *Familial granulocytopenia* with associated immunoglobulin abnormalities has been described in three brothers. Fatal infections occurred in the three patients who had constant severe neutropenia with low levels of IgG and IgA.

Neutropenia can be induced by a variety of drugs such as aminopyrines, phenothiazines, thioureas and sulfonamides. Chloramphenicol is an antibiotic which leads to aplastic anemia and agranulocytosis at a relatively high frequency. The onset of infection in drug-induced neutropenia is quite sudden. High, spiking temperatures are associated with the infections, while signs of localized infection and pus formation in the lesion are lacking because of the absence of leukocytes. Bone marrow examination usually shows a decrease in the neutrophilic precursors.

Neutropenia can be a manifestation of various disorders affecting the bone marrow. Leukemia, lymphomas and disseminated neoplasms lead to myelophthisic neutropenia with consequent infection and generalized sepsis. Leukopenia is also associated with many collagen diseases, particularly systemic lupus erythematosus. Transient depression of bone marrow with neutropenia occurs in viral and bacterial infections. Leukopenia is frequently encountered in diseases associated with marked splenomegaly. In these conditions, leukopenia is ascribed to peripheral sequestration of the cells in the spleen.

Chronic idiopathic neutropenia, a recently described entity, is *not* associated with an increased frequency of infections. The patients described had severe neutropenia of 1 to 19 years duration, but no hypoplasia of the bone marrow or splenomegaly. It is a benign condition that requires no treatment.

The diagnosis of the above conditions is predicated on the history of severe infections, the finding of neutropenia during these episodes and bone marrow histology. Treatment consists of prompt therapy of the infection with antibiotics and, above all, removal of any agent responsible for the neutropenia. The need for vigorous therapy becomes more eminent in the presence of septicemia which is associated with a 25 percent mortality in these cases. The choice of antibiotics is based on the organism isolated and its sensitivity pattern. Long term management consists of avoidance of the sensitizing agent. The use of prophylactic antibiotics in recurrent neutropenia is not recommended.

Qualitative Defects. Recognition of diseases characterized by recurrent serious bacterial infection due to specific metabolic defects of the leukocyte is a recent event. The first disease to be so classified was described as a clinical entity in 1957. It was not until about a decade thereafter that the underlying pathogenetic mechanism was defined as the inability of the patient's polymorphonuclear leukocyte to effect intracellular killing of the organisms following phagocytosis. Based on recently acquired knowledge of the metabolic processes involved in the intraphagocytic killing of batceria, defects in the enzymes responsible for these processes have been described to account for this finding.

"Chronic granulomatous disease of childhood" is the current name for the syndrome representing the prototype of this disease. The clinical manifestations of chronic granulomatous disease are characteristic. The patient is a child who, during the early months of life, suffers from severe protracted infections with concomitant febrile episodes. Examination of the patient reveals the presence of infected eczematoid lesions and suppurative draining adenitis, together with evidence of chronic pulmonary infection. Hepatosplenomegaly, associated with hepatic abscesses, and osteomyelitis can occur in addition to the above. The white blood cell count and differential are normal or elevated. X-ray studies of the chest show the presence of acute and chronic bronchopneumonias, with characteristic pneumonias that are discrete, homogenous and round in contour. These have been labeled "encapsulating" pneumonias. Marked hilar lymphadenopathy is usually seen. When osteomyelitis is present, it usually involves the small bones of the hands and feet. The lesions show little evidence of acute destruction, with absence of sclerotic reaction.

In contrast to the bacterial etiology encountered in patients with neutropenia, the organisms isolated from the lesions of patients with chronic granulomatous disease are of low virulence. Coagulase-positive staphylococci and gram-negative organisms, such as *Serratia marcescens, Escherichia coli* and species of Enterobacteriaceae are most commonly involved. Virulent organisms such as group A streptococci and pneumococci are not found. Studies of the immunological status of these individuals reveals that they have adequate amounts of immunoglobulins in their serum and normal levels of total complement and complement components. Challenge with a variety of antigens elicits a normal humoral and cell-mediated immune response. Studies of the local inflammatory response by the skin window technique show normal migration of leukocytes to the site of injury. Histological studies of the involved tissue reveal a granulomatous reaction at the site of infection. This type of tissue response to infection is characteristic of this disease.

Initial studies on the pathogenesis of this disease have led to the establishment of specific diagnostic tests. Studies on the phagocytic capacity of the leukocytes from patients with chronic granulomatous disease for the organisms responsible for the infection, *Staphylococcus aureus* and *Serratia marcescens,* have revealed that, although phagocytosis of the organism occurred normally, the ingested bacteria were not killed. Thus, while a 2 log (99%) decrease in the number of viable organisms occurred 2 hours after phagocytosis by normal leukocytes, leukocytes obtained from patients with chronic granulomatous disease do not produce a significant decrease in the number of viable organisms during this interval. In contrast to the decreased capacity of the defective leukocytes to kill *S. aureus* and *S. marsescens,* streptococci and pneumococci are as effectively killed by the leukocytes from patients with this disease as by normal leukocytes.

Another test that has been used in the diagnosis of this disease is the inability of the leukocytes from patients with chronic granulomatous disease to reduce nitroblue tetrazolium dye (NBT). As outlined above, the metabolic events that are associated with intracellular killing following phagocytosis include a shift to the hexose-monophosphate shunt, utilizing the cyanide-insensitive NADH oxidase. The ability of normal leukocytes to reduce NBT dye to purple formazan during phagocytosis *in vitro* has been ascribed to NADH oxidase activity. The defective NBT reduction that has been found in the leukocytes of patients is probably a reflection of an abnormality in the NADH oxidase system, correlating well with the lack of bactericidal capacity of these leukocytes. The NBT test is now used as a screening test in identifying patients with this disease and their carrier parents and siblings. The test can be performed as a quantitative test or as a simple micro-method slide test. It should be pointed out that the NBT test is not reliable in patients on steroid therapy.

"Chronic granulomatous disease of childhood" is a familial disease, transmitted either as an X-linked or an autosomal recessive trait. Leukocytes from parents and siblings of patients with the disease show partial defects in the reduction of NBT. While the lack of bactericidal activity and depressed reduction of the NBT dye by the leukocyte suggest an abnormality in the hexose-monophosphate pathway, the precise nature of the defect has not been definitely established. Various studies have suggested a deficiency in NADH oxidase and lack of production of H_2O_2, an iodination defect following phagocytosis, a deficiency of myeloperoxidase or lability of the glucose-6-phosphate dehydrogenase as underlying metabolic defects. The particular association of infection with and the specific inability of leukocytes to kill primarily organisms that produce catalase suggests that the defect is strongly related to hydrogen peroxide production either by the leukocyte or the ingested organism. The absence of the production of H_2O_2 by either results in the lack of activation of the myeloperoxidase-mediated bactericidal system of the leukocyte.

Clinical variants of the X-linked chronic granulomatous disease have been described recently. Several female patients with the clinical and pathological findings of the disease have been reported. The metabolic defect in these patients' leukocytes consists of a reduction or absence of the glutathione peroxidase. Deficiency of myeloperoxidase has been described in another patient with repeated candida infection. The patient's leukocytes showed inability to kill candida organisms *in vitro*. A peculiar defect has also been reported in a patient with recurrent staphylococcal infections. His leukocytes showed defective killing of the staphylococcal organism but were capable of exerting normal bactericidal activity on gram-negative organisms.

Job's syndrome is another variant of chronic granulomatous disease described by Davis and his associates. It occurs in red-haired, fair-skinned girls and is autosomal recessive. It manifests clinically by the formation of recurrent cold staphylococcal abscesses, occurring from birth. Leukocytes from these patients cannot kill staphylococci or reduce NBT but can destroy ingested streptococci. In one report, a patient's sister also showed defective NBT dye reduction.

Another syndrome associated with leukocyte abnormality in which recurrent and sometimes fatal bacterial infections occur is the Chediak-Higashi syndrome. This syndrome shows an autosomal recessive pattern of inheritance. It is characterized by partial oculo-cutaneous albinism, granulocytopenia and the presence of giant granules, or lysosomes, in the leukocytes. Generalized mononuclear infiltration of organs is seen in these patients. The granulocytopenia has been ascribed to increased sequestration in the enlarged spleen, together with destruction of the cells in the medulla of bone.

Deficiency of the Fixed Phagocytes of the Reticuloendothelial System

The role of the reticuloendothelial system in the clearance of organisms from the blood stream is a vital one. Studies have shown that the liver and spleen are the major organs involved. In immune experimental animals, the liver is the organ responsible for the clearance of bacteria from the blood-stream, whereas the spleen assumes the primary role in the clearance of organisms from the blood of the non-immune animal. These findings are supported by clinical experience in which rapidly fulminating infections with pyogenic organisms occur in patients with absent or non-functional spleens, especially early in life.

Congenital absence of the spleen occurs in association with cardiac malformation. The presence of target cells, spherocytosis, Howell-Jolly or Heinz inclusion bodies in the red cells would suggest the occurrence of asplenia. *Familial splenic hypoplasia* has been described, in which condition the patients had diminutive spleens and severe fulminating bacteremia. *Functional reversible asplenia* has been described in association with sickle cell disease. Decreased opsonins for pneumococci have been described in patients with the latter disease and are thought to contribute to the increased susceptibility of these patients to serious infections by this organism. Surgical removal of the spleen for hypersplenism, the correction of hematological abnormalities or following trauma, carries a high risk for overwhelming sepsis in infants and younger children. The risk is also high when the underlying diseases are Thalassemia major, Wiskott-Aldrich syndrome and reticuloendotheliosis. Traumatic rupture, hereditary spherocytosis and idiopathic thrombocytopenic purpura carry a lower risk. The course of sepsis in the asplenic patients is very rapid, with death occurring within 24 hours from onset. For this reason, splenectomy for hematological problems should not be performed before the age of five years unless deemed highly indicated.

Generalized involvement of the reticuloendothelial histiocytes, or fixed macrophages, has been described in a family by Ford and his co-workers. This familial condition is characterized by *lipochrome pigmentation of histiocytes* from various organs. The patients suffered from severe recurrent infections. Arthritis was present in one patient. All had pulmonary infiltration, splenomegaly and hyperglobulinemia. The reason for the increased susceptibility of these patients to infection is thought to be due to the presence of the lipid in the histiocytes and consequent blockading of the reticuloendothelial system.

The diagnosis of asplenia is suggested by the presence of inclusion bodies and abnormal morphology of the red blood cells in the peripheral smear. Confirmation can be obtained by radiological examination and radioactive scintillation scan studies. The diagnosis of lipochrome histiocytosis is made by histological studies of a lymph node or liver tissue. The phagocytic capacity of the reticuloendothelial system can be assessed by measuring the clearance of colloidal radioactive gold from the blood-stream. The clearance of radioactive-labeled bacteria from the bloodstream has also been used for the measurement of phagocytic activity by the reticuloendothelial organs in experimental animals.

Investigation of Patients with Suspected Deficiency of Phagocytic System

Defective phagocytosis should be suspected in patients with recurrent bacterial infections, with persistent infections associated with granuloma formation and in patients with a familial history of recurrent infections. Because of the overlap in the clinical manifestations and the occurrence of dual humoral and phagocytic deficiencies in certain diseases, investigation of both the humoral and cellular mechanisms are carried out initially.

In the study of these deficiency states it is advisable to start with simple, expedient and easily available screening tests. The techniques for studying humoral and cell-mediated immune mechanisms have been outlined in Chapter 5. Of those, quantitative determination of immunoglobulins and isohemagglutinins, the Schick and Dick skin tests yield prompt answers to the level and activity of the immunoglobulins. Candida and streptokinase-streptodornase skin tests can also be easily performed to test the cell-mediated immune function. White blood cell counts and differentials during the episodes of infections and remissions, with examination of the smear for abnormal morphology of the granules or inclusion bodies, will yield information regarding the presence of quantitative defects, qualitative defects or splenic dysfunction. Abnormality of the leukocyte metabolism and intraphagocytic bactericidal activity is readily tested by using the NBT slide test.

The performance of the above studies can yield concrete information regarding the nature of the underlying defect in a patient with recurrent infection. More definitive tests should be performed to confirm and define the nature of abnormalities that will be suggested by these studies. Such tests, which are somewhat elaborate, can be performed in any hospital setting with adequate laboratory facilities.

The definition of the underlying nature of a quantitative defect in leukocytes is based on a study of both the peripheral blood and the bone marrow. A *bone marrow aspiration* for culture and morphological studies should be carried out on such patients.

Assessment of humoral factors involved in phagocytosis involves assay of *opsonins,* specific and non-specific, to the organisms responsible for the recurrent infections. This is usually performed as part of the phagocytosis test using the patient's fresh plasma in one tube and pooled normal plasma in another. Measurement of levels of *complement,* either as total complement activity or as individual component activity, can be performed on the patient's plasma. If deficient levels are found, their role in phagocytosis can be assessed by adding the individual component to the phagocytic test.

Studies of the response of peripheral leukocytes to an inflammatory stimulus are performed using the "Skin Window Technique" described by Rebuck. This is carried out by applying a glass cover slip over an abraded area of the skin and examining the morphology of the exudate that accumulates on the cover slip at various intervals. This test allows the *in vitro* study of chemotaxis, a test that can also be performed *in vitro* using specially designed chambers.

The basis for the use of the nitroblue tetrazolium (NBT) dye in testing for intraphagocytic bactericidal activity was detailed above. The procedure consists of adding the dye to the phagocytic system *in vitro*. Reduction of the dye to a blue formazan pigment occurs following phagocytosis and intraphagocytic digestion. The slide test consists of determining the percentage of granulocytes which contain the dark blue formazan. In normal individuals, no less than 30 percent of the polymorphonuclear leukocytes show the reduced formazan. In the quantitative test the dye is extracted from equal numbers of resting and phagocytizing leukocytes and the optical density of the extract measured. Normal adults should show a rise of about 0.200 in the O.D. between resting and phagocytizing samples if the phagocytosis mixture is incubated for 15 minutes. Younger individuals might show lower differences.

The *in vitro* phagocytic and bactericidal capacity of leukocytes for the organisms associated with the infections in the patient is the most definitive test for determining the presence of any specific phagocytic defects. An optimal number of organisms are added to a tube containing the patient's leukocytes suspended in fresh normal serum, and the tube is rotated at 37°C to allow for phagocytosis. Aliquots are obtained at 0 hr., 30 min., 1 hr. and 2 hr. and the leukocytes ruptured by diluting the sample in distilled water. Measured amounts of these dilutions are spread on agar plates which are incubated for 24 hours or more, then counted for the number of colonies formed. The bactericidal activity is measured as a decrease in the number of viable colony forming organisms during the above intervals. Normal leukocytes kill at least 90 percent of the organisms 2 hours after phagocytosis, while defective leukocytes show no more than 50 percent reduction in viable organisms during this interval.

Another *in vitro* technique for studying phagocytosis and intraphagocytic degradation utilizes radiolabeled bacteria. Phagocytosis is assessed by the decrease of radioactivity in the supernate. Intraphagocytic digestion is measured by the release of dialyzable radioactivity by the phagocytizing leukocytes.

Determination of specific metabolic defects in the leukocytes can be carried out by assaying the level of the enzymes known to be involved in the phagocytic and bactericidal activity. NADH-oxidase, myeloperoxidase, glutathione peroxidase and glucose-6-phosphate dehydrogenase, all are examples of enzymes which have been assayed and found to be defective in leukocytes with decreased phagocytic and bactericidal activity. It can be surmised that the list for these enzymes is not final. It probably constitutes only the beginning of a growing catalogue for specific deficiencies that we have just started to enunciate in attempting to explain what was, less than 10 years ago, an unexplained phenomenon associated with some mysterious disease.

SELECTED REFERENCES

Alper, C. A., Abramson, N., Johnston, R. B., Jr., Jandl, J. H., and Rosen, F. S.: Complement defect associated with increased susceptibility to infection. New Eng. J. Med., *282*:349, 1970.

Ayoub, E. M., and Wannamaker, L. W.: The fate of Group A streptococci following phagocytosis: *In vitro* phagocytic studies of isotope-labeled streptococci. J. Immunol., *99*:1099, 1967.

Ayoub, E. M., and White, J. G.: Intraphagocytic degradation of Group A streptococci: Electron microscopic studies. J. Bacteriol., *98*:728, 1969.

Baehner, R. L., and Nathan, D. G.: Leukocyte oxidase: defective activity in chronic granulomatous disease. Science, *155*: 835, 1967.

Baehner, R. L., and Karnovsky, M. L.: Deficiency of reduced nicotinamide-adenine dinucleotide oxidase in chronic granulomatous disease. Science, *162*:1277, 1968.

Baehner, R. L., and Nathan, D. G.: Quantitative nitroblue tetrazolium test in chronic granulomatous disease. New Eng. J. Med., *278*: 971, 1968.

Bellanti, J. A., Cantz, B. E., and Schlegel, R. J.: Accelerated decay of glucose-6-phosphate dehydrogenase activity in chronic granulomatous disease. Pediat. Res., *4*:405, 1970.

Bridges, R. A., Berendes, H., and Good, R. A.: A fatal granulomatous disease of childhood: the clinical, pathological and laboratory features of a new syndrome. Amer. J. Dis. Child., *97*:387, 1959.

Carson, M. J., Chadwick, D. L., Brubaker, C. A., Cleland, R. S., and Landing, B. H.: Thirteen boys with progressive septic granulomatosis. Pediatrics, *35*:405, 1965.

Cohn, Z. A., and Hirsch, J. G.: Isolation and properties of the specific cytoplasmic granules of rabbit polymorphonuclear leukocytes. J. Exper. Med., *112*:983, 1960.

Cohn, Z. A., and Hirsch, J. G.: The influence of phagocytosis on the intracellular distribution of granule-associated components of polymorphonuclear leukocytes. J. Exper. Med., *112*:1015, 1960.

Davis, S. D., Schaller, J., and Wedgwood, R. J.: Job's syndrome: recurrent, "cold," staphylococcal abscesses. Lancet, *1*:1013, 1966.

Davis, W. C., Douglas, S. D., and Fudenberg, H. H.: A selective neutrophil dysfunction syndrome impaired killing of staphylococci. Ann. Intern. Med., *69*:1237, 1968.

DeDuve, C.: Lysosomes, new group of subcellular particles. In: *Subcellular Particles:* A symposium held during the meeting of the Society of General Pathologists at the Marine Biological Laboratory, Woods Hole, Mass., 1958. Edited by Hayashi, T., Ronald, New York, 1959.

Ford, D. K., Price, G. E., Culling, C. F. A., and Vassar, P. S.: Familial lipochrome pigmentation of histiocytes with hyperglobulinemia, pulmonary infiltration, splenomegaly, arthritis and susceptibility to infection. Am. J. Med., *33*:478, 1962.

Gifford, R. H., and Malawista, S. E.: A simple rapid micromethod for detecting chronic granulomatous disease of childhood. J. Lab. Clin. Med., *75*:511, 1970.

Hirsch, J. G., and Cohn, Z. A.: Degranulation of polymorphonuclear leukocytes following phagocytosis of microorganisms. J. Exper. Med., *112*:1005, 1960.

Holmes, B., Park, B. H., Malawista, S. E., Quie, P. G., Nelson, D. L., and Good, R. A.: Chronic granulomatous disease in females: a deficiency of leukocyte glutathione peroxidase. New Eng. J. Med., *283*:217, 1970.

Kaplan, E. L., Laxdal, T., and Quie, P. G.: Studies of polymorphonuclear leukocytes from patients with chronic granulomatous disease of childhood: bactericidal capacity for streptococci. Pediatrics, *41*:591, 1968.

Karnovsky, M. L: Metabolic basis of phagocytic activity. Physiol. Rev., *42*:143, 1962.

Klebanoff, S. J.: Myeloperoxidase-halide-hydrogen peroxide antibacterial system. J. Bacteriol., *95*:2131, 1968.

Klebanoff, S. J., and White, L. R.: Iodination defect in the leukocytes of a patient with chronic granulomatous disease of childhood. New Eng. J. Med., *280*:460, 1969.

Kritzler, R. A., Terner, J. Y., Lindenbaum, J., Magidson, J., Williams, R., Preisig, R., and Phillips, G.: Chediak-Higashi syndrome: cytologic and serum lipid observations in a case and family. Am. J. Med., *36*:583, 1964.

Kyle, R. A., and Linman, J. W.: Chronic idiopathic neutropenia: A newly recognized entity? New Eng. J. Med., *279*:1015, 1968.

Lehrer, R. I., Hanifin, J., and Cline, M. J.: Defective bactericidal activity in myeloperoxidase-deficient human neutrophils. Nature, *223*:78, 1969.

Miller, D. R., and Kaplan, H. G.: Decreased nitroblue tetrazolium dye reduction in the phagocytes of patients receiving prednisone. Pediatrics, *45*:861, 1970.

Miller, M. E., and Ulf, R. N.: A familial deficiency of the phagocytosis-enhancing activity of serum related to a dysfunction of the fifth component of complement (C_5). New Eng. J. Med., *282*:354, 1970.

Pearson, H. A., Spencer, R. P., and Cornelius, E. A.: Functional asplenia in sickle-cell anemia. New Eng. J. Med., *281*:923, 1970.

Quie, P. G., White, J. G., Holmes, B., and Good, R. A.: *In vitro* bactericidal capacity of human polymorphonuclear leukocytes: diminished activity in chronic granulomatous disease of childhood. J. Clin. Invest., *46*:668, 1967.

Schulkind, M. L., and Rabins, P.: Effect of purified rabbit anti-*Salmonella typhimurium* antibodies on the fate of intravenously injected bacteria. Infection and Immunity, *3*:154, 1971.

Southam, C. M., and Levin, A. G.: A quantitative Rebuck technique. Blood, *27*:734, 1966.

Suter, E.: Multiplication of tubercle bacilli within mononuclear phagocytes in tissue cultures derived from normal animals and animals vaccinated with BCG. J. Exp. Med., *97*:235, 1953.

Ward, P. A., and Schlegel, R. J.: Impaired leucotactic responsiveness in a child with recurrent infections. Lancet, *2*:344, 1969.

Windhorst, D. B., Page, A. R., Holmes, B., Quie, P. G., and Good, R. A.: The pattern of genetic transmission of the leukocyte defect in fatal granulomatous disease of childhood. J. Clin. Invest., *47*:1026, 1968.

Wolfson, J. J., Quie, P. G., Laxdal, S. D., and Good, R. A.: Roentgenologic manifestations in children with a genetic defect of polymorphonuclear leukocyte function. Radiology, *91*:37, 1968.

Wood, W. B., Jr.: Phagocytosis with particular reference to encapsulated bacteria. Bacteriol. Reviews, *24*:41, 1960.

Chapter 3

THE CIRCULATORY ANTIBODY SYSTEM

Normal persons usually recover from acute infectious diseases, and following recovery are frequently resistant to re-infection. For example, pneumococcal pneumonia is an acute febrile illness progressing almost relentlessly if not treated with antibiotics, but after 7 to 14 days, defervescence occurs promptly (crisis) and the patient then recovers rapidly. Subsequently, these individuals are insusceptible to re-infection by the type of pneumococcus responsible for their earlier disease. This process of recovery from infection may be attributed to production of specific serum antibody. Acquired resistance to re-infection is almost always attributed to cellular or humoral immune mechanisms. Use of these principles has been responsible for the development of methods for prophylactic immunization and has served as an important stimulus to our understanding of immunology. Protection against infectious disease, however, may not be the primary function of the immune system. Control of aberrant cell growth by continuous immunological surveillance of the host's tissues may be equally, if not more important than protection against infection in maintaining the integrity of the body.

The immune response is divisible into 1) production of serum or circulatory antibody; 2) production of secretory antibody; and 3) altered reactivity of lymphocytes and macrophages (the cellular immune system). The secretory immune system and the cellular immune systems are discussed in Chapters 4 and 5. Here, discussion will be limited largely to the serum or circulatory immune system.

Characteristics of Serum Antibody

Antigens are the substances which induce antibody production in the host and which react specifically with those antibodies. The bond between antigen and antibody results from the action of weak forces such as hydrogen bonds, van der Waals forces and electrostatic interactions. The antibodies induced by microorganisms and other antigens have unique specificity for the antigens or for molecules which are structurally closely related.

The first time an individual is inoculated with an antigen, 7 to 10 days are usually required to achieve peak amounts of antibody in the serum, and this is referred to as a *primary response.* The next time the individual is injected or infected with the same antigens, a *secondary response* occurs, characterized by higher antibody levels achieved usually in a shorter period of time.

Antibodies are serum proteins referred to as immunoglobulins (Ig). They are among the slowest moving proteins during electrophoresis of serum at an alkaline pH, but may extend through the gamma, beta, and alpha globulin regions. The immunoglobulins are best defined by their amino acid sequences or antigenic characteristics, but also have been classified by their electrophoretic properties, sedimentation coefficients, molecular weights, and biological activities (e.g., "skin fixing", complement fixing, precipitating, etc.). They have been subdivided into five major classes based upon their antigenic specificity, as assayed with antibody induced with the immunoglobulins in a heterologous animal species (e.g., human immunoglobulin used to immunize rabbits). The physical and biological properties of these five classes of immunoglobulins are listed in Table 3.1. The variations between the immunoglobulins are related to structural differences and are best illustrated by considering the structure of immunoglobulin G (IgG).

IgG is a symmetrical molecule for which Porter has proposed the classic straight stick model shown in Figure 3.1. The molecule consists of two pairs of different chains of amino acids, called the Light (L) and Heavy (H) chains. These chains are linked by disulfide bonds and can be separated by chemical reduction and fractionation. These L and H chains vary from molecule to molecule because of differences in amino acid sequences. The N terminal$\sim$107 residues of these chains exhibit the greatest variation in sequence and hence are called the variable or V regions. The remaining portions of the chains exhibit less variation and are, therefore, called the constant or C regions.

Fragmentation of IgG molecules by proteolytic enzymes or chemical cleavage results in two fragments referred to as Fab and Fc (Fig. 3.1). The Fab region is composed of the L chains and the amino terminal half of the H chain. This fragment retains the antigen combining site of the antibody. The Fc fragment retains the sites responsible for complement fixation, attachment to cell membranes and other biological properties.

The differences between immunoglobulin classes (IgG, IgE, IgA, IgM,

TABLE 3.1
Physical and biological properties of immunoglobulins

Class	IgG				IgM		IgA		IgD	IgE
Subclass	IgG_1	IgG_2	IgG_3	IgG_4	IgM_1	IgM_2	IgA_1	IgA_2	IgD	IgE
Molecular weight	160,000				900,000		160,000-serum 370,000-secretory		160,000	200,000
Sedimentation coefficient	7S				19S		7S-serum 11S-secretory		7S	8S
Molecular weight of heavy chain	51,600	51,600	59,000	?	~70,000		56,600	51,900	60,000	75,500
Mg% in serum (% subclass)	800–1680 70–80%	13–18%	6–8%	3%	50–190 65%	35%	140–420 93%	7%	0.3–40	0.02
Body distribution (% in I.V. pool)	48–62				65–100		40 (serum)		63–86	?
Half life (days)	23				4–5		4–5 (serum)		3	?
Site of synthesis	spleen, lymph nodes				spleen, lymph nodes		mucus membrane of gut, lung, lymph nodes		spleen, lymph nodes	mucus membranes
Cross placenta	Yes				No		No		No	No
Fixation of complement	+	+	++	0	++++		0		0	0
Alternate pathway	+	+	+		+		+			±
Ability to fix to human mast cells	No				No		No		No	Yes
Major function	Protection in interstitial & intravascular spaces by toxin neutralization, opsonization and lysis gram-negative bacilli in presence of complement				Protection in intravascular spaces		Protects mucous membrane surfaces by virus neutralization		?	Makes man miserable with allergies

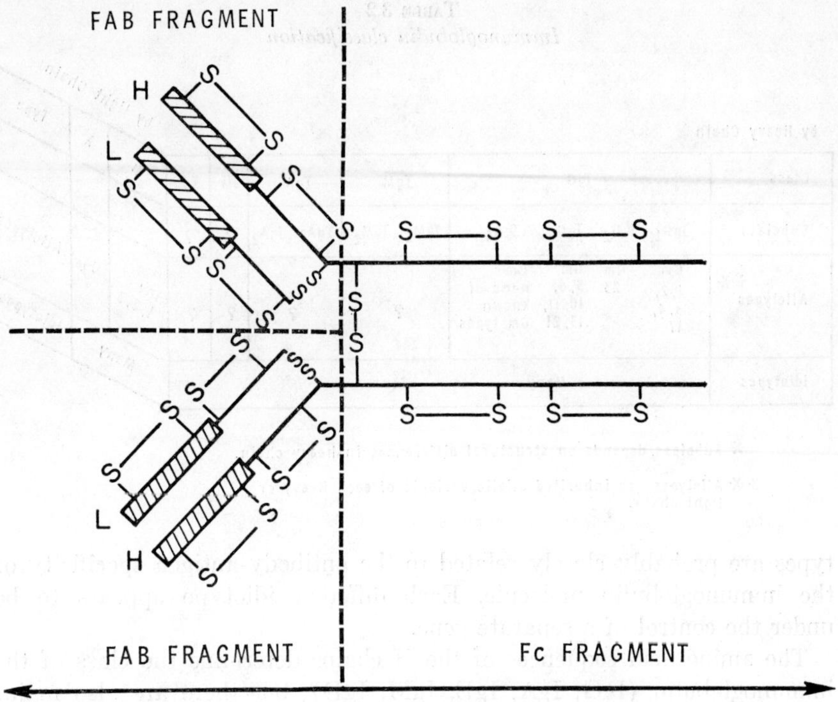

FIG. 3.1. "Straight stick" model for IgG.

Shaded area represents the variable region; the non-shaded area depicts the constant regions. The interchain (L-H and H-H) disulfide bonds vary in number and/or position with subclass (see Fig. 3.2), but the intrachain disulfide bonds are common to all IgG subclasses.

IgD) are related to the amino acid sequences of the constant regions of the H chains. These constant (C) regions are similar within an immunoglobulin class but differ from class to class.

Determination of the amino acid sequences and corresponding antigenic characteristics of the H and L chains of immunoglobulins from the same or different individuals have allowed more detailed classification (see Table 3.2). The L chains are divisible into two types, called kappa (κ) and lambda (λ). A given individual has both types, but not in the same immunoglobulin molecule. The synthesis of these two types of L chain are under the control of separate genes, as indicated by the different amino acid sequences of their C regions. The κ and λ chains can be subdivided into different allotypes, called Inv 1,2,3, or O_z. The allotypic markers are alleles and an individual does not have more than two different allotypes of the κ and two allotypes of the λ Light chains. The allotypes of the L chains can be further subdivided into idiotypes based upon the amino acid sequences or resulting antigenic sites of their V regions. The idio-

Table 3.2
Immunoglobulin classification

by Heavy Chain

Class	IgG				IgM		IgA		IgD	IgE
Subclass *	IgG_1	IgG_2	IgG_3	IgG_4	IgM_1	IgM_2	IgA_1	IgA_2	?	?
Allotypes **	Gm 1, 2, 3, 4, 17	Gm 23	Gm 5, 6, 10, 11, 13, 21	Gm none of known Gm types	?		?		?	?
Idiotypes	Many									

by Light Chain

Type	μ	λ
Allotypes	Inv 1, 2, 3	Oz
Idiotypes	Many	

* Subclass depends on structural differences in heavy chain.

** Allotypes are inherited allelic variants of each heavy or light chain.

types are probably closely related to the antibody-antigen specificity of the immunoglobulin molecule. Each different idiotype appears to be under the control of a separate gene.

The amino acid sequences of the H chains determine the class of the immunoglobulin (IgG, IgA, IgE, IgM, IgD), but there are also major differences in their overall structure, as shown in Figure 3.2. Heavy chains of a given class are named by the Greek letter corresponding to the class name, i.e., IgA has α heavy chains. The H chains of most immunoglobulin classes can be subdivided into subclasses based on their amino acid sequences and antigenic characteristics. For example, IgG has been subdivided into four subclasses (Table 3.2), and an individual has IgG from all four subclasses. The synthesis of each of the subclasses is under control of separate genes. The subclasses can be further subdivided into allotypes and idiotypes as with the L chains.

Genetic Basis for Antibody Heterogeneity

Extensive amino acid sequence studies of many different L chains have led to a clearer understanding of the genetic basis for antibody heterogeneity. This work has been summarized and interpreted by Hood and Talmage, and the reader is referred to their article for a more detailed treatment of the following concepts.

How many genes control the structure of a single immunoglobulin molecule? According to the hypothesis of one gene per polypeptide chain one would surmise two genes: one for L chains and one for H chains. However, genetic control of immunoglobulins is more complex and it seems that four genes is the right answer: one for the V region of the L chain, another

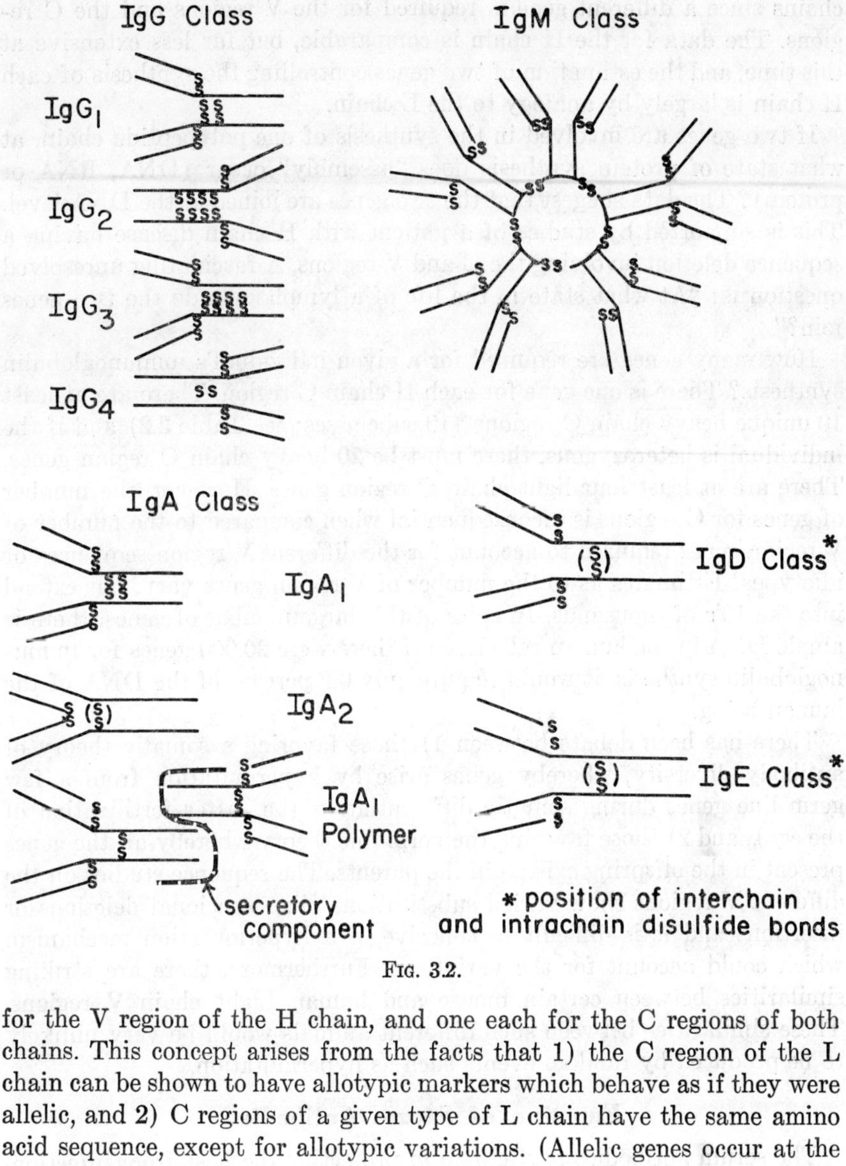

FIG. 3.2.

for the V region of the H chain, and one each for the C regions of both chains. This concept arises from the facts that 1) the C region of the L chain can be shown to have allotypic markers which behave as if they were allelic, and 2) C regions of a given type of L chain have the same amino acid sequence, except for allotypic variations. (Allelic genes occur at the same locus on the chromosome. An animal heterozygous for a given characteristic will have two alleles, but a population of animals can have many.) Hence, the C region seems to be under the control of one gene. Sequence analysis of the V regions of over 40 Kappa type light chains demonstrates 3 major and many more minor groups. Since all three major groups are found in one individual, they cannot be allelic, and must be controlled by more than one gene. At least 2 genes are required for the L chains since a different gene is required for the V regions and the C regions. The data for the H chain is comparable, but far less extensive at this time, and the estimation of two genes controlling the synthesis of each H chain is largely by analogy to the L chain.

If two genes are involved in the synthesis of one polypeptide chain, at what state of protein synthesis does "assembly" occur (DNA, RNA or protein)? The data suggest that the two genes are joined at the DNA level. This is supported by studies of a patient with H chain disease having a sequence deletion involving the C and V regions. A fascinating unresolved question is: "At what state in the life of a lymphocyte do the two genes join?"

How many genes are required for a given individual's immunoglobulin synthesis? There is one gene for each H chain C region. There are at least 10 unique heavy chain C regions (10 subclasses; see Table 3.2) and if the individual is heterozygous, there must be 20 heavy chain C region genes. There are at least four light chain C region genes. However, the number of genes for C regions is inconsequential when compared to the number of V region genes required to account for the different V region sequences or idiotypes! Estimates as to the number of V region genes vary, but extend into the 10's of thousands. In spite of this large number of genes, there is ample DNA in the human cell. Even if there were 20,000 genes for immunoglobulin synthesis, it would require only 0.2 percent of the DNA of the human being.

There has been debate between 1) those favoring a somatic theory of antibody diversity, whereby genes arise by hypermutation from a few germ line genes during somatic differentiation (i.e., after fertilization of the egg), and 2) those favoring the germ line theory whereby all the genes present in the offspring existed in the parents. The sequence studies on the different V regions show varied substitutions plus occasional deletions or insertions and it is difficult to conceive of a hypermutation mechanism which could account for the variations. Furthermore, there are striking similarities between certain mouse and human Light chain V regions. These similarities between such different animals would be very unlikely to be produced by random events such as hypermutation.

Function of Serum Antibodies

The serum antibodies participate in protecting the host from infection, but also are responsible for certain injurious effects. These effects of antibody are termed immunity when beneficial or protective, and hypersensitivity or allergy when harmful to the host. These designations, however, do not imply different mechanisms or different immunoglobulins responsible for these two events, and a single antibody may have both effects when reacting with a particular antigen.

IgG accounts for about 75 percent of serum immunoglobulins in man

(Table 3.1). Antibodies of this immunoglobulin class are responsible for acquired resistance or immunity to infection by many viruses and gram-positive bacteria, and protection against microbial exotoxins such as those of diphtheria and tetanus. Maternal IgG immunoglobins are transported across the placenta to the fetus, and these antibodies are important in protecting the newborn infant from infection until its own synthetic mechanisms are established between two to six weeks of life. Other immunoglobulins are excluded from the fetal circulation. Interaction of IgG with specific antigen activates the complement system (see Chapt. 6), leading to release of several chemical mediators including factors causing chemotaxis of leucocytes, enhancing phagocytosis, and causing immune adherence, as well as anaphylatoxins and permeability factors which initiate inflammation and hypersensitivity reactions. These results of interaction of IgG with microbial antigens are of great importance in controlling pyogenic infection. IgG is widely distributed in the interstitial and intravascular spaces. Therefore, its potential role in acquired resistance is considerable.

IgA comprises about 15 percent of the serum immunoglobuins, but is prodominant in secretions from mucous membranes and is considered an important part of the secretory immune system (Chapt. 4).

IgM accounts for 5 to 10 percent of the serum immunoglobulins, and phylogenetically is the most primitive. It is the first immunoglobulin antibody synthesized by the newborn infant. Its large molecular weight restricts IgM largely to the intravascular spaces. A single molecule attached to a specific antigen, such as a gram-negative bacillus, avidly fixes complement and thereby initiates a lesion in the cell membrane leading to cell lysis, as in bacteriolysis. IgG also may fix to cell surfaces but at least two molecules must be attached to "neighboring sites" to produce cell lysis after fixation of complement. The bactericidal activity of human serum against gram-negative bacteria, therefore, is mainly dependent upon IgM antibodies.

The function of IgD immunoglobulin is a mystery, but it is found in high levels in serum of pregnant black women at the time of delivery.

IgE, like IgA, is a secretory immunoglobulin (Chapt. 4), and is found in serum in minute amounts. It fixes to mast cells ("skin sensitizing"), and upon reaction with specific antigen, causes release of histamine, slow reacting substance of anaphylaxis (SRS-A) and bradykinins from these cells, leading to acute allergic reactions. Its role in acquired resistance to infection has not yet been proven. It has been postulated that IgE may serve to control parasitic infections, perhaps by producing an inflammatory reaction to the parasite at its site of lodgement. Persons with parasitic diseases are reported to have high levels of serum IgE.

Bacteriolysis, inflammation, enhancement of phagocytosis and toxin neutralization are the principle processes initiated by the immunoglobulins responsible for protection or immune effects in bacterial infection. These elements provide the means for killing microorganisms after a specific immunoglobulin antibody has interacted with cell surface antigens of the pathogen. Protection against viral infection also is dependent upon interaction of specific antibody with viral antigen, preventing attachment of virus to host cells.

Immune Deficiency States

Defects in various components of the immune system may profoundly affect resistance to infection. Such defects can be physiological, acquired or heritable. They have provided both severe challenges and great insight into the relative roles of the cellular and humoral immune systems.

Physiological hypogammaglobulinemia is a normal condition developing within 4 to 12 weeks after birth. The maternally transferred IgG is catabolized and the infants production of immunoglobulin will not have developed adequately to maintain antibody levels. The serum concentrations of immunoglobulin usually fall to 300 to 500 mg. percent, but may fall as low as 75 to 100 mg. percent. Infants with particularly low levels may experience repeated infections until their own immunologically responsive cells become more active during the second to fourth month of life.

Acquired hypogammaglobulinemia may occur at any age and in both sexes as a result of either decreased synthesis or increased loss of immunoglobulins. Decreased synthesis sometimes develops spontaneously and for unexplained reasons, becoming manifest by recurrent episodes of pneumonia or other respiratory infections. At other times these patients may have lymphoma or leukemia. The lymphoid tissues, as in familial hypogammaglobulinemia, reveal absent plasma cells, and the follicles may be atrophic or hypertrophied. IgG, IgM, and IgA are all affected, but serum immunoglobulin levels are not as low as in familial hypogammaglobulinemia, often between 100 to 200 mg. per 100 ml.

Hypogammaglobulinemia also may be secondary to excessive protein loss in feces or urine. The *nephrotic syndrome*, for example, is characterized by marked proteinuria; and this may be associated with decrease in serum levels of IgG and albumin although levels of IgA and IgM are usually normal. Lymphoid tissue is normal in these patients, for they have no defect in immunoglobulin production, and antibody formation following immunization is normal. *Exudative enteropathy*, as in patients with malabsorption syndrome, may result in diminution of all serum proteins, including IgG, IgA, and IgM, leading to protein loss in feces.

Primary or Familial Immune Deficiency Diseases

Over the last several decades a group of pediatric patients have been recognized with congenitally impaired immune defenses and severe recurrent acute infections often caused by antigenically identical microorganisms. Intensive study of these patients, summarized in a recent book entitled *Immunologic Deficiency Diseases in Man,* is increasing our immunologic knowledge and leading to dramatic new forms of therapy.

These diseases are best understood as resulting from impaired development of the lymphoid system. Figure 3.3 depicts the sequential development of stem cells into granulocytes, thymus dependent cells which mediate cellular immunity, or "bursal" dependent plasma cells (or lymphocytes) responsible for antibody synthesis. This scheme is derived in part from experiments with very young chickens wherein ablation of the bursa of Fabricius eliminates immunoglobulin synthesis while thymectomy destroys cellular immunity. The mammalian equivalent of the bursa is unknown. In Figure 3.3 genetic defects are postulated to explain the various combinations of immune defects.

In evaluation of such patients it is crucial to assay each component of the patient's immune system. Cellular reactions can be induced with skin sensitizing agents like fluorodinitrobenzene (FDNB) if delayed skin reactivity to tuberculin, mumps or to tetanus toxoid are negative. Immunoglobulin levels can be readily determined and serum antibody responses can be evaluated using either the natural antibodies to blood group substances or other antigens like tetanus toxoid.

Reticular Dysgenesis is a rare fatal disease characterized by a total lack of granulocytes, lymphocytes, and immunoglobulins. The only possible single lesion to produce all three deficiencies must be prior to stem cell differentiation into either the granulocytic series or the lymphoid series, as suggested in Figure 3.3.

Patients with *Swiss type agammaglobulinemia* show marked inhibition of delayed hypersensitivity, lymphopenia, low levels of all immunoglobulins and absence of antibody response to antigenic stimulation, but do have granulocytes. Hence, it is postulated that there is a genetic alteration which interferes with the differentiation of the lymphoid precursor cell. The familial pattern suggests that this genetic lesion is recessive and affects an autosomal gene. A sex-linked form of *lymphopenic hypogammaglobulinemia* has also been reported which is not as severe as the autosomal recessive disease, but again involves defects of both cellular and humoral immunity.

Two forms of cellular immune deficiency with normal immunoglobulin levels have been reported which are both associated with thymus abnormalities. Di George has described a syndrome associated with parathyroid and thymic aplasia and with absence of cellular immunity, while Nezelof has reported patients with normal parathyroids but vestigial thymus glands and no cellular immunity. Antibody responses in both types of patients are diminished in spite of the normal immunoglobulin levels.

Familial hypogammaglobulinemia was first described in 1952 by Bruton

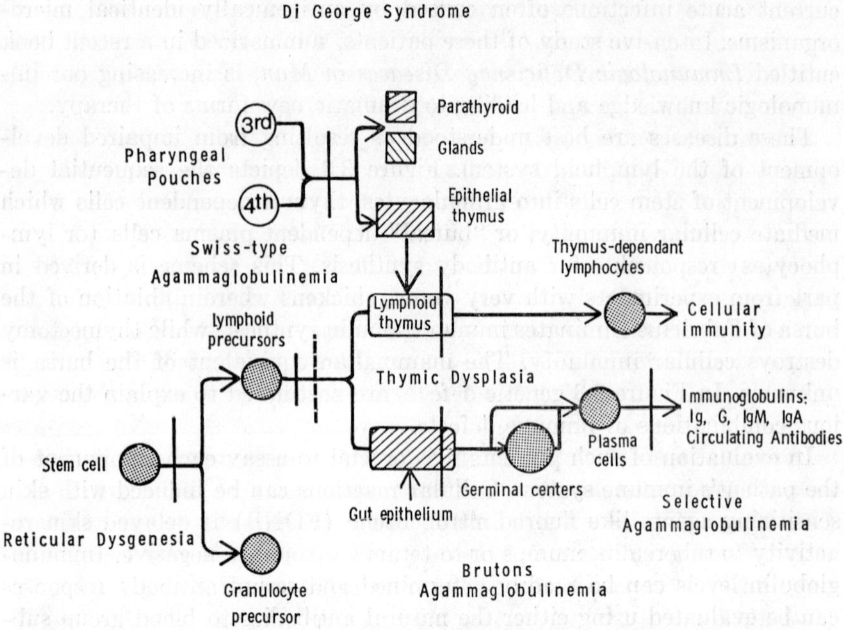

FIG. 3.3. Schematic diagram of normal lymphoid development including presumed developmental defects for various immune deficiency diseases (slightly modified from Hoyer *et. al.* (pg. 101) in *Immunologic Deficiency Diseases in Man.*

in a child with recurrent infections of the respiratory system. This disorder is inherited as a sex-linked recessive characteristic. All serum immunoglobulin classes are markedly decreased, total levels in serum are 50 mg. percent or less. Repeated infections develop in the first two years of life and administration of concentrated human globulin at regular intervals to those affected has been useful in controlling infection and prolonging life. They do not, however, develop serum antibody upon active immunization, except occasionally in very low titer. Patients with familial hypogammaglobulinemia do not have plasma cells or germinal centers in their lymph nodes, spleen, or bone marrow.

Most of the clinical manifestations of hypogammaglobulinemia are a direct consequence of impaired host resistance resulting in increased susceptibility to infections, with development of recurrent bouts of pneumonia, otitis media, sinusitis, meningitis, septic arthritis and pyogenic skin infections. The microorganisms responsible for these infections are usually indigenous, including the pneumococci, streptococci, and staphylococci, and also hepatitis virus, generalized vaccinia, pneumocystis carinii and cytomegalovirus.

Patients with familial hypogammaglobulinemia have developed recurrent non-pyogenic arthritis and various collagen-vascular disorders. In addition, some patients with idiopathic acquired hypogammaglobulinemia have developed leukopenia, thrombocytopenia and anemia. In both these types of hypogammaglobulinemia there has been an increased frequency of lymphoma and possibly other forms of neoplasia.

Selective immunoglobulin deficiencies occur, some of which may be heritable, but which may be unassociated with increased susceptibility to infection, probably indicating that host resistance to an infection is not the exclusive function of one immunoglobulin class.

Selective or generalized immunoglobulin deficiencies may be observed in patients with leukemia, reticulum cell sarcoma, multiple myeloma, and macroglobulinemia. These patients may or may not have recurrent infections and the immunoglobulin deficiency may be recognized incidentally.

The importance of understanding these various diseases is no longer an "academic exercise." Within the last few years two groups have been able to reconstitute the deficient lymphoid systems of two patients with cells from closely related relatives, and thereby restore these patients to health. This dramatic breakthrough heralds a new era in management of genetically determined disease. In addition, restoration of cellular immune responses has been possible by use of transfer factor (Chapt. 5).

SELECTED REFERENCES

Bergsma, D.: *Immunologic Deficiency Diseases in Man. Birth Defects: Original Article Series.* National Foundation-March of Dimes. 1968.

Cohen, S. and Melstein, C.: Structural activity of immunoglobulins. *Advances in Immunology. 7*:1, 1967.

Frangione, B., Milstein, C. and Pink, J. R. L.: "Immunoglobulins." Nature, *221*:145, 1969.

Good, R. A., ed.: *Immunobiology.* Senauer Associates, Inc., 1971.

Grubb, R.: *The Genetic Markers of Human Immunoglobulins.* Springer-Verlag, New York, 1970.

Hood, L. and Talmage, D. W.: Mechanism of antibody diversity: germ line basis for variability. Science, *168*:325, 1970.

Chapter 4

SECRETORY IMMUNOLOGIC SYSTEM

The concept of local immunity was first proposed by Besredka about 40 years ago. His concept, that there were immune mechanisms resident on mucosal surfaces distinct from circulating antibody, was not widely accepted. The antibody activity that was measured in external secretions was generally thought to be a result of spillover from serum antibody. Most immunologists felt that, although antibody on mucosal surfaces might be important, the easiest way to stimulate this antibody production was to simply raise the level of antibody in the serum. This opinion prevailed despite the excellent work of Walsh in the 1930's, which showed that antibody in the respiratory tract was locally produced. Fazekas de St. Groth in 1950 showed, in mice infected with influenza virus, that protection was related to bronchial secretion antibody and not serum antibody, and that the most effective method of stimulating bronchial secretion antibody was by administering the live or killed influenza virus by nose drops.

In recent years there has been a resurgence of interest in the concept of a local immune system, mainly because the concept of spillover of serum antibody has been largely disproven. This began with the findings of Hanson and Tomasi that the predominant immunoglobulin in external secretions is IgA, a relatively minor immunoglobulin in serum. Furthermore, it was found that this IgA in external secretions had a significantly different structure than did serum IgA. Serum IgA has a molecular weight of around 170,000 and a sedimentation coefficient of 7. Most of the IgA in secretions has a molecular weight of 380,000 and a sedimentation coefficient of 11. In addition, IgA in secretions has an additional antigenic component which is present in only minute amounts in relationship to serum IgA. This additional antigenic component is now called secretory compo-

This paper was also published in Postgraduate Medicine, Nov. 1971, McGraw-Hill, Inc.

nent, and has formerly been called transport piece, T piece or secretory piece.

Production of Secretory IgA

The data indicate that secretory IgA is predominantly locally synthesized and does not come by either transport or passive diffusion from serum. Histochemical studies have indicated that secretory IgA is synthesized in two different sites. The dimerized IgA is synthesized in plasma cells which lie beneath the epithelium of secretory surfaces. This dimerized IgA passes between epithelial cells or through intracellular channels to reach the mucosal surface. The secretory component is synthesized in the epithelial cells and also passes onto the epithelial surface. It is at this surface that the combination of secretory component with the dimerized IgA occurs, resulting in the secretory IgA molecule.

Role of Secretory IgA

The function of secretory component is unknown. As can be ascertained from its former name, "transport piece," it has been postulated that it serves a transport function. However, the more recent data, which indicates that secretory component does not combine with the dimerized IgA molecule until the IgA reaches the epithelial surface, militates against that hyopthesis. The other postulated function is to stabilize the molecule. It is obvious that the milieu in which secretory IgA finds itself is not as favorable as the milieu of intravascular spaces. Proteolytic enzymes abound in most secretions. Studies have indicated that secretory IgA is slightly more stable than is serum IgA, which in turn is much more stable than is IgG in the presence of proteolytic enzymes. Other functions, such as one of helping in a complement-like reaction, have not been ruled out.

Other Immunologic Modalities

In addition to secretory IgA, there are other important immunologic modalities which have been identified in secretions. Other immunoglobulins are present. Although IgG and IgM are present in lower concentrations than in serum, they still may be functionally important, especially in certain circumstances. It has yet to be proven that secretory IgA is bacteriocidal. Since it has been shown that IgG and IgM can be bacteriocidal, these immunoglobulins, although present in small amounts, may be functionally important for protection against diseases such as the bacterial enteritides.

Another immunoglobulin class which may play an important role on secretory surfaces is IgE. IgE-producing lymphoid cells are present in much larger relative numbers in the submucosae of secretory tissues than are present in spleen or lymph nodes. IgE in secretions probably is not different from serum IgE; i.e., it is present in the monomeric form and not associated with secretory component. Its role in protection against and as a cause of illness is speculative at the present time. However, it is surely to be an area of importance in the next several years.

Cell-mediated immunity has also been demonstrated on secretory surfaces, especially the respiratory tract. It has been demonstrated in several model systems that cell-mediated immunity in the respiratory tract is relatively independent of systemic cell-mediated immunity. Furthermore, it has been shown that, in the case of experimental tuberculosis infection, cell-mediated immunity in the respiratory tract correlates better with resistance to respiratory challenge than does systemic cell-mediated immunity, as measured by sensitized lymphocytes being present in the circulation or in the spleen.

A final immunologic modality that has been demonstrated in secretions is the presence of interferon following viral infections. The role of interferon in protection against viral infections of the secretory surfaces, as is the case with the role of interferon elsewhere, is a matter of intense investigative work at the present time.

Antibodies Containing Secretory IgA

Secretory antibody is locally produced in the secretory mucosa. Most of the antibody to *Herpesvirus hominis* is found in lacrimal secretions; to respiratory syncytial virus, rhinovirus, parainfluenza virus, polio virus, influenza virus and diphtheria toxoid, in respiratory secretions; to *Vibrio cholera* cell wall antigens and polio virus, in the gastrointestinal secretions; and to *Candida albicans* antigens, in the female genital tract, to name a few, all have been shown to be IgA immunoglobulins. In many of these studies subcutaneous immunization has been shown to stimulate serum antibody to virtually the same level as actual infection; however, this route of immunization stimulated very little secretory antibody.

In studies with influenza virus, neither subcutaneous immunization nor local application of infective or inactivated virus was very efficient in stimulating neutralizing antibody activity in saliva, an external secretion that contains similar quantities of secretory IgA as does nasal secretions and sputum. This lends support to the hypothesis that secretory IgA antibody is locally produced and stimulated, for the salivary glands are not stimulated directly by antigen during influenza infection nor following aerosol or subcutaneous immunization.

Selective Reactions to Antigens

One antibody producing site of the secretory IgA system is probably not induced to produce specific antibody following application of antigen to another site, although this is somewhat controversial. As mentioned above, antibody production into nasal secretions and sputum was not accompanied by a corresponding response in saliva. Humans with double-barreled colostomies, immunized with poliovirus antigen into one limb of the large intestine, produced specific antibody in that limb but not elsewhere. Administration of influenza virus vaccine into the upper respiratory tract induces better nasal secretion antibody response than if administered into the lower respiratory tract. The converse is true for antibody in sputum. This suggests that secretory IgA antibody is produced locally when antigen is applied to that site.

In contrast, however, respiratory challenge with live rhinovirus has shown antibody production in lacrimal secretions in the absence of detectable virus replication there. Conceivably, viral replication was undetected or enough antigen was absorbed to stimulate production of secretory antibody in the lacrimal glands. Parenterally administered antigens have been shown in several studies to stimulate the production of secretory antibody, but not as efficiently as local application of antigen. Killed influenza virus, parainfluenza, polio, rhinovirus, diphtheria toxoid and tetanus toxoid given subcutaneously stimulate high levels of serum but low levels of respiratory secretion antibody. On the other hand, the local application of antigen leads to the production of much higher levels of respiratory secretion antibody.

Secretory IgA Antibody and Protection

The presence of respiratory secretion IgA antibody and protection against infection are not necessarily synonymous. To test the ability of antibody to protect, field trials have been carried out to test aerosol immunization in naturally occurring influenza epidemics. In three such reported field trials the aerosol route of immunization rendered protection rates of between 70 to 80 percent. There were differences primarily in the protection rates afforded by subcutaneous immunization. It appears that poorer protection results from subcutaneous immunization in individuals with pre-existing serum antibody. In the 1967–68 field trial the pre-existing titer against the classical A_2 influenza virus was about 1:40 whereas the 1968–69 trials the pre-existing antibody titer against the A_2/Hong Kong virus was $<1{:}4$. It is conceivable that anything which interferes with antigen reaching the secretory mucosa, such as pre-existing systemic antibody binding the antigen, reduces the secretory antibody response to parenteral antigen. The presence of secretory IgA antibody correlates with protection against illness; this indication is supported by studies with rhinovirus and parainfluenza virus, revealing that nasal secretion antibody against the challenge virus is more closely related to protection than is serum antibody.

Secretory IgA antibody may be less specific than is serum IgG antibody. Dowdle and co-workers demonstrated significant rises in nasal secretion antibody to previous influenza A strains following A_2 influenza virus immunization, but little or no rise in serum antibody. In another study, immunization by aerosol with an Asian strain of inactivated influenza virus vaccine prior to the appearance of the A_2/Hong Kong variant induced antibody rise against the vaccine strain in both respiratory secretions and serum, but no rise in serum antibody to the heterologous strains, A/PR_8 and A_2/Hong Kong influenza. However, there was a significant rise in IgA antibody to these heterologous strains.

Clinical Correlations

What is the clinical importance of the secretory immunologic system, defining this system in its broadest terms; that is, including all the modalities which have been discussed above? At the present time the clinical importance is mainly the recognition that the secretory immunologic system exists. In the past, physicians were concerned primarily about serum antibody when thinking about immunity against infectious agents; or occasionally were concerned with cellular immunity. However, it has become apparent that the secretory immunologic system must be considered whenever infections occur on secretory surfaces or whenever infectious agents enter the body through secretory surfaces. This obviously includes most infectious agents.

If the mechanisms concerned with the secretory immunologic system are important in protecting secretory surfaces, then one would expect that a deficiency in one or more of the components results in an increased incidence of infections of the surfaces. Cellular immune mechanisms on secretory surfaces in patients with a deficiency of the thymus-dependent lymphocytic population have not been studied. Fortunately, no patients are known to have interferon production deficiency. In immunoglobulin deficiency states, the immunoglobulin content of external secretions correlates with that of the systemic system; that is, in IgA deficient individuals, secretory IgA is deficient in the external secretions. IgA deficiency is the most common isolated immunoglobulin deficiency. There are no known cases of secretory IgA deficiency in patients with normal IgA serum levels. There are only one or two cases in which secretory IgA has been demonstrated in patients with serum IgA deficiency. Since serum IgA comes from mucosally synthesized IgA in normals, it is not surprising that generally IgA levels in serum and secretions are related.

The clinical picture in patients varies. Some patients with IgA deficiency are perfectly normal, with no increase in mucosal infections. It has been postulated that another immunoglobulin class takes over the function of IgA in the external secretion. The class most commonly involved is IgM.

Some patients with IgA deficiencies have either severe respiratory or gastrointestinal tract difficulties. Most of the patients with respiratory difficulties have IgA deficiency associated with hereditary ataxia telangectasia. Clinically these patients may have severe recurrent viral and bacterial infections of the respiratory tract, resulting in eventual chronic bronchitis and bronchiectasis.

It is impossible at this time, however, to strictly link the IgA deficiency and the propensity to respiratory infections. Many of these patients have other concomitant immune abnormalities, such as deficiency of IgE or of the cellular immune mechanism.

Several syndromes involving the gastroinestinal tract have been associated with IgA deficiencies. A group of patients with diarrhea, steatorrhea and *Giardia lamblia* infection, severe IgA and IgM deficiencies and with moderate deficiency of IgG has been reported. Small intestinal biopsies in these patients showed a nodular lymphoid hyperplasia. Another group of patients showed isolated IgA deficiencies and malabsorption with a clinical picture resembling non-tropical sprue and a clinical response to a gluten-free diet.

In a series of patients with tropical sprue, 2 of 28 showed IgA deficiencies. In both the tropical and non-tropical sprue patients, the immunoglobulin abnormalities apparently persist despite correction of the clinical symptomatology. The relationship of the IgA deficiency to the gastrointestinal disease is not clear. With the exception of the *Giardia lamblia* infestation, IgA deficiency has not been related to known infections of the gastrointestinal tract. Of course, non-tropical and tropical sprue have been postulated to be due to (an) infectious agent(s). It is tempting to hypothesize that in non-tropical sprue there is local IgG, IgM or IgE antibody production to wheat gluten, whereas in normals, IgA antibody to gluten is produced. This IgA antibody might be considered as "blocking" antibody, since IgA antibody does not cause cellular damage, as does IgG and IgM antibody through the complement system, and IgE through the release of histamine and other vasoactive substances. Definite data supporting this postulated local hypersensitivity reaction has not been obtained.

As mentioned above, IgA deficiency is not uncommon, with a frequency of about 1 in 700. Although many of these show no increased incidence of infectious diseases, there is an unusually high incidence of auto-immune diseases and malignancies. Also, IgA deficiency has been reported with increased incidence in patients with disseminated lupus erythematosus, Still's disease, cirrhosis, idiopathic pulmonary hemosiderosis, and in mentally retarded patients with congenital abnormalities and a defect of chromosome #18. In none of these disorders is the relationship between the disease and the IgA deficiency known.

This relationship of IgA deficiency and auto-immune diseases has another facet also. Auto-antibodies have been found in secretions in pernicious anemia, and the possible role of salivary and gastric auto-antibodies to an intrinsic factor in the etiology of the disease is currently a subject of investigation. In ulcerative colitis, colon-reactive antibodies have been found in the regional lymph nodes of the colon but not in the small intestinal glands of the same individual.

Finally, mention should be made of physiological IgA deficiency; i.e., the situation in infants. The IgA system slowly matures with age. In the neo-natal period no IgA containing plasma cells are found in the gastrointestinal tract. Some of the diseases of the gastrointestinal and respiratory tracts occurring in early childhood may be attributable to delayed maturation of the local secretory IgA system. It has been postulated that in the newborn the IgA antibody in colostrum and milk may be an important method of passive immunity for the gastrointestinal tract. However, there is no clinical data indicating that gastrointestinal infections are more common in the neo-natal period in non-breast-fed infants as compared to breast-fed infants.

SELECTED REFERENCES

Besredka, A.: *Local Immunization,* Williams and Wilkins, Baltimore, Md., 1927.

Chodirker, W. B. and Tomasi, T. B.: Gamma-globulin: Quantitative relationships in human serum and nonvascular fluids. Science, *142:*1080, 1963.

Crabbe, P. A. and Heremans, J. F.: The distribution of immunoglobulin-containing cells along the human gastrointestinal tract. Gastroenterology, *51:* 305, 1967.

Dayton, D. H., Jr., Small, P. A., Jr., Chanock, R. M., Kaufman, H. E., and Tomasi, T. B., Jr., eds., *The Secretory Immunologic System.* U. S. Government Printing Office, 1969.

Fazekas de St. Groth, S. and Donnelley, M.: Studies in experimental immunology of influenza IV. The protective value of active immunization. Austral. J. Exp. Biol. Med. Sci., *28:*61, 1950.

Ogra, P. L. and Karzon, D. T.: Poliovirus antibody response in serum and nasal secretions following intranasal inoculation with inactivated polio vaccine. J. Immunol., *102:* 15, 1969.

Ogra, P. L. and Karzon, D. T.: Distribution of poliovirus antibody in serum, nasopharynx and alimentary tract following segmental immunization of lower alimentary tract with poliovaccine. J. Immunol., *102:*1423, 1969.

Smith, C. B., Bellanti, J. A. and Chanock, R. M.: Immunoglobulins in serum and nasal secretions following infection with type 1 parainfluenza virus and injection of inactivated vaccines. J. Immunol., *99:*133, 1967.

Tomasi, T. B. and Bienenstock, J.: Secretory immunoglobulins. Advances in Immunology, *9:*1, 1968.

Tomasi, T. B., Jr., Tan, E. M., Soloman, A., and Prendergast, A. L.: Characteristics of an immune system common to certain external secretions. J. Exp. Med., *121:* 101, 1965.

Waldman, R. H. and Henney, C. S.: Cell-mediated immunity and antibody responses in the respiratory tract after local and systemic immunization. J. Exp. Med., *134:* 482, 1971.

Waldman, R. H., Kasel, J. A., Fulk, R. V., Mann, J. J., Togo, Y., Hornick, R. B., Heiner, G. T., Dawkins, A. T.: Influenza antibody in human respiratory secretions following subcutaneous or nasopharyngeal immunization with inactivated vaccine. Nature, *218:*594, 1968.

Chapter 5

ACQUIRED CELLULAR RESISTANCE

Exposure of the animal host to an infecting microorganism begins a number of processes which not only influences the host's response to that infection, but may alter his response to subsequent infection by the same microorganism. These altered responses are mediated by altered physiologic states defined as delayed hypersensitivity, macrophage activation, the production of physiologically important chemical mediators, and the induction of immediate hypersensitivity leading to antibody formation. As the latter will be considered in another section, it is the purpose of this chapter to review the mechanics of the former phenomena, to inter-relate them when possible, and to discuss and document their significance to the host during the course of an infectious disease. These phenomena have in common an intimate association with cells, particularly those of the lymphocytic and phagocytic series.

Delayed Hypersensitivity

Functional differentiation of hypersensitivity into immediate and delayed types in the intact animal is a reflection of postulated differences in developmental anatomy. Studies in avian species have demonstrated different developmental anlage for those tissues ultimately responsible for the integrity of the different systems. Thus, the Bursa of Fabricius, located near the cloaca, is responsible for the development of antibody producing cells, while the thymus gland has its primary role in the development and integrity of cells mediating delayed hypersensitivity. The mammalian analogue of the Bursa of Fabricius is most probably reticuloendothelial tissue scattered through the gastrointestinal tract and lymph nodes. The effect of neonatal thymectomy in experimental animals has demonstrated the importance of the thymus to the integrity of delayed hypersensitivity. A body of evidence suggests that there are definite inter-relationships between these two systems, though they may be of different embryological origin, as documented by the multiple heritable disorders in which combined deficits of both antibody production and delayed hypersensitivity occur. While the extent and significance of these inter-relationships have not yet been fully explored, there are many similarities between the two. Enough differences exist, however, to emphasize the concept that each may have a unique functional significance to the normal individual.

Transfer of Delayed Hypersensitivity

Following injection of specific antigen into the skin of an animal with the appropriate delayed hypersensitivity, an erythematous, indurated skin reaction evolves reaching a maximum at 24 to 48 hours. While there has been some disagreement as to the nature and significance of the cellular response associated with this reaction, it is generally agreed that the early phase (up to 10 hours) involves primarily polymorphonuclear leukocytes and that subsequently a preponderance of mononuclear cells develops. This increase may be due either to specific local accumulation or to the more rapid emigration of polymorphonuclear cells, resulting in a relative enrichment of round cells at the site.

When experimental animals are passively immunized in delayed hypersensitivity by the transfer of lymphocytes, only a small percentage of cells found at the skin test site can be shown to originate from the donor animal. This suggests that there is either a recruitment of previously non-immunized cells or that non-specific leukotactic factors exert a profound influence on the histology of the reaction. The transfer of serum from the immunized donor is largely ineffective in transferring delayed hypersensitivity. The ability of immune lymphocytes to accomplish this transfer is in agreement with the predominance of mononuclears in the local cellular response, indicating this type of cell as the one of importance in delayed hypersensitivity.

Two systems have been described in which soluble factors alone may accomplish transfer of delayed hypersensitivity. Lawrence and his coworkers have demonstrated a dialysable leukocyte extract which is susceptible neither to DNAase nor RNAase and which can transfer delayed hypersensitivity from the immunized to the nonimmunized patient. Within hours after the administration of such an extract, delayed hypersensitivity specific to the immune status of the donor can be demonstrated and may persist for a number of years. This "transfer factor" is also able to sensitize nonimmunized lymphocytes *in vitro*. Lawrence has suggested that the transfer factor converts a limited number of lymphocytes to an antigen-responsive state, and that the propogation of delayed hypersensitivity in the host results from continuing proliferation of these specifically converted cells. A similar factor has not been found in extracts of leukocytes from experimental animals. Good and his associates, however, have demonstrated the ability to transfer delayed hypersensitivity in guinea pigs passively with a plasma factor migrating electrophoretically in the albumin-prealbumin regions. This material has the ability to sensitize nonimmune splenic lymphocytes *in vitro* and therefore could represent the non-human analogue of transfer factor.

Specificity of Delayed Hypersensitivity

As with immediate hypersensitivity, one of the outstanding and uniform characteristics of delayed hypersensitivity is its remarkable specificity. Thus, only chemically definable antigens identical or nearly identical to the immunizing material can elicit the reaction. Compared with information defining chemical characteristics of materials active in the elicitation of antibody, relatively little is known concerning structural characteristics of similar molecules active in delayed hypersensitivity systems. It is clear, however, that small molecules (haptens) are not effective unless chemically conjugated with larger ones such as proteins or polypeptides (carriers). Important differences have been shown with respect to the specificity of haptenic determinants in delayed as opposed to antibody mediated hypersensitivity. Whereas antibodies directed solely against the haptenic grouping can be demonstrated, the primary specificity in delayed hypersensitivity resides in an area of the molecule involving both the hapten and the adjacent part of the carrier. This is true even when the carrier protein is native to the recipient animal and implies that some alteration in structure of the carrier occurs with its conjugation to the hapten.

Antibodies with similar specificity seem to occur only in the earliest phases of antibody response. If the carrier protein is foreign to the recipient animal, it also serves as an antigenic determinant in addition to fulfilling its role in the hapten-carrier site for delayed hypersensitivity. Leskowitz has shown that conjugation of hapten onto polyamino acids may elicit strict hapten specificity, but this observation seems to be unique to haptens on synthetic carriers.

It is also of interest that polysaccharide antigens which may elicit excellent antibody response will fail to produce detectable delayed hypersensitivity in the same host, while proteins are effective in eliciting hypersensitivity of both types. Borek and his coworkers have found that if polysaccharide antigens are attached as haptens to protein carriers they may participate in the specificity of delayed hypersensitivity, though specificity for the polysaccharide itself is poor. This is of great interest in view of the ubiquitous occurrence of polysaccharides in the cell walls and capsules of many of the bacteria which cause infection of man. A correlary to the role of hapten carrier systems in the elicitation of delayed hypersensitivity may lie in the function of antigen-antibody complexes as antigens. In this case, some alteration in configuration of the antibody molecule as a consequence of its interaction with antigen is undoubtedly involved, though the molecular alteration is not adequate to elicit an antibody response. Such complexes could conceivably play an important role in the induction of delayed hypersensitivity to microbial antigens. The specific chemical or structural traits which make a molecule antigenic in delayed hypersensitivity are poorly understood. Size alone may be a limiting factor, but suggestive evidence also exists that structural characteristics of the molecule as a whole are critical. Thus, studies of penicillin congeners have demonstrated specificity to the basic ring structures as well as the influence of side chain charge in determining antigenicity.

Antigen Recognition in Delayed Hypersensitivity

Whereas the interaction between specific antibody and its antigen in liquid medium is a well-studied phenomenon, the means by which the antigen in delayed hypersensitivity is recognized by the body is as yet incompletely understood. It is clear that the immunologically competent lymphocyte or one of its derivatives is almost certainly involved at an early stage. It has been suggested that a highly avid antibody of the classical sort, possibly cytophilic and thereby primarily attached to cells, may be the important moderator of the recognition phenomenon. Levine has calculated binding affinities for antigens in immediate and delayed hypersensitivity systems and can demonstrate very high values in the latter, compatible with the concept of a highly avid antibody acting in this system. At this time, however, evidence that such an antibody functions in delayed hypersensitivity remains circumstantial, and recent data have supported the concept that immunologically competent cells have receptors on their surface which bind antigen and start the chain of events involved in this form of hypersensitivity.

In addition to skin tests of the living animal, a number of other *in vitro* and *in vivo* methods for the detection of delayed hypersensitivity exists. Rich and Lewis recognized that the emigration of immunized macrophages from tissue in the presence of specific antigens was impaired; George and Vaughn, David, and others have adapted this observation for the demonstration of delayed hypersensitivity. Basically the system utilizes free living cells, often from peritoneal exudates, harvested into a capillary tube and allowed to grow in a liquid medium in the presence or absence of specific antigen. The normal fanlike migration of macrophages from the tip of the capillary tube can be specifically inhibited by the appropriate antigen. It has been shown that two cell populations are involved: a small percentage of immune lymphocytes acting as the antigen detectors and migrating macrophages acting as the indicator cells. Modifications of this test may be applied to humans either by preliminary cultivation of lymph node cells, changing them into a migratory population, or by using supernatants obtained from human lymphocytes cultured in the presence of antigen to inhibit the migration of guinea pig macrophages in the usual capillary tube technique.

Cultivation of lymphocytes from immunized donors in the presence of specific antigen will cause these cells to become larger and to assume a blast-like appearance. This morphologic change is associated with alteration in the histochemical and fine structural characteristics of the cell. Turk and his coworkers have demonstrated that this morphologic alteration is a nonspecific cell response to sublethal stimuli, but with appropriate controls it can be used to detect delayed hypersensitivity. During the course of this morphologic change, net DNA synthesis occurs when the inciting stimulus is delayed hypersensitivity. It can be monitored by the uptake of radio-labelled nucleic acids into cell nuclei or DNA. The test is influenced by the quantity of antigen used and may be negative when either too little or too much is present. There also appears to be variation between different individuals as to the optimal antigen range at which appropriate responses are elicited.

Two additional procedures have specialized use in the study of delayed hypersensitivity. It has been demonstrated that the time necessary for rejection of organ grafts from genetically dissimilar members of the same animal species is dependent upon prior exposure of the recipient animal to tissue antigens of the donor. Prior "immunization" of this sort produces an accelerated rejection of the graft. And secondly, Rosenow and others have demonstrated that immunized lymphocytes will adhere to and subsequently lyse genetically dissimilar tissue cells to which the lymphocytes had been previously immunized. It has been suggested that attachment of lymphocyte to target cell is immunologically specific but that the actual lytic process is non-specific and possibly mediated by humoral factors. The efficacy of the system in studies of tissue antigens in delayed hypersensitivity is well defined, but a comparable interaction between immunologically competent cells and microorganisms has not been shown.

Non-specificity of Cellular Reactions

It is clear that delayed hypersensitivity is but one of a number of stimuli which may institute a set of cellular reactions of similar if not identical types. As mentioned earlier, the distinctive aspect which delayed hypersensitivity offers is its antigenic specificity. The classic examples of non-specific stimuli eliciting these common cellular responses are the phytomitogens. These substances are included in a group of plant lectins of poorly defined nature each of which is probably a complex mixture, and of which phytohemagglutinin (PHA), pokeweed mitogen and extracts from various beans and peas are examples. Such compounds in appropriate concentrations can induce lymphocytes to mimic essentially all of the effects resulting from their stimulation by specific antigen following immunization. Thus, blast transformation, DNA synthesis, RNA synthesis and morphologic alteration including histochemical and fine structural changes are observed. They may also induce cell culture cytolysis. In some instances the time course of these reactions differs when compared with those due to delayed hypersensitivity, though the possibility of quantitative differences as an explanation for this altered time course must be entertained.

Lymphocyte responsiveness to phytomitogens may parallel clinically demonstrable delayed hypersensitivity in patients with a variety of diseases. Thus, PHA induced transformation may be diminished in patients with Hodgkin's disease and sarcoidosis. The mechanism whereby mitogens affect lymphocytes and other cells is unclear, but it has been related to their ability to alter cell membranes. Their activity supports the concept that the cellular changes we recognize to be associated with delayed hypersensitivity are probably non-specific responses appropriate to multiple inciting stimuli.

Macrophage Activation

In his book, *The Pathogenesis of Tuberculosis*, Arnold Rich noted "...we can observe directly that following the introduction of an equal number of bacilli into the normal and the tuberculous or vaccinated body, markedly fewer will be found in the tissues of the latter after any given lapse of time...." There has as yet appeared no better summary of the phenomenon by which certain infections, particularly those caused by primarily intracellular organisms, can favorably influence the ability of the host to phagocytose and kill invading microorganisms. From the work of Mackaness and others it is now clear that exposure of the living host to infection with such organisms as *M. tuberculosis, Listeria monocytogenes,* or brucella alters the characteristics of host macrophages. In addition to enhanced phagocytic activity, they are able to kill ingested bacteria more effectively, to migrate more rapidly to sites of inflammation and infection, and they have certain intrinsic morphologic and metabolic alterations which include increased numbers of mitochondria and lysosomes, an increased frequency of mitosis, and an increased glucose uptake and enzyme content. Collectively, these alterations are responsible for the state called "macrophage activation." The development of these physiologic and morphologic alterations occurs simultaneously with the increasing ability of the host to clear the infecting bacteria, and their presence is responsible for host resistance to subsequent infection by the same organisms.

TABLE 5.1

Some characteristics of acquired resistance to infection mediated by activated macrophages

1. Resistance inducible by intracellular microbes infecting macrophages *in vivo.*
2. Killed microbial vaccines largely ineffective in inducing resistance.
3. Resistance non-specific during initial infection, specific on re-infection or after passive transfer.
4. Development of resistance temporally associated with the development of delayed hypersensitivity to antigens of the infecting microbe.
5. Cell of importance is the short lived lymphocyte which can passively transfer resistance.

A characterization of the state of enhanced cellular resistance is presented in Table 5.1, which summarizes the basic observations concerning macrophage activation. It is clear that acquired resistance of this sort is usually inducible by intracellular microbes infecting the host macrophages *in vivo.* By and large, killed microbial vaccines are ineffective, though they may be quite effective in producing delayed hypersensitivity. The development of cellular resistance is temporally associated with the development of delayed hypersensitivity to antigens of the infecting microbe. Whereas the delayed hypersensitivity can be shown to be quite specific for these antigens, the host at this time demonstrates an increased resistance to infection by both the original bacterium and by other unrelated intracellular organisms. Following recovery from the inciting infection, cellular resistance wanes over a period of a few weeks. If the host is subsequently rechallenged by infection with a number of such intracellular microbes, he can be shown to have a relative resistance only to infection by the original inciting microbe. That is, the resistance has now become specific.

If one harvests splenic cells from infected hosts and transfers them to the previously unexposed recipient, the recipient can be demonstrated to have increased resistance to infection. In this instance, as opposed to the primary infection of the donor, the resistance is also specific to that bacterium which was used to infect the donor originally. Studies involving thoracic duct cannulation have demonstrated that not all lymphocytes are effective in achieving this transfer. It is the short-lived lymphocyte which is capable of transferring this type of resistance, rather than the long-lived, thymus-derived cell which represents the major population of lymphocytes circulating in the blood and in which the phenomenon of immunologic memory resides.

The mechanism whereby information is transferred from short-lived lymphocytes to macrophages is not clear. It has been shown that certain of the chemical mediators known to be effective in the interaction between lymphocyte and macrophage in delayed hypersensitivity (as described below) cause many of the effects on the macrophage demonstrable during the course of macrophage activation. Thus, increased metabolic activity and phagocytic capability result from exposure of macrophages to migration inhibition factor, though evidence that bactericidal capability of the macrophages is similarly enhanced has not been presented. It is appealing to believe, therefore, that mediators are also important in the process of increasing cellular resistance by macrophage activation and, in fact, that these mediators may be similar or identical to those active in delayed hypersensitivity reactions.

Comparisons Between Delayed Hypersensitivity and Macrophage Activation

It is clear that a number of similarities exist between the phenomena associated with delayed hypersensitivity and those of increased cellular resistance due to macrophage activation. The development of the two processes during the course of active infection is coincident. Following reinfection of the actively exposed host, or following infection of the passively activated recipient, both systems are specific to the original antigen or microbe. In both systems recognition is mediated through a lymphocyte while effector phenomena are expressed by macrophages. Due to such similarities a number of workers believe that the two processes are identical. A number of distinct differences between them are apparent, however. While killed vaccines are most effective in inducing delayed hypersensitivity, they are largely ineffective in the induction of cellular resistance by macrophage activation. While antigenic specificity is the hallmark of delayed hypersensitivity, the initial state of cellular resistance induced by active infection in the host is characteristically nonspecific and extends to resistance against infection by a number of microbes. It is very clear that the long-lived, thymus-derived lymphocyte, which is the seat of immunological memory in delayed hypersensitivity systems and which responds to antigenic stimulation *in vitro,* is apparently not critical to the development of cellular resistance in the form of macrophage activation.

In addition to these basic observations, a number of experiments have suggested dissociation between the phenomena of cellular resistance and delayed hypersensitivity. Thus, Wells and Wylie, working with BCG, demonstrated that cellular resistance may be retained after delayed hypersensitivity has disappeared. Both Raffel working with the tubercle bacillus and Ackerman working with Listeria organisms were able to obtain bacterial extracts effective in the induction of delayed hypersensitivity but ineffective in inducing cellular resistance to infection by those organisms. Wilson working with the tubercle bacillus and again Ackerman were able to demonstrate desensitization of the actively immunized host to the point

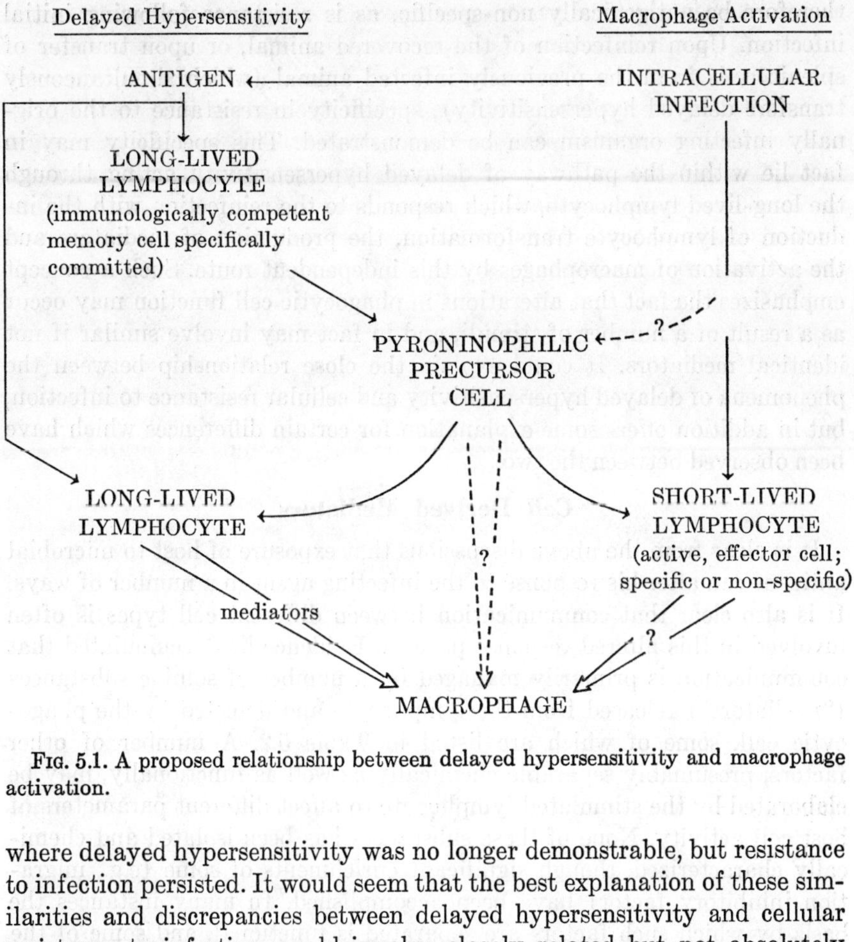

FIG. 5.1. A proposed relationship between delayed hypersensitivity and macrophage activation.

where delayed hypersensitivity was no longer demonstrable, but resistance to infection persisted. It would seem that the best explanation of these similarities and discrepancies between delayed hypersensitivity and cellular resistance to infection would involve closely related but not absolutely identical processes. Such a correlative scheme is presented in Figure 5.1 and may be explained as follows.

It is very clear that active infection with intracellular organisms can serve as a source of antigen for immunization. This is proved by the development of classical delayed hypersensitivity and even antibody formation following such infections. It may be postulated that following initial infection with such organisms there is, in addition, a direct effect of the infection either upon the pyroninophilic precursor cell or directly on the population of short-lived lymphocytes which is a function of the infection per se and unrelated to delayed hypersensitivity or the antigenic composition of the infecting organisms. As a result of this effect, mediators are released which cause the phenomenon of macrophage activation with enhanced resistance to the infecting microbe. This phenomenon would therefore be antigenically non-specific, as is resistance following initial infection. Upon reinfection of the recovered animal, or upon transfer of splenic cells from the previously infected animal (which simultaneously transfers delayed hypersensitivity), specificity in resistance to the orignally infecting organism can be demonstrated. This specificity may in fact lie within the pathway of delayed hypersensitivity acting through the long-lived lymphocyte, which responds to the reinfection with the induction of lymphocyte transformation, the production of mediators and the activation of macrophages by this independent route. Such a concept emphasizes the fact that alterations in phagocytic cell function may occur as a result of a number of stimuli, and in fact may involve similar if not identical mediators. It could explain the close relationship between the phenomena of delayed hypersensitivity and cellular resistance to infection, but in addition offers some explanation for certain differences which have been observed between the two.

Cell Derived Mediators

It is clear from the above discussions that exposure of host to microbial antigens can alter his response to the infecting agent in a number of ways. It is also clear that communication between different cell types is often involved in this altered response pattern. Evidence has accumulated that communication is primarily managed by a number of soluble substances ("mediators") released from the lymphocyte and detected by the phagocytic cell, some of which are listed in Table 5.2. A number of other factors, presumably separable chemically as well as functionally, may be elaborated by the stimulated lymphocyte to affect different parameters of host cell activity. None of these substances has been isolated and chemically characterized, though significant enrichments of some (e.g., migration inhibitory factor) have been accomplished. In many instances the basis by which such factors are separated is functional, and some of the described activities may ultimately prove to reside in the same mediator molecule.

Chemotactic factors directed at both the tissue macrophage and the blood neutrophil have been described and can be dissociated from the migration inhibition factor by disc electrophoresis. David has shown that as a result of the elaboration of migration inhibition factor, the lympho-

TABLE 5.2

A listing of some soluble factors released from lymphocytes by delayed hypersensitivity or other stimuli

1. Chemotactic factor(s)	4. Non-lethal cell inhibition factor(s)
2. Migration inhibition factor	5. Skin reactive factor(s)
3. Interferon	6. Blastogenic factor

cyte can influence many macrophages, a cascade effect in the mediation of hypersensitivity. Interferon may be released from body cells by viral invasion, and from lymphocytes by mitogens or delayed hypersensitivity as well. Its appearance correlates with the clearance of viremia, and it may therefore represent a primary defense mechanism against continuing cell invasion by the virus. A number of factors which can reversibly inhibit cell functions have been described, releasable by both delayed hypersensitivity and often by mitogens, and resulting in the inhibition of cell cloning, cell proliferation and DNA synthesis. On the other hand, cytotoxic factors lethal to a variety of tissue types may be released during delayed hypersensitivity or mitogenic stimulation. An element of tissue specificity has been ascribed to some of these, contrasting with the non-specific nature of the majority of mediators now known. Factors producing morphologic and histologic changes in the skin similar to those associated with the antigen-induced delayed hypersensitivity reaction are also known, as well as a factor which may induce the transformation of the cell which classically starts all of these events, the lymphocyte.

It is clear that at least three of these substances may have activities appropriate to their proposed role in resistance to infection. Thus, the macrophage chemotactic factor which attracts macrophages to the site of inflammation, and the migration inhibition factor which stabilizes macrophages at the site of inflammation and increases their phagocytic activity, could have quite obvious functions in helping the host combat infection. Similarly, interferon, which increases cell resistance to viral invasion, may be a most important defense mechanism. Immune lymphocytes excited by delayed hypersensitivity are known to release these mediators, including interferon and the cytotoxic, cell inhibiting, chemotactic and mitogenic factors. The fact, however, that production of mediators such as cytotoxic and cell inhibiting factors and interferon may be induced by phytomitogens or other non-specific stimuli suggests that this class of chemicals represents a communication system to which a number of different inciting processes have access.

The Role of Delayed Hypersensitivity in Infection

Evidence from studies of experimental animals presented in the preceeding section supports the concept that acquired cellular resistance as a consequence of macrophage activation exerts a strong influence on the living animal's resistance to intracellular infections. It would also seem from clinical evidence that delayed hypersensitivity as mediated by the long-lived, thymus-dependent lymphocyte can play at least an adjunctive role in this resistance by its ability to activate macrophages and to stimulate the production of chemical mediators.

Heritable disorders such as the thymic alymphoplasias associated with selective impairment of thymically-controlled delayed hypersensitivity are subject to recurrent infections. These patients classically have recurrent episodes of infection by Candida as well as the cytomegalovirus and herpes virus, and are susceptible to progressive vaccinia and disseminated BCG infection following immunization. While other infections may occur, the striking association between these diseases and infection with predominantly intracellular organisms supports the concept that delayed hypersensitivity may mediate at least a part of resistance in the normal and intact human. A number of diseases, however, such as intestinal lymphangectasia, sarcoidosis, acute viral infections and even uremia may be associated with evidence of impaired delayed hypersensitivity without an apparent increase in susceptibility.

Recent observations have suggested that defects in delayed hypersensitivity may occur at different points in the chain reaction associated with this event. It is therefore probable that our assessment of "deficiency" in this system is subject to false positive as well as false negative interpretations, and little is known to indicate the degree of deficiency necessary before increased infections occur. When assessing the role of delayed hypersensitivity in infections caused by extracellular pathogens, greater difficulty is found. It is very clear that delayed hypersensitivity to microbial antigens develops almost universally following infection in the immunologically competent host. In fact, delayed hypersensitivity to antigens of over 30 microbes known to be pathogenic in man has been demonstrated. The role of delayed hypersensitivity in resistance to or recovery from infection in these instances is unclear and, in fact, one may suspect that the development of delayed hypersensitivity represents mainly immunization as by isolated antigens rather than a functionally important host response to the infecting microbe.

Evidence from a variety of sources does indicate that delayed hypersensitivity significantly influences the *manifestations* of infection in man. Rich has summarized the evidence demonstrating that the extent and destructiveness of a tuberculous lesion is directly related to the virulence of the organism, the number of organisms, and the hypersensitivity state of the host, and is inversely related to the resistance of the host. This formulation recognizes two important aspects of host response to intracellular infection. The first is that host resistance and host hypersensitivity may be separable phenomena. The second is that the extent and degree of tissue destruction resulting from an infectious process may be related to the degree of delayed hypersensitivity existing in the infected animal.

Other examples of this concept exist. Lymphocytic choriomeningitis is a highly lethal viral infection of mice. If the animals are thymectomized at birth and subsequently infected with the virus, viral invasion and replication in the central nervous system are demonstrable, but the animal remains clinically well. If competence in delayed hypersensitivity is restored by thymic transplants, these mice quickly become ill and die. There is no known infection in man which is so singularly dependent in its manifestations upon the presence or absence of delayed hypersensitivity, but a number of examples suggest that manifestations of human infection are probably related to delayed hypersensitivity mechanisms. It has been postulated for some time that the rash associated with viral exanthems in man may be based upon host hypersensitivity to the virus. This association has been drawn from the facts that the exanthem occurs at a long enough time after viral invasion to allow the establishment of a delayed hypersensitivity state and is often associated with a second phase dissemination of the virus (antigen). It has also been demonstrated that desensitization of the immunized experimental animal with antigens causing delayed hypersensitivity can result in the development of a skin rash which is morphologically similar to those seen during viral exanthems, and histologic findings in the two situations are comparable.

Recent experimental evidence has also suggested that some granulomas associated with parasitic infestation are related to delayed hypersensitivity mechanisms. In the area of alterations in body physiology, Rich, Stead, and others have postulated that pleural effusions occurring during the course of tuberculous infection in man may be due to or contributed to by delayed hypersensitivity to tuberculous antigens rather than actual infection of the pleural space. This suggestion has been supported by the frequent absence of demonstrable tubercle bacilli in these effusions, the self limited nature of the lesion, its occasional association with significant systemic symptoms and transient cutaneous anergy to tuberculoprotein, and its rapid resolution upon the administration of steroids.

Recently, experiments in experimental animals have supported the concept that pleural effusion may develop as a result of a pure delayed hypersensitivity mechanism without the necessity of active infection, and that the reaction is associated with a distinctive physiologic aberration in protein movement through the pleural space.

Conclusions

Available evidence demonstrates that the cellular aspect of host resistance to infection resides primarily in enhanced function of the macrophage. This enhancement can be triggered by delayed hypersensitivity, by an intracellular infection, and possibly by other inflammatory stimuli. It is communicated primarily via soluble mediators released from the lymphocyte in amounts which often reflect the lymphocytes' previous experience or immune state. In addition, manifestations of infectious disease may be significantly influenced by alterations of the immunological or activation status of body cells, though the cellular and chemical pathways mediating these effects are not yet known.

SELECTED REFERENCES

Bloom, B. R., and Chase, M. W.: Transfer of delayed-type hypersensitivity. A critical review and experimental study of the guinea pig. Progr. in Allergy, *10*:151, 1967.

David, J. R.: Lymphocytic factors in cellular hypersensitivity. Hosp. Practice, *6*:79, 1971.

David, J. R.: Macrophage migration. Fed. Proc. *27*:6, 1968.

Green, J. A., Cooperband, S. R., and Kibrick, S.: Immune specific induction of interferon production in cultures of human blood lymphocytes. Science, *164*:1415, 1969.

Humphrey, J. H., and White, R. G.: *Immunology for Students of Medicine*, 3rd ed., 1970, F. A. Davis Co., Philadelphia.

Mackaness, G. B.: Cell-mediated immunity to infection. Hosp. Practice, *5*:73, 1970.

Mackaness, G. B.: Resistance to intracellular infection. J. Infect. Dis., *123*:439, 1971.

Rich, A. R.: The Pathogenensis of Tuberculosis, 1944, Charles C Thomas, Springfield, Ill.

Rosenau, W.: Target cell distruction. Fed. Proc. *27*:34, 1968.

Turk, J.L.: Delayed hypersensitivity, in *Frontiers of Biology,* Neuberger, A., Tatum, E. L., Eds., 1967, American Elsevier Publishing Company, Inc.

Chapter

6

THE IMMUNOLOGIC CONSEQUENCES OF INFECTION

Thucydides and Hippocrates observed that certain communicable diseases such as plague conferred upon the survivors a lifelong resistance to further encounters with the disease. During the past century our understanding of the biologic processes underlying this host resistance has mushroomed. Furthermore, we now realize that these protective mechanisms do not always produce results beneficial to the host; rather they may elicit tissue injury and death. The purpose of this paper is to discuss some of these immune phenomena which are deleterious to the host. To do this more effectively I will initially discuss the general immune response to foreign materials such as microbial agents. Subsequently, I will review some of the specific pathologic consequences of the interaction between this immune response and individual infectious agents.

The Immune Response

Antibodies

Initial contact between host and microbe usually stimulates production of antibodies to a variety of antigens resident within the microbial structure. Currently, antibody activity is thought to reside in immunoglobulins belonging to five distinct classes: IgG, IgM, IgA, IgE, and IgD. Since we know nothing of the biological role of IgD, we will no longer consider it. Most commonly, infectious agents provoke formation of antibodies belonging to more than one of these immunoglobulin classes. However, certain factors such as time, the route of invasion used by the pathogen, and type of infectious agent may determine the production of a predominant

This paper was also published in Postgraduate Medicine, Nov. 1971, McGraw-Hill, Inc.

immunoglobulin type. For instance, IgM antibodies are customarily the first to appear during an infection, followed in a few days by the emergence of IgG antibodies. Agents which enter the body via the respiratory or GI tracts elicit IgA antibodies which appear in the respiratory and GI secretions. Parasites, such as the helminths, stimulate the appearance of IgE antibodies; gram-negative bacterial infection, on the other hand, results in a predominantly IgM response.

Antibodies elicited by a single antigen have other than immunoglobulin class differences. For instance, detection of antibody response utilizes several immunochemical and biological techniques such as complement fixation, hemagglutination, precipitation, etc. The unitarian theory of antibody production, first proposed by Zinsser, held that antibody to specific antigen could perform all these different immunochemical functions providing the appropriate quantities of antibody and antigen were present. This theory stated that such antibodies were chemically homogeneous. Studies in the past decade have repudiated this notion. It has been clearly demonstrated that antibodies produced in response to a single antigen are not homogeneous but rather a mixture of heterogeneous molecules with differing physicochemical characteristics. Such antibodies vary both in their binding affinity and binding specificity for the antigen. In general, antibodies first produced by the host have great specificity but relatively poor binding affinity for antigen. Antibodies subsequently produced have less specificity but much greater binding affinity for the antigen. Undoubtedly, these physicochemical differences account for both the immunochemical dissimilarities and for some of the bizarre and occasionally devastating responses to microbial agents.

The interaction between antibody and microbial antigen can produce several possible results. The microorganism may be localized to its inoculum site; it may be phagocytized and digested by host cells; or it may be lysed extracellularly. Such outcomes are regarded as protective to host and referred to as host immunity. Occasionally, the organism may be totally unaffected by antibody; and least frequently, antibody-antigen interaction produces tissue damage—a process referred to as hypersensitivity.

There are three types of antibody mediated hypersensitivity reactions. 1) Anaphylaxis, or immediate hypersensitivity which is triggered by antigen which in turn combines with cell-bound IgE antibody. Chemical mediators such as histamine and slow reacting substance of anaphylaxis (SRS-A) are discharged, resulting in increased vascular permeability and smooth muscle contraction. Clinically, mediator release is manifested by shock, asthma and urticaria.

2) Cytotoxic reactions which develop more slowly and which occur when antibodies destroy cells by direct interaction with antigen on a cell surface. These reactions via the activation of the complement system re-

lease chemotactic factors which attract polymorphonuclear cells. These cells in turn release a host of enzymes and permeability factors which can injure normal tissue.

3) Serum sickness, or immune complex reactions. These occur when complexes, formed by antigen and antibody in moderate antigen excess, become deposited in small capillaries. This deposition results in an Arthus type of response with subsequent damage of the adjacent tissues.

The biological results produced by antibody-antigen interaction are mediated through the complement system and through non-protein, small molecular sized, vasoactive chemicals. It is appropriate to review our current knowledge of these substances.

Complement

The complement system is composed of nine serum proteins (designated, in order of their reactivity, C1, C4, C2, C3, C5, C6, C7, C8 and C9) which interact, in sequential fashion, in a manner reminiscent of the clotting cascade. Each protein exists in body fluids in a precursor form which has to be activated or enzymatically altered before it can participate in the sequence. Activation of the complement system results in the generation of several biologically active compounds: 1) Three polymorphonuclear leucocyte chemotactic factors and one eosinophile chemotactic factor are produced when C3, C5, and a complex of C5, 6, and 7 become involved; 2) Anaphylatoxins—small molecular weight compounds which have the capacity of releasing histamine from mast cells—are released from splitting of C3 and C5; 3) The attachment of a large molecular weight piece of C3 to cells imparts to those cells an adherent property so that the C3-cell complex can readily stick to erythrocytes, polymorphonuclear leucocytes or macrophages. This property of the C3 molecule, called immune adherence, probably enhances opsonization and phagocytosis of microbial agents; 4) Attachment of C8 and C9 to a microbe may lead to membrane damage and cell lysis.

There are several methods by which the complement system may be activated. Classically, antibodies of either the IgG or IgM class, when combined with antigen, can activate and attach the C1 molecule. C4 and C2 are subsequently linked to the immune complex and form an enzyme which allows for the splitting and attachment of C3. The terminal five components are sequentially involved. Other serum factors, such as kallikrein and plasmin can similarly activate C1.

Recently it has been recognized that the participation of the first three components (C1, C4, and C2) is not always necessary for the generation of the biological activities produced by the C3 through C9 steps. Rather, several bacterial products—such as endotoxin from gram-negative bacteria or proteinases from *Serratia marcescens* or Group A streptococci—can bypass the C1,4,2 steps, directly cleave C3 and thus fire off the terminal portion of the complement reaction. Clinically, this bypass production of anaphylotoxin and chemotactic factors probably contributes to the shock and leucocytosis seen in patients with endotoxemia.

Chemical Mediators of the Immune Response

Several low molecular weight vasoactive compounds are thought to participate in these immune reactions. Histamine has been the most extensively studied. It is capable of constricting veins, dilating venules and increasing vascular permeability. Clinically these effects are seen in angioedema, urticaria and shock. It is released from tissue mast cells and circulating basophiles upon interaction of IgE attached to the cell membrane and an appropriate antigen.

The second chemical mediator is slow reacting substance of anaphylaxis (SRS-A)—so named because it was originally released by challenge of sensitized guinea pig lung with antigen and produced a delayed, sluggish contraction of an antihistamine-treated guinea pig ileum. In man it is thought to be a potent stimulator of bronchiolar smooth muscle contraction which is responsible for the bronchospasm in patients with extrinsic asthma.

Serotonin and bradykinin have been postulated as mediators of the immune response. Serotonin can be released from the mast cells of rats after an appropriate immune challenge. However, it has never been shown to play a role in the inflammatory response of man. Bradykinin is a nonapeptide which is formed by the action of kallikrein upon its alpha-2-globulin precursor, kininogen. It has the capacity to dilate arterioles, increase vascular permeability and lower blood pressure. When injected intradermally into man it causes pain, erythema, and wheal formation. The effects of bradykinin and histamine on vascular permeability are additive. Unfortunately, its exact biologic role in mammalian tissues has yet to be determined.

The Polymorphonuclear Leucocyte

Polymorphs are thought to play major roles in immune responses to microbial agents and in the tissue injury induced by Arthus or immune complex type hypersensitivity reactions. These cells are attracted to the site of antigen—antibody binding by chemotactic factors derived from complement and other polymorphonuclear cells. The compounds responsible for their activity are enclosed in the lysosomes which contain approximately 25 digestive enzymes, phagocytin, bacteriocidal proteins, hemolysin, endogenous pyrogen, chemotactic factors, proteins which degranulate mast cells and at least four compounds (one of which is inhibitable by antihistamines) that increase vascular permeability. Acid cathepsins A, D, and E and a neutral collagenase can attack basement membranes. An elastase is capable of disrupting the internal elastic lamellae of small arterioles and venules. The activities of the cathepsins and the elastase result in the pathologic lesions of serum sickness and the Arthus phenomenon, respectively.

Cell Mediated Immunity

Many viruses, fungi, bacteria and protozoa stubbornly resist the humoral defense mechanisms that have just been discussed. Host survival upon challenge with such microorganisms depends upon development of cell-mediated immunity. Two cell types are involved in this mechanism: The first is a small, short lived, non-circulating lymphocyte. Invasion by one of these microorganisms (such as the tubercle bacillus) stimulates the multiplication and attraction of these small cells. Contact of these cells with specific microbial antigen causes the release from the lymphocytes of 1) a factor which is chemotactic for a second cell type—the phagocytic macrophage; and 2) migratory inhibitory factor (MIF) which retains the attracted phagocytes at the site of cell-antigen interaction. This phagocytic macrophage is metabolically altered by the small lymphocyte in such a manner that it can ingest and destroy the invading pathogen.

Induction of cell-mediated immunity simultaneously results in induction of hypersensitivity to the antigen and subsequent tissue destruction. The consequences of this type of hypersensitivity will be elaborated upon in the discussion of tuberculosis.

Immunologic Consequences of Individual Microbial Agents

Streptococcal Disease; Rheumatic Fever

The relationship between group A, beta hemolytic streptococcal disease and the development of rheumatic fever is firmly established. The latent period that intervenes between the pyogenic manifestations of streptococcal disease and the onset of signs of rheumatic fever is compatible with the idea that an immune mechanism, requiring the production of antibody, is involved. Furthermore, a rise in titer of antibody directed to at least one of the several streptococcal antigens is detected in almost every case of acute rheumatic fever. Recently, Kaplan has published extensively on his observation that antigens present in group A streptococci cross react with sarcolemma and subsarcolemmal sarcoplasm in cardiac myofibers. These antigens are probably constituents of both the streptococcal cell wall and cell membrane. At least one of them is closely associated with the M protein—the virulence factor of the group A streptococcus. He found these cross reacting antibodies in 55 percent of patients with active rheumatic fever, in 58 percent of patients with rheumatic heart disease, and in 24 percent of patients with recent streptococcal disease. In contrast, he could detect these antibodies rarely in patients with rheumatoid arthritis, systemic lupus erythematosus and a variety of other chronic disorders.

Using a variety of immunopathological techniques, he found gamma-globulin bound to myofiber, endocardium, and smooth muscle of coronary vessel walls in biopsy specimens taken from the auricular appendages of 18 percent of patients with clinically inactive disease. He observed gammaglobulin and C3 deposited diffusely throughout the myocardium of hearts taken from five children who died of fulminant rheumatic fever. Since each child had demonstrated rapidly progressive congestive heart failure with EKG evidence of diffuse myocardial injury, he proposed that these deposits were related pathogenetically to the clinical picture.

In contrast, the immunopathologic findings in the heart valves of rheumatic fever patients differed from those in the myocardium. IgG globulin with only a minimum amount of complement was observed. Furthermore, the antibody that was present was distributed throughout the connective tissue and was not limited to the myofibers within the valve leaflet. This suggests that the immune mechanisms responsible for the myocardial lesions differ from those responsible for the valvular lesions.

Post-Streptococcal Glomerulonephritis

Clinically, several observations support the concept that immune pathways, different from those involved in acute rheumatic fever, are operative in the tissue damage observed in post streptococcal glomerulonephritis: 1) the case attack rate of nephritis following outbreaks of group A streptococcal infection varies from 0.3 to 60 percent; in acute rheumatic fever it remains a constant 3 percent; 2) a very limited number of group A strains predispose the patient to nephritis; all strains, however, can predispose to rheumatic fever; and 3) antibodies that cross react with the kidney and the streptococcus have been found with only one of the nephritogenic streptococcal strains (Type 12). Antibodies to streptococcal antigen that cross react with cardiac muscle have been found in a variety of streptococcal strains.

Dixon has proposed that the deposition of immune complexes in the renal glomeruli is the primary etiologic event in post-streptococcal nephritis. The ratio between antigen and antibody is important in establishing localization in the glomerular capillaries. Small complexes formed in great antigen excess remain soluble and circulating. Complexes formed at equivalence or slight antigen excess precipitate and are rapidly phagocytized. Complexes, intermediate in size, formed in moderate antigen excess retain their solubility but are subject to entrapment by the glomerular capillaries.

The deposition of immune complexes results in the local activation of complement and generation of its chemotactic factors. Polymorphonuclear leucocytes migrate to the glomeruli, discharge their lysosomal proteolytic enzymes and thereby damage the vessels and basement membrane of the glomerulus. Experimental observations that antibody and complement can be eluted from glomeruli of patients with post-streptococcal glomerulonephritis and the electron microscopic demonstrations of collections of electron dense material along the basement membrane support Dixon's hypothesis.

The Fungi and Allergic Pulmonary Diseases

Considerable recent interest has focused on the relationship between the common fungi and pulmonary disease. Since illnesses due to a variety of species of Aspergillus have been studied most fully, the following comments will be directed to them. It appears, however, that other fungi—such as candida—produce respiratory symptoms by the same mechanisms.

Aspergilli are common commensals in the human respiratory tract and are prevalent in the environment, particularly in moldy hay and in other moist organic materials. Inhalation may be responsible for pulmonary disease. They can produce three types of hypersensitivity lung disease: 1) an asthmatic like syndrome; 2) Allergic alveolitis, which includes Bronchopulmonary aspergillosis and farmer's lung; and 3) a rare, tuberculoid type of pneumonitis. Clinically the mycetoma and suppurative pneumonitis caused by aspergilli are more common entities; but these diseases are thought to be non-immune and will not be considered.

The first syndrome, that of reversible bronchiolar constriction, is quite common and is associated with an immediate type wheal and flare reaction upon intradermal challenge of the patient with Aspergillus antigen. Inhalation of the antigen produces asthmatic symptoms 15—20 minutes after aerosol challenge. This entity is thought to be mediated through the release of slow reacting substance of anaphylaxis by the union of antigen with cell bound IgE.

The second immunologic syndrome, allergic alveolitis, is characterized by a biphasic clinical picture; the early phase (occurring 10—20 minutes after antigen inhalation) is characterized by wheezing; the later phase, appearing after 6—8 hours, by the development of systemic symptoms of fever, chills, malaise, transient pulmonary infiltrates, and blood eosinophilia. This syndrome depends upon the presence of antibodies belonging to two immunoglobulin classes—IgE and IgG—which act in concert to produce the syndrome. The early phase is mediated by IgE and resembles classic anaphylactic bronchoconstriction. The later phase, mediated by IgG, pathologically resembles the Arthus reaction. Intradermal challenge with antigen also produces a bimodal response. In 10 to 20 minutes a typical wheal and flare results. Four to eight hours later this is replaced by edema, erythema and tenderness which on biopsy histologically mimics the Arthus phenomenon.

Farmer's lung, a disease related to the inhalation of moldy hays, represents an allergic response to thermophillic actinomycetes and is apparently mediated by immune complexes in the lung interstitium formed between the inhaled antigens and circulating IgG antibody. Cell-mediated immunity may also play a role.

The third syndrome, which can be confused with pulmonary tuberculosis, is mediated by cellular hypersensitivity but will not be discussed here.

Allergic Response to the Helminth Infections

Diseases caused by intestinal worms are frequently accompanied by urticaria, angioedema, asthma and a marked eosinophilia. The reasons for these allergic complications are now evolving.

The worm structure incorporates dozens of different antigens which provoke antibodies of all major immunoglobulin classes. Most fascinating is their capacity to stimulate high titers of IgE antibodies. The union of cell-bound IgE with worm antigen promotes the release of histamine and SRS-A which act upon end organ receptors in venule walls and bronchiolar smooth muscle to effect increased vascular permeability and bronchoconstriction. Thus, when the trichinella cyst migrates to the muscles and tissues about the eye, periorbital angioedema appears; when the ascaris larvae migrate through the lung, bronchoconstriction and wheezing occur.

The eosinophilia observed in patients with these infections is probably explained by the recent discovery of an eosinophile chemotactic factor whose production is also IgE mediated.

Tuberculosis and Cell-Mediated Hypersensitivity

Tuberculosis is the prototype disease in which immunity and hypersensitivity (both processes develop simultaneously) are dependent upon the interaction of two cell types—the small lymphocyte and the mononuclear macrophage. Many other infectious agents—bacteria, viruses, fungi, protozoa and parasites—promote this phenomenon. Even the streptococcus, pneumococcus, and staphylococcus stimulate delayed hypersensitivity; however, humoral factors probably play a much more important role in the normal response to these pyogenic microorganisms.

Tubercle bacilli introduced into an unsensitized individual will slowly proliferate and migrate. Ten to fourteen days after infection occurs, the host develops hypersensitivity and immunity to the organism. Clinically, this is manifest by a positive tuberculin skin test, and histologically by formation of the tubercle. This results in decrease in the number of viable bacilli, in cessation of bacillary migration, and eventually in necrosis of the tissues enclosing the tubercles containing viable bacteria. Ultimately, the tubercles solidify, calcify and markedly suppress further bacterial multiplication. In this instance hypersensitivity is apparently beneficial to the host.

Hypersensitivity may also be deleterious. In overwhelming, rapidly progressing tuberculous caseation, liquefaction and cavitation may appear. These processes occur only in hypersensitive individuals and their precise mechanism is unknown. They result in marked tissue destruction, promote bacillary proliferation and interfere with normal host phagocytosis.

Hypersensitivity to tuberculin antigen accounts for two cutaneous lesions encountered clinically. First is the local necrosis and slough at the site of a tuberculin skin test or at the site of accidental cutaneous autoinoculation by a laboratory worker. Secondly are the lesions of erythema induratum. These appear as indurated nodules with a proclivity for ulceration on the calves of young women with tuberculosis. Biopsies reveal granuloma formation, local panniculitis, and perivascular inflammation; no tubercle bacilli are found. The inciting cause of this condition is unknown.

Syphilis and the Appearance of Auto-antibodies

Treponema pallidum stimulates the production of several interesting antibodies. Many of these, such as the *Treponema pallidum* immobilization antibody, are directed against the organism itself. More interesting are those directed towards determinants found in normal host tissues—the antibody to Wasserman antigen and the Donath-Landsteiner antibody.

The Wasserman antigen is a cardiolipid which occurs in the mitochondria of many mammalian tissues. Classically, antibody to it will react with alcoholic extracts of human liver or heart. Antigenically, similar material occurs in bacteria, mycoplasma and yeast. As a result of its wide distribution in nature, antibody to the Wasserman antigen appears in a variety of infectious diseases—such as leprosy, infectious hepatitis, infectious mononucleosis and after smallpox vaccination, thus accounting for the "false positive" serological tests for syphilis occasionally noted in these diseases.

The Donath-Landsteiner cold-warm hemolysin antibody is seen occasionally in syphilitic patients. At low temperatures this antibody combines with a specific antigen found on erythrocytes, platelets and perhaps other body cells to produce agglutination of the cells. Upon subsequent warming, the agglutinated cells are lysed in the presence of complement. It is speculated that the antigenic stimulus arises from tissue changes incidental not only to infections with *T. pallidum* but also to infection by viruses.

The relationship between these antibodies and the clinical manifestations of syphilis—particularly the late stages of cardiovascular and neurosyphillis—remains mysterious. However, the increased incidence of Wasserman antibodies in systemic lupus erythematosus, in rheumatoid arthritis, and in Hashimoto's thyroiditis and the pathologic findings in tertiary syphilis of focal, vascular and connective tissue injury are such that these manifestations may represent an autoimmune phenomenon.

Autoimmune Phenomena Related to Infectious Agents

Animals can produce antibodies to their own tissues when exposed to antigens which are similar, though not identical to their own body constituents or when their own antigens are structurally distorted. Microorganisms may provoke an autoimmune response in several ways. 1) Following cell damage, which exposes intracellular components, normally protected by the cell membrane, to the immune system; 2) alteration of normal tissues by bacterial enzymes or other bacterial products; for instance *Mycoplasma pneumoniae* can alter the I antigen of red blood cells. This may result in the production of cold agglutinins seen in this disease; 3) linking microbial antigens to normal tissue material to produce a compound that is immunologically recognized as foreign; 4) stimulation of antibodies to microbial antigens that cross react with several tissue antigens. We discussed this mechanism in considering post-streptococcal rheumatic fever.

Other examples exist. Children with ulcerative colitis will frequently produce antibodies both to their own colonic mucosa and to *E. coli* 014. 5) Microorganisms may act as adjuvants. In experimental animals the injection of foreign material in emulsions with mycobacteria can increase the resulting antibody titer and alter the type of antibody response produced. Many other microorganisms have similar activities. No evidence exists that such adjuvant activity of microbial agents plays a role in human disease; however, such a relationship has been postulated for a few disorders such as lupus erythematosus and rheumatoid arthritis. 6) Stimulation of rheumatoid factor production. Rheumatoid factors are antibodies directed toward the host's own gammaglobulins. Many infectious diseases —such as tuberculosis, subacute bacterial endocarditis, leprosy, infectious mononucleosis, infectious hepatitis and trypanosomiasis can be associated with positive rheumatoid factor tests.

Slow Virus Infection and Autoimmunity

Investigations in the past decade have suggested that at least two neurological disorders—Kuru and Jacob-Creutzfeldt disease—are caused by "slow virus" infection. Such infections have incubation periods of months or years during which period the virus maintains its viability despite normal host defenses. After this prolonged latent period, a relatively rapid phase of cellular destruction occurs with the clinical evidence of a fulminant disease. The course of these illnesses questions how the virus can be tolerated for so long without host injury and then suddenly produce widespread tissue damage. Hotchkin has proposed that the slow virus particle, by nature of surface antigens closely related to the host, is immunologically unrecognized as foreign and the normal immune response to this foreign agent is silenced. The virus can proliferate in cells for years. Then this tolerance mysteriously disappears—perhaps by alterations of host cell constituents, so that they become recognized as foreign antigens. Subsequently, the transformed cell constituents are attacked by the immune system and cell death ensues. Extrapolation of these concepts to other neurological disorders and to so-called "auto-immune" disorders raises the possibility of exciting future research into these diseases.

Therapeutic Considerations

The treatment of the immunologic events that complicate the infectious diseases has been difficult. Ideally, therapy should be directed towards the prevention, rather than the cure of the immunologic injury. Thus, post-streptococcal glomerulonephritis, rheumatic fever, or the late complications of syphilis can be prevented by adequate penicillin therapy early in the course of the infection. Adequate anti-tuberculous therapy will eliminate the cell-mediated hypersensitivity reactions to the tubercle bacillus. In fact, 70 percent of tuberculin positive patients will convert to the tuberculin negative state after one year of INH therapy. The reactions to the helminths are cured by eradicating the parasite. The allergic pulmonary manifestations of the fungi can be prevented by avoidance of the areas that are contaminated by the mold.

Theoretically, interfering with antibody formation should interrupt the immunolgic event in which it is involved. Many agents—among them are 6-mercaptopurine, azathioprine (Imuran), the folic acid antagonists, and the alkylating agents such as cyclophosphamide—inhibit proliferation or differentiation of antibody forming cells and thus impede antibody synthesis. Trials of these agents in post-streptococcal glomerulonephritis, in rheumatic fever, or in immune complex nephritis have been disappointing.

The steroids are the most widely used agents for suppressing the immune response. Their pharmacologic mechanism is largely unknown. They do suppress white cell chemotaxis and allegedly stabilize lysosomal membranes, thereby interfering with enzyme release. In this fashion they may diminish the leucocytic contribution in such entities as immune complex glomerulonephritis. They have not been shown to alter the course of rheumatic fever, post-streptococcal glomerulonephritis or tertiary syphilis. They will control the asthmatic symptoms, transiently, in allergic alveolitis or helminth disease (supposedly by reducing intrabronchial inflammation which contributes to bronchoconstriction). They will reduce the symptoms of patients with serum sickness but will not alter the outcome of the illness. They have been tried as a means of reducing the cell-mediated inflammation which accompanies tuberculosis—such as in tuberculous meningitis—but the results, as measured by patient salvage, are inconclusive.

Recently anti-lymphocyte serum or globulin has been used to control the rejection of transplanted organs. Since all patients treated with this agent have been receiving other immunosuppressive drugs, it is most difficult to evaluate its role in suppressing the immune response. Furthermore there is no experience of its use in controlling the immunological complications of the infectious diseases in humans.

SELECTED REFERENCES

Asherson, G. L.: The role of microorganisms in autoimmune disease. Progr. Allerg., *12*:192, 1968.

Bloch, K. J., Kourilsky, F. W., Ovary, Z., and Benacerraf, B.: Properties of guinea pig 7S antibodies. III. Identification of antibodies involved in complement fixation and hemolysis. J. Exp. Med., *117*:965, 1963.

Cannafax, G. R., Norins, L. C., and Gillespie, E. J.: Immunology of syphilis. Ann. Rev. Med., *18*:471, 1967.

Chapitis, J., Ward, P. A., and Lebow, I. H.: Generation of chemotactic activity from human serum and purified components of complement by Serratia proteinase. Presented at the Fourth Complement Workshop, January 28, 1971

Cluff, L. E. and Johnson, J. E., II.: Poststreptococcal Disease, in *Immunological Diseases* (Ed. by M. Samter), Little, Brown, Co., 1965, p. 416.

Cochrane, C. G.: Immunologic tissue injury mediated by neutrophilic leucocytes. Advances Immunol., *9*:97, 1968.

Dixon, F. J.: The pathogenesis of glomerulonephritis. Am. J. Med., *44*:493, 1968.

Gewurz, H., Shin, H. S., and Mergenhagen, S. E.: Interaction of the complement system with endotoxic lipopolysaccharide. Consumption of the six terminal complement components. J. Exp. Med., *128*:1049, 1967.

Gigli, I., Kaplan, A., and Austen, K. F.: Enhancement of the hemolytic activity of activated first component of human complement by a fragment apparently derived from kallikrein. Presented at the Fourth Complement Workshop, January 27, 1971.

Hersh, E. M. and Body, G. P.: Leukocytic mechanisms in inflammation. Ann. Rev. Med., *21*:105, 1970.

Hotchin, J.: Immune and autoimmune reactions in the pathogenesis of slow virus disease. in *Slow, latent, and temperate virus infections,* (Gajdusek, D. C., Gibbs, C. J., Jr., Alpers, M., eds.) U. S. Govt. Print. Office, Washington, D. C., 1965.

Humphrey, J. H. and White, R. G.: *Immunology for Students of Medicine*, Philadelphia, F. A. Davis Company, 1970, p. 430.

In vitro correlates of delayed hypersensitivity. Intersociety symposium. Fed. Proc., *27*:3, 1968.

Kaplan, M. H.: Autoimmunity to heart and its relation to heart disease. Progr. Allerg., *13*:408, 1969.

Kay, A. B., Stechschulte, D. J., and Austen, K. F.: in press. Levine, V., Celano, M. J.

and Faikowski, F.: The specificity of the antibody in paroxysmal cold hemoglobinuria. Ann. N. Y. Acad. Sci., *124*:456, 1965.

Mackaness, G. B. and Blanden, R. V.: Cellular immunity. Progr. Allerg., *11*:89, 1967.

Mackaness, G. B.: The influence of immunologically committed cells on macrophage activity *in vivo*. J. Exp. Med., *29*:973, 1969.

Müller-Eberhard, H. J.: Chemistry and reaction mechanisms of complement. Advances Immunol., *8*:1, 1968.

Orange, R. P., and Austen, K. F.: Slow reacting substance of anaphylaxis. Advances Immunol, *10*:106, 1969.

Orange, R. P., and Austen, K. F.: Chemical mediators of immediate hypersensitivity. Hosp. Prac., *6*:79, 1971.

Pepys, J. *Hypersensitivity diseases of the lungs due to fungi and organic dusts*. Monographs in Allergy. Vol. 4. Eds.: P. Kallos, M. Hasck, T. M. Inderbitzen, P. A. Miescher and B. H. Waksman. S. Karger, Basel, 1969.

Watson, D. W. and Johnson, A. G.: The clinical use of immunosupression. Med. Clin. N. Amer., *53*:1225, 1969.

Webster, M. E.: The kinin System—a review, in *Cellular and Humoral Mechanisms in Anaphylaxis and allergy*. Ed. by H. Z. Movat. Karger, Basel/New York, 1969, p. 207.

SECTION TWO

GENERAL PROBLEMS OF INFECTIOUS DISEASES

Chapter 7

INTRODUCTION

Many of the manifestations of infectious diseases are non-specific. These non-specific manifestations may dominate, and the role of infection may be overlooked. In the preparation of this introduction, an attempt was made to itemize some of these manifestations. The list began with anemia, included congenital heart disease, malabsorption syndrome, cholelithiasis, pneumothorax, subarachnoid hemorrhage, peripheral neuropathy, hypertension, adrenal insufficiency, abortion, sterility, exfoliative skin disease, skin depigmentation, and ended with fractures. No system or organ escapes involvement and a complete description of all features of infectious diseases would itself become a textbook of medicine. *This explains why every physician must be knowledgeable about infectious diseases and why the specialist in infectious diseases must remain a generalist.*

Infectious diseases influence human behavior. Venereal disease, leprosy, and tuberculosis have social, cultural, and even religious overtones which frequently influence attitudes and actions of the afflicted and unafflicted. These and other infections may be resultants as much of socio-economic and cultural forces as they are of the pathogens themselves. Pandemics or epidemics of infection have changed the course of history by determining the victor in war or economic productivity and artistic or scientific effort. Literature is replete with examples of the effects of infection upon individuals, families and social groups.

In the past few years the threat of infection for the hospitalized patient has produced fear in the public, renewed efforts at infection control, and stimulated a wave of investigation to define more clearly the microbiological, environmental, and clinical determinants of the problem. Much has been learned, public concern now is less, but the problem remains. Epidemic hospital infections have been reduced or eliminated, but nosocomial infections continue to occur with distressing frequency. The advances in treatment of patients with formerly hopeless diseases have carried with them new threats of infection in hospitalized patients. Constant attention and alertness to inadequacies of prevention and control always will be required. Awareness that most deaths are caused by infection following transplant surgery or during treatment with drugs impairing host resistance should force us to regularly assess the acceptibility or risk of our "scientific" advances. The importance of nosocomial infections is fully documented in this section, and principles of isolation needed to control the problem are covered in Chapter 8.

Anemia and fever are not diseases but are manifestations of an underlying disorder. Fever often is erroneously interpreted as pathognomonic of infection. Anemia, on the other hand, often is not considered an important manifestation of infection. In fact, fever has causes other than infection, and many instances of anemia are caused by chronic or acute infection. These features may be the only objective manifestations of illness and present difficult diagnostic dilemmas. Intensive clinical and experimental studies in the past few years have clarified the pathogenesis of fever and anemia. Similarly, the clinical evaluation of perplexing fevers and the interpretation of anemia in infection has been better defined. Recently, a sizable amount of information also has been obtained on abnormalities of the coagulation system of the blood in infection, explaining some poorly understood manifestations and indicating potentially valuable new therapeutic methods.

The impressive developments in antimicrobial drug therapy over the past 25 years have contributed probably the single most important advance to control of disease. Antimicrobial drug treatment, however, is not necessarily followed by recovery from the manifestations of an infectious disease. The pathophysiological processes initiated by infection may progress without interruption even though the microorganism is eliminated; they may resolve slowly or result in permanent injury. Interest has been emerging and efforts are increasingly being made to understand some of the effects of infectious diseases. Without such understanding we may acquire new and better antimicrobial drugs but remain unable to influence the course of disease.

Some persons are susceptible to certain infections while others are insusceptible. The factors influencing this susceptibility are often related to the mechanisms of resistance discussed before. At times other factors are involved. Transient bacteremia, for example, is ordinarily a harmless event. In patients with congenital or acquired valvular heart disease, however, transient bacteremia may have devastating effects. Furthermore, some patients developing bacteremia develop shock which may result in death despite effective antimicrobial drug treatment. This may be related at times to microbiological determinants, but often it is not. The influence of bacteremia upon cardiovascular function, coagulation factors and upon cell activity is now becoming clear, and management of afflicted patients is becoming more rational.

New approaches to the study of infectious diseases in the future, therefore, must include greater attention to the pathophysiologic consequences of infection, including effects on the blood, cardiovascular system, muscles, nervous system, and metabolism. Until such new understanding is available, we will be faced with the possibility of putting out fires but not knowing how to assist in rebuilding the house.

This section, therefore, deals with three most important types of problems in infectious diseases. *First,* the insidious, endemic problems of nosocomial infection are discussed, highlighting their importance but also pointing to efforts we can make to reduce the risk of infection in the hospitalized patient. These patients are often the most predisposed to infection and the hospital should not be as hazardous to them as it often turns out to be.

Second, two important pathophysiological events of infection, hematological manifestations and shock, are discussed, highlighting the importance of understanding host reactions to infection, and indicating that their control requires measures other than those just directed towards elimination of the microorganisms. If we are to increasingly control disease as well as infection, we must acquire such an understanding.

Finally, the problem of recovery from infectious illness is discussed, with particular attention to symptomatic recovery, emphasizing the importance of understanding that emotional settings also affect responses to disease and influence our effectiveness in treating sick persons. Recovery from disease is a multifactorial process and the physician's responsibility does not end with termination of infection, but extends through the period required for restoration of health. Follow-through is as important in medicine as it is in golf or tennis.

Chapter 8

NOSOCOMIAL INFECTIONS

Introduction

According to recent estimates, 5 to 10 percent of patients admitted to general hospitals in the United States develop infections while there. The more serious the disease requiring hospitalization, the more likely an infection will complicate it. About three percent of patients undergoing surgery develop post-operative wound infections, but the frequency varies according to the operative procedure, and rates as high as 40 percent are associated with some kinds of abdominal surgery. Roughly three percent of hospitalized persons develop urinary tract infections, usually as a consequence of catheterization, instrumentation or surgery upon the urinary tract. Pneumonia develops in about two percent of patients, and as many as one percent of hospitalized persons develop septicemia or bacteremia. Some persons will die because of their infection. Fortunately, this tragic outcome is an uncommon event. Most people dying from any cause in hospitals will develop an infection during their terminal illness, but death in most of these patients is due to the progression of the underlying disease, and not to infection. While accurate figures have been impossible to obtain, one estimate is that approximately one of every 5000 patients entering American hospitals dies as a consequence of an infection contracted there. When these deaths are viewed as consequences that must be anticipated when advances in medicine and surgery are made generally available, it will be appreciated that they are far outweighed by the lives saved by these innovations. In so far as they are preventable, however, these unfortunate and sometimes tragic occurrences are worthy of our most careful study and attention.

Gram-negative enteric bacteria now account for about two-thirds of all infections developing in hospitalized patients. Staphylococci were the most troublesome organisms about a decade ago, but they now account for only about one-quarter of the infections. Oftentimes, the offending organism is one of the patient's own, but in the majority of instances the offender is not brought into the hospital by the patient. Instead he acquires the organism at some normally colonized site during hospitalization, only to develop a clinically significant infection with it when his resistance later declines because of his underlying disease and its treatment, or because of the surgical procedure performed. Attention has been called to the fact that hospital food may be the source of some antibiotic-resistant pseudomonas, *E. coli* and klebsiella strains later found in the feces of patients treated with antibiotics. One way to reduce the spread of these organisms is to discourage unnecessary antibiotic therapy, and another is to pay more attention to bacteria in the food, drink and medicines consumed by patients.

In addition to the lives lost and to the suffering experienced by patients because of nosocomial infections, the enormous cost to society in general must be acknowledged. A great deal of time is spent by physicians and nurses in attempting to prevent as well as to manage these infections. Hospitals spend enormous sums of money on their control. This is an important factor contributing to the high cost of medical care and to the shortage of skilled health personnel. Certain medical advances, such as kidney and heart transplants, have been hindered or delayed by the infectious consequences that commonly complicate them. These must be prevented if such advances are to become truly successful and practical.

It is unlikely that nosocomial infections will ever be completely prevented. Medical and surgical advances have always been two-edged swords, and they will continue to be so in the future. Whenever we prolong the lives of highly-susceptible patients, serious infections will inevitably occur. In fact, there is reason to believe that future medical advances will probably further accentuate this problem. One authority has remarked that if we should ever reach the point where all bacterial, viral, protozoal, and fungal infections have been successfully controlled, then highly susceptible patients will become infected with mushrooms. While largely facetious, this statement was intended to emphasize by exaggeration the virtual impossibility of preventing all contact between susceptible persons and opportunistic organisms which find their vulnerable tissues a favorable site for implantation and growth. For these reasons, much more attention needs to be paid to possible ways to correct those factors that compromise resistance to infection.

Factors Associated with an Increased Frequency of Infection

Infections occur frequently in hospitalized patients because their usually sterile tissues may come into contact with potential pathogens, and because their tissues have impaired resistance to infection. Examples in the former category include surgery, burns or severe dermatitis, urinary or intravenous catheterization or cutdowns, contaminated injections, and the inhalation of contaminated aerosols generated by respirators and inhalation therapy devices. As an example of the latter category, one of the most important factors is a delayed and deficient granulocyte acute inflammatory reaction because of agranulocytosis, leukemia, hypotension, the effects of certain anesthetic agents on leukocyte mobility, and the similar effects of edema, hematomas, foreign bodies, diabetic or uremic acidosis, and adrenal steroid or immunosuppressive therapy. Defective macrophage function and impaired cellular immunity may be associated with Hodgkin's disease, terminal malignancies, and adrenal steroid or immunosuppressive therapy, and is often associated with fungal infections. Gamma globulin deficiencies also contribute to the development of infection, particularly in patients with leukemia, lymphoma, or multiple myeloma. It should be pointed out that the emergence of especially pathogenic or virulent species of microorganisms is not an important factor in nosocomial infections. Indeed, many of them are caused by saprophytic or commensal organisms.

Post-operative Wound Infections (see also Chapt. 18)

It is trite but true that good surgical techniques continue to afford the best assurance of a low rate of wound infections. The importance of handling tissues gently, of avoiding dead spaces, of preventing hematomas, and of all the other factors that make up what is widely referred to as the skills of the surgeon, all cannot be overemphasized. Even so, the appearance of infection does not necessarily indicate that bad technique has been used. For one thing, the duration, extensiveness and complexity of the procedure, along with the degree of contamination of the operative field by bacteria from the patient must be taken into consideration.

Prophylactic Antibiotics

After many years of argument, it is still clear that prophylactic antibiotics are not very worthwhile for preventing surgical wound infection. Too many potential pathogens are involved, and their susceptibility to antibiotics is too variable for any antibiotic regimen to be consistently effective, especially over a long period of time. The emergence of resistant organisms ultimately limits this measure. Following most kinds of surgery, prophylactic antibiotics merely alter the character of the infecting organisms. All too often they eliminate the patient's normal flora, encouraging the overgrowth of antibiotic-resistant hospital pathogens, and thus ensuring that when infections do occur they will be caused by stubborn organisms.

There is also the possibility that by eliminating relatively non-pathogenic organisms (such as *Streptococcus viridans,* Diphtheroids, and Lactobacilli), from the body surfaces and encouraging their replacement with virulent organisms (Klebsiella, Pseudomonas, and Staphylococcus), the frequency of infection may actually be increased by the use of prophylactic antibiotics. On a neurosurgical unit in Glasgow a serious outbreak of cross-infection due to Klebsiella which may exemplify this possibility was reported recently. About 25 percent of the patients on this service developed Klebsiella respiratory infections, and more than 10 percent had Klebsiella in their urine, usually in association with catheters. Serious post-operative wound infections were also noted. Four-fifths of the patients with these infections had received previous chemotherapy, usually with ampicillin or other antibiotics to which the Klebsiella strains were resistant. Isolation of infected cases, environmental measures, and treatment or prophylaxis with massive doses of antibiotics failed to control the outbreak. Finally, the use of all antibiotics was discontinued on that ward. This drastic measure was accepted as an alternative to closure of the neurosurgical unit. This course of action was followed by an immediate reduction in the frequency of Klebsiella infection. Within four weeks, the organism was not found to cause urinary tract infection and the chest infection rate had fallen to two percent. Total infections were also reduced in number. It seems clear that this extreme measure is not a permanent or widely applicable measure for preventing nosocomial infections, for there are many patients who should and must be treated with antibiotics. It is strong testimony, however, to the wisdom of withholding antibiotics in hospitalized patients unless there is a clear need for their use. More documentation of the effects of restriction of the use of antibiotics in special circumstances such as this needs to be obtained.

Urinary Tract Infections

Nosocomial urinary infections continue to be related primarily to the frequency of instrumentation and catheterization of the urinary bladder, with attendant introduction of organisms the occasional but inevitable consequence (see Chapt. 24). There is ample evidence that the maintenance of a closed sterile drainage system with or without a continuous bladder rinse with an antibacterial solution by means of a triple-lumen catheter is very effective in preventing infection of patients undergoing continuous bladder drainage. The problem is that the maintenance of a closed sterile system is easier said than done, and continued education and supervision of involved personnel must be undertaken if breaks in techniques are to be the exception rather than the rule.

A thought-provoking account from the University of Minnesota Hospitals details the isolation of an unusual number of strains of the pseudomonad EO-1 (*Ps. kingii*) from urine cultures at that institution in the Fall of 1969. This microbacteria is probably identical to those described in other outbreaks as *Ps. cepacia,* or *Ps. multivorans.* It was found that all patients from whom these strains were isolated had undergone a recent urethral catheterization with the use of a commercially packaged and sterilized catheter tray. When items from the kits were cultured, the unusual organism was isolated frequently from the cleansing germicidal solution. All the contaminated solutions were clear and could not be distinguished visually from sterile samples. This uncommon organism seemed to be of low pathogenicity. Only two of the thirteen patients from whom the organism was isolated were symptomatic, and the organism usually disappeared from the urine without treatment when the indwelling catheter was removed. This problem apparently has been corrected by the manufacturer, and all contaminated kits have been recalled. Nonetheless, the incident emphasizes the very real problem of guaranteeing the sterility of prepackaged items.

Under some conditions, sterilization of plastics and other materials which may come in contact with susceptible human tissues is not always certain with ethylene oxide or other common sterilizing agents. Various common hospital disinfectants, such as benzalkonium chloride, can support the growth of Pseudomonas strains, which are notorious for their ability to survive and grow in water. The need for more rigid quality control checks of prepackaged items to detect contamination is evident, and more consideration in the future needs to be given to the importance of these items in the development of nosocomial infection.

Respiratory Infections

Pneumonia caused by Klebsiella, Pseudomonas, or *Serratia marcescens* is becoming an increasingly important problem in debilitated hospitalized patients, particularly those with tracheostomies (Chapt. 14). Colonization of the trachea and bronchi by these organisms is a frequent antecedent to the development of pneumonia, and is difficult to treat or prevent with antibiotics (although some success with use of antibiotic aerosols has been reported in preliminary studies). It has been reported recently that the prevalence of gram-negative bacilli among the oral pharyngeal flora rises markedly in patients with severe illnesses, and this phenomenon does not seem to be entirely explainable by consideration of prior antibiotic or inhalation therapy.

An intrinsic deficiency in undefined bacterial clearance mechanisms in very sick persons has been invoked as an additional explanation. However, aerosols generated by contaminated inhalation therapy equipment are probably more important in the genesis of these infections. Devices such as positive pressure breathing machines, humidifiers and nebulizers may become heavily colonized with Pseudomonas or Serratia organisms, particularly in areas of moisture, and they can be responsible for the transmission of organisms in large numbers to susceptible patients. Contaminated solutions should always be a suspect source when infections with these and other organisms that thrive in water become prevalent. Anesthetic jelly, bottles of medications for aerosol use, and colonized nebulizer reservoirs have been incriminated. Copper mesh is antibacterial, and if placed in nebulizer reservoirs, may prevent their heavy colonization by Pseudomonas. Further work, however, needs to be done on the efficacy and safety of this measure. The routine daily decontamination of inhalation therapy equipment containing nebulizer reservoirs with 0.25 percent acetic acid has been recommended and shown to be effective and practical in routine hospital use. Fine particle humidifiers are difficult to disinfect, and if found to be a source of trouble are best eliminated. Solutions used to store and rinse tracheal catheters may be heavily colonized and a dangerous source of these organisms.

Lowbury and his colleagues recently reported their studies of infection in patients with tracheostomy in an intensive care unit. Eight outbreaks occurred in which patients had tracheal infection with pseudomonas. It was uncommon for strains to be present in the environment prior to their isolation from tracheal mucus. Of the numerous sources from which the organisms were isolated and from which patients might become infected, the hands of nurses and other members of the staff seemed to present a special hazard. Other potentially important sources were sinks, plastic washing bowls, food, and the suction apparatus. Frequent handwashing, the use of disposable plastic gloves for a wide range of nursing procedures, and attention to wash bowls, solutions, suction techniques, and inhalation therapy devices, all seemed to be important.

Bacteremia

Hospital patients who are at special risk of developing bacteremia include those with extensive burns, leukemia, agranulocytosis, intravenous catheters, or following cardiac surgery with insertion of foreign bodies (Chapt. 9). The considerable risk of local and systemic infection associated with cutdowns or polyethylene intravenous catheters needs repeated emphasis, since these useful procedures and devices are more and more frequently employed. Because mild phlebitis is very common with their use, while serious phlebitis is uncommon, those who use them most commonly may fail to appreciate the hazard of bacteremia and death associated with them. However, careful study of patients who develop bacteremia usually reveals that polyethylene intravenous catheters are one of the most important factors associated with preventable and sometimes fatal bacteremia in hospitalized patients. The organisms usually implicated are Staphylococci, Pseudomonas, Serratia, Herellea and Candida. To minimize infections, these devices should be inserted using careful sterile technique; they should be securely anchored to prevent movement back and forth in the vein; and they should be inspected daily for signs of inflammation and removed at once when this is detected.

Application of an antibacterial ointment daily to the site of the catheter wound may delay the development of local infection, but certainly does not prevent it indefinitely. The use of such antibacterial ointments containing neomycin and polymyxin favors acquisition of resistant organisms, and may be one reason why *Candida* fungemia has been noted so frequently recently in association with intravenous catheters.

All studies indicate that the longer these catheters are left in, the more likely that phlebitis and bacteremia will occur. They should practically never be used in the leg because of the attendant high frequency of bacterial contamination and septic embolization. Ideally, they should be removed after 48 to 72 hours of use. If this is not possible, they should be removed when the patient develops unexplained fever or local phlebitis.

Phlebitis may be chemically induced and is not a sure sign of local infection. When infection ensues, removal of the catheter is the most important therapeutic measure, although antimicrobial agents are also usually indicated. Anticoagulants are rarely needed, but surgical excision of the involved segment of vein followed by delayed wound closure may be necessary to control suppurative thrombophlebitis in an occasional patient, particularly those with burns.

Infection in Burn Patients (see also Chapt. 18)

Bacteremia from the site of intravenous catheterization, or more commonly in association with suppuration in the burn wound surface, is one of the most important causes of death in severely burned persons. Prophylactic penicillin seems useful in preventing the streptococcal infections that occur so commonly in the first week or two following burns, but prophylactic antibiotics are less useful in preventing the staphylococcal or gram-negative infections that occur later.

Many agents have been used topically on the burn wound to prevent colonization, suppuration and sepsis. With these agents it is usually found that the frequency of serious infections can be reduced initially but that eventually organisms resistant to the topical agents become prevalent in the burn unit environment. The frequency of infection then gradually returns to its former level, but with a therapeutically more formidable organism. In addition, topical antibiotics are of little use in the treatment of burn wound infection once it has become established. Thus, topical therapy with ordinary antibiotics is severely limited by the development of resistant organisms. However, topical antibacterial solutions or ointments containing sulfonamides, silver nitrate or silver sulfadiazine seem promising. These have a definite but limited place. Further studies will probably lead to improved and more practical preventive measures using such agents.

Because Pseudomonas infections are so frequent in severely burned patients, the utility of Pseudomonas vaccines has been explored. A completely proven and satisfactory vaccine is not yet available. It seems likely that a vaccine containing more than one antigen will have to be used to protect against Pseudomonas strains, and there is an additional problem in that burn patients do not seem to make protective antibodies as soon as and as well as do normal persons. Thus, it may be necessary to passively immunize burn patients with antiserum obtained from healthy hyperimmunized donors. This is an area of great interest, and it is one that requires further careful study.

Burn wound infection with viral organisms has not been given much attention until recently when six patients were reported who had burn wound infection with *Herpesvirus hominis,* principally in areas of healing partial-thickness burns. Two patients died of disseminated herpetic infection, with hepatic and adrenal involvement. It was suggested that these patients were experiencing their primary herpetic infection, and that they had no antecedent neutralizing antibodies. It is also possible that dissemination was the result of immunoglobulin deficiencies, which have been reported in burn patients. All of the patients had burns involving the face, the most common area of latent herpes virus infection. The burn wound infection was frequently complicated by secondary bacterial infection with conversion to a full-thickness skin loss, which seemed to predispose to Pseudomonas infection. It was not possible to treat the herpetic infections in these patients, and indeed frequently the infections were not recognized antemortem. The evidence suggested that the herpetic infections contributed to the fatal outcome of these patients, and this is clearly an area worthy of further study.

Hepatitis

Because of the relatively long incubation periods of both recognized types of viral hepatitis, accurate epidemiologic studies of the frequency of hepatitis acquired in the hospital are not available. Hepatitis transmitted by blood, blood products or needles is probably of greater incidence in hospitals than is hepatitis transmitted by fecal contamination or contact with oral secretions from infected patients. The use of pooled blood products has been curtailed justifiably because of increasing awareness of its hazards. Whole blood obtained from commercial sources remains one of the most important vehicles for transmitting this virus, and routine testing of all blood for transfusion for the presence of hepatitis antigens (Australia, Au, HA antigen) will probably result in a considerable reduction in the frequency of serum hepatitis. Further studies of the nature of this antigen will probably lead to additional important preventive measures. We can anticipate new problems in dealing with patients (and their blood), physicians, nurses, and other healthy hospital employees who are found to be carriers of this antigen, so intimately related to the hepatitis virus.

Pneumocystis Carinii Pneumonitis

The advent of effective chemotherapy with pentamidine isethionate has emphasized the need for the early diagnosis of Pneumocystis pneumonitis. Our understanding of this disease is limited by insufficient knowledge of the causative organism and by our inability to cultivate it. Most patients with Pneumocystis pneumonia have either leukemia, lymphoma, renal transplants, hypogammaglobulinemia, or connective tissue disorders, and are being treated with antibiotics, adrenal steroids, immunosuppressives or cytotoxic chemotherapy.

The disease is most frequently related to long-term prednisone therapy, in doses of 40 milligrams per day or greater. The infection is characterized by an insidious onset, with dry cough, cyanosis, moderate fever, bilateral patchy pulmonary infiltrates, especially at the lung bases, and blood gas studies compatible with an alveolar-capillary block. Coexistent pulmonary infections with other organisms such as fungi or cytomegalovirus are common.

Infection has been diagnosed before death by identifying the organism in stained smears of tracheal exudates, but a lung biopsy is usually necessary. About one-half of those treated with pentamidine have recovered, but the drug is not innocuous and can cause azotemia, local reactions, and changes in liver function. It may have caused death in two patients. Pentamidine is obtainable in the U.S. only from the National Communicable Disease Center.

Cytomegalovirus Infection

Patients with renal transplants or leukemia occasionally develop severe cytomegalovirus (CMV) infection. Clinically the infection in adults is primarily that of pneumonitis. CMV infection also has been associated with cardiopulmonary bypass, where it may cause the so-called post-perfusion syndrome. This is an infectious mononucleosis-like illness occurring after cardio-pulmonary bypass, or less frequently after blood transfusion for other reasons. Fever, splenomegaly, lymphocytosis and lymphadenopathy are the usual manifestations, and occur two to six weeks after cardiac surgery. The complete clinical spectrum of this illness has not been defined. The evidence suggests that CMV infection can induce a variety of clinical and immunological abnormalities in post-perfusion patients, including a lymphocytic leukemoid reaction, hemolytic anemia with erythrocyte auto-antibodies, and the development of rheumatoid factor, antinuclear antibodies, cold agglutinins, and cryoglobulins. Evidence of infection with the Epstein-Barr virus has also been noted following open-heart surgery, but the clinical delineation and significance of this infection are not yet certain.

Systemic Mycoses

Fungi are being encountered more and more frequently as invaders of the compromised host. The organisms most frequently implicated are Candida, Phycomycetes (Rhizopus, Mucor), Cryptococcus, Aspergillus, and Torulopsis. The infections are most frequently associated with extensive surgery, leukemia, Hodgkin's disease, disseminated neoplasms and homotransplantation. Granulocytopenia and azotemia adversely influence survival rates following infection. Intravenous therapy, antibiotics, adrenal steroid and cytotoxic drug therapy are important predisposing conditions, as is diabetes mellitus. The success of treatment with amphotericin has been correlated with the ability of the physician to control the underlying and predisposing disease process.

The appearance of unexplained fever, pulmonary infiltrates, central nervous system signs and symptoms, or simply unexplained clinical deterioration in a compromised host should suggest infection with opportunistic fungi. The definitive diagnosis of deep fungal infection is usually difficult because it necessitates demonstration of the normally saprophytic organism at a deep site unexposed to external contamination. Blood cultures are particularly helpful, as is examination of the cerebrospinal fluid. The finding of pseudohyphal forms of Candida in addition to the less significant yeast forms in stained smears of exudates is highly suggestive of tissue invasion. Some patients with Candida septicemia require prolonged treatment with amphotericin, while others with candidiasis do not need to be treated for very long, or even at all. Further experience is needed to determine guidelines, but most experts recommend beginning therapy with amphotericin if the patient is clinically deteriorating.

Special Problems of Antimicrobial Resistance

It is very likely that the development and recent wide use of semi-synthetic penicillins resistant to penicillinase has had a good deal to do with the apparent decline in the relative frequency of staphylococcal cross-infection in hospitalized patients, as well as with the increasing prevalence of gram-negative and fungal infections. In Sweden, staphylococci resistant to methicillin have been detected with alarming frequency in certain hospitals and regions, and concomitantly an increase in the severity and frequency of staphylococcal infections in patients has been noted. Such organisms are very common in certain parts of Great Britain and Europe, and yet they are relatively uncommon in the United States. The reasons for the differences in their prevalence are not certain and seem attributable only in part to regional differences in habits of antibiotic usage and sensitivity testing methods. Great effort should be made to limit the spread of these organisms if they should become more frequent in the United States. They are noteworthy not only for their resistance to methicillin, but also because of frequent cross-resistance with oxacillin, cloxacillin, nafcillin and the cephalosporins. Patients with serious infections caused by such strains are usually best treated with either vancomycin or a combination of an aminoglycoside such as gentamicin or kanamycin with a cephalosporin derivative.

During the past 10 years there has been clear evidence all over the world of a fascinating and rapidly increasing frequency of antibiotic resistance in salmonella, shigella and other gram-negative enteric organisms. This resistance is determined by transmissible factors (R factors) which are extra-chromosomal genetic factors (episomes) passed between bacterial species during conjugation. R factors are capable of transferring resistance between common intestinal bacteria as well as to very unrelated organisms such as Pseudomonas and Pasteurella, and they may mediate resistance to as many as nine antibacterial agents. The resistant progeny in turn then become potential donors of their newly acquired R factors. R factors seem to be the predominant cause of clinically significant antibiotic resistance in gram-negative bacilli, and they are a serious threat to the usefulness of our existing antibiotic armamentarium. One mechanism by which they frequently operate is by conveying the ability to synthesize an enzyme that inactivates the antibiotic.

The epidemiology of the spread of these R factors has not been completely worked out, but attention has been focused primarily upon their transfer within the gastrointestinal tract, where enteric organisms might find an environment favorable for the exchange of these factors between species, especially under the selective pressure of antibiotics. It seems likely that selection by antibiotics of resistant organisms with subsequent colonization of patients with a strain carrying an R factor is of far greater epidemiologic significance than is transfer of R factors within the gastrointestinal tract of each patient. By whatever means, however, a hospital population of enteric bacilli with accumulated resistant genes might be expected to emerge eventually, as did the so-called hospital staphylococci under the selective pressure of intensive antibiotic usage. Thus far this has not been shown to be the case to any significant degree.

Despite occasional reports suggesting a modest trend towards increasing resistance among the common enteric organisms, marked shifts have not been common, and in fact a trend towards increasing sensitivity has been noted in some studies. Nonetheless, further attention to this problem is warranted, and a surveillence system designed to detect changes in antibiotic sensitivity patterns and geographic clusters of resistant isolates is worthwhile. This would permit early detection of nosocomial outbreaks due to organisms containing R factors, thus permitting intensive efforts to prevent their dissemination.

Conclusion

This brief survey of the current status of nosocomial infections should make it clear that the problem will be with us for a long time. This is a problem that by its variety and seriousness demands attention by basic scientists and clinicians from many different disciplines. It should also be abundantly clear that an even more vigorous and aggressive application of antimicrobial agents as a preventive measure is not likely to be a satisfying solution. In fact, evidence is accumulating that this problem is in large part attributable to the excessive use of antibiotics in hospitals. This is reminiscent of our experience with hospital staphylococci about 10 years ago, but now the emphasis has shifted to the gram-negative bacteria and to other opportunistic microbes. Since it is most unlikely that antibiotics able to successfully combat all of these organisms will become available, we need to devote more attention to understanding the host-factor deficiencies that are so important in the pathogenesis of these infections. Measures designed to prevent the spread of these organisms from one person to another are worthwhile in preventing outbreaks. However, such measures are not likely to be totally rewarding because all of us normally carry organisms capable of causing mischief in hospitals.

SELECTED REFERENCES

Deane, R. S., Mills, E. L., and Hamel, A. J.: Antibacterial action of copper in respiratory therapy apparatus. Chest, *58*:373, 1970.

Editorial: Bacteria in Faeces and Food. Lancet, *2*:805, 1970.

Editorial: Prophylactic antibiotics, The Lancet, *2*:1231, 1970.

Foley, F. D., Greenawald, K. A., Nash, G., and Pruitt, B. A.: Herpesvirus infection in burned patients. N. Eng. J. Med., *282*:652, 1970.

Grieble, H. G., Colton, F. R., Bird, T. J., Torgo, A., and Griffith, L. G.: Fine-particle humidifiers. N. Eng. J. Med., *282*:531, 1970.

Hardy, P. C., Ederer, G. M., and Matsen, J. M.: Contamination of commercially packaged urinary catheter kits. N. Eng. J. Med., *282*:33, 1970.

Hart, P. D., Russell, E. J., and Remington, J. S.: The compromised host and infection; II. Deep fungal infection. J. Inf. Dis., *120*:169, 1969.

Kantor, G. L., Goldberg, L. S., Johnson, B. L., Derechin, M. M., and Barnett, E. V.: Immunologic abnormalities induced by postperfusion cytomegalovirus infection. Ann. Int. Med., *73*:553, 1970.

Lowbury, E. J. L., Thom, B. T., Lilly, H. A., Barb, J. R., and Whithall, A.: Sources of infection with *Pseudomonas aeruginosa* in patients with tracheostomy. J. Med. Microbiol., *3*:39, 1970.

Pierce, A. K., Sanford, J. P., Thomas, G. D., and Leonard, J. S.: Long-term evaluation of decontamination of inhalation therapy equipment and the occurrence of necrotizing pneumonia. N. Eng. J. Med., *282*:528, 1970.

Price, D. J. E., and Sleigh, J. D.: Control of infection due to *Klebsiella aerogenes* in a neurosurgical unit by withdrawal of all antibiotics. Lancet, *2*:1213, 1970.

Rifkind, D., Marchioro, J. L., Waddell, W. R., and Starzl, T. E.: Infectious diseases associated with renal homotransplantation. JAMA, *189*:397, 1964.

Western, K. A., Perera, D. R., and Schultz, M. G.: Pentamidine isethionate in the treatment of pneumocystis carinii pneumonia. Ann. Int. Med., *73*:695, 1970

Chapter 9

BACTEREMIA AND BACTEREMIC SHOCK

Bacteremia

Bacteremia occurs frequently, and may be asymptomatic, produce fever and chill or lead to shock and death. The term septicemia has been used to define bacteremia with clinical manifestations of infection, but is imprecise and will not be used here. Bacteremia usually signals an uncontrolled infection, but it also can occur when microorganisms are introduced directly into the bloodstream, as in administration of contaminated transfusions. Some types of infection (e.g., typhoid, brucellosis) are regularly accompanied by bacteremia while in others (e.g., streptococcal pharyngitis, shigellosis), bacteremia is uncommon.

Bacteremia by indigenous, moderately pathogenic microorganisms (staphylococci, Pseudomonas, Proteus, coliform bacilli, etc.) is most often observed in patients with serious underlying or associated diseases responsible for diminished resistance to infection, and usually is associated with fever and may produce shock. Asymptomatic bacteremia by organisms with low pathogenicity (e.g., *Streptococcus viridans*) frequently occurs following procedures such as dental extraction. Consideration of bacteremia, therefore, must include discussion of its mechanisms, the settings when it occurs, its diagnosis, its clinical features and its management.

Bacteria enter the bloodstream through the lymphatic system, except during intravascular infections (endocarditis, endarteritis, septic thrombophlebitis) and with contaminated intravascular injections. Therefore, invasive infections spreading through tissues and into lymphatics, or anatomical and mechanical factors facilitating lymphatic drainage or flow from a focus of infection, are important in the pathogenesis of bacteremia. Group A streptococcal skin infection and pneumococcal pneumonia are examples of invasive infection by virulent bacteria frequently associated with bacteremia. Extraction of a tooth, urethral catheterization, and incision, drainage or manipulation of an abscess, all are examples of mechanical and anatomical factors facilitating occurence of bacteremia.

Bacteremia may be *transient* and self limited, *intermittent*, or *continuous*.

Transient Bacteremia

Transient bacteremia most often accompanies manipulation of abscesses or infected tissues, and may be induced by seemingly benign events such as chewing, or follow surgical, positional or manual procedures. Instrumentation of the urinary tract, other endoscopic procedures, and dental extractions frequently result in transient bacteremia.

The danger of transient bacteremia is related to the responsible microorganisms and the presence or absence of underlying disease. Transient bacteremia by gram-negative bacilli, as following urethral instrumentation, may produce chill, fever, and hypotension in 30 to 60 minutes, and is usually but not invariably self limited. Transient bacteremia by *Staphylococcus aureus* may lead to development of metastatic abscesses in bone or kidney. *Streptococcus viridans* bacteremia resulting from dental manipulation almost never causes difficulty except in patients with valvular heart disease, congenital cardiac malformations or vascular aneurysms leading to bacterial endarteritis or endocarditis.

Transient bacteremia may occur during the initial stage of some infections, as in pneumococcal pneumonia. Persistence of bacteremia in these circumstances is related to progression and extension of the local infection and may lead to or be indicative of metastatic infection.

Introduction of exotic as well as common bacteria into the circulation by narcotic addicts has resulted in serious infection; e.g., gonococcal and candida endocarditis, hepatitis, and malaria.

Although transient bacteremia is often benign, it may under certain conditions induce serious consequences. Awareness of these situations provides the basis for using antimicrobial drugs immediately before and for a short time after procedures likely to induce bacteremia (Table 9.1). For example, bacteremia by *Streptococcus viridans* is most common during dental extraction, and penicillin administered an hour before and for a day following the extraction is recommended in patients with rheumatic or congenital heart disease. Bacteremia by *Streptococcus fecalis* or enterococcus may occur during urethral or pelvic instrumentation, and prophylaxis with ampicillin is recommended in those patients with valvular heart disease. Bacteremia by *Staphylococcus aureus* probably occurs frequently during incision and drainage of staphylococcal abscesses of the skin and

TABLE 9.1
Settings when prophylaxis recommended in patients with congenital or rheumatic heart disease

1. Any dental manipulation	Penicillin: 1.2 mill. units IM one hour before and next day
2. Urethral instrumentation of uninfected urinary tract	Ampicillin: 0.5 gm. IM one hour before and 1.0 gm. next day
3. Labor and delivery (parturition)	Penicillin as in dental manipulation
4. Surgery under general anesthesia	Methicillin: 2 gm. IM one hour before and next day
5. ? Bronchoscopy	Penicillin as in dental manipulation

subcutaneous tissues. A penicillinase resistant antibiotic (methicillin, oxacillin, cloxacillin, cephalothin, cephalexin) is recommended in patients with such infections to prevent development of metastatic infection.

Specific antimicrobial therapy probably should be given before, during and after surgery upon or manipulation of infected tissues. Total excision of an infected area requires antimicrobial treatment before and after surgery; but if the infection is confined to the excised tissue, treatment may not be prolonged. On the other hand, if the infection is usually associated with widespread dissemination, as in tuberculosis or histoplasmosis, treatment should be continued as if surgery were not done. For example, complete removal of a tuberculous lung lesion will not reduce the 12 to 18 months of desired treatment for the disease. Again, the objectives are to prevent, if possible, the consequences of transient bacteremia and provide treatment of the infection.

Intermittent Bacteremia

Recurrent bacteremia, in which consecutive blood cultures are intermittently positive, is characteristic of abscesses and a few specific infections. It should be recognized that recurrent bacteremia also may be induced by repeated manipulations responsible for transient bacteremia. Furthermore, the intermittent bacteremia associated with pyogenic infections can often be related to manipulation, positional change, or instrumentation (probing) of abscesses. Patients with perirectal or prostatic abscess, for example, may have bacteremia following defecation or rectal examination. Similarly, patients with perinephric abscess may experience bacteremia following flank trauma, bending or even from vigorous palpation of the affected kidney. Intermittently obstructed drainage of an abscess, such as of the urinary tract, sinus tract, or biliary tract (*Charcot's intermittent fever*), may result in intermittent bacteremia. A large majority (85 percent) of patients with bacteremia from a staphylococcal abscess will have intermittent bacteremia. The occurrence of intermittent bacteremia is often associated with rapidly rising fever followed by rapid defervescence and chill or rigor, producing a hectic, septic or intermittent fever. It is important to recognize, however, that administration of aspirin or other antipyretic to febrile patients also can produce chill and intermittent or hectic fever without bacteremia.

Chronic meningococcemia and gonococcemia are specific infections characterized by intermittent bacteremia accompanied by recurrent fever and bacteremia without apparent abscesses. Brucellosis, as a recurrent febrile disease, might also be classed as causing intermittent bacteremia; but during febrile periods, which may last for many days, blood cultures are usually always positive. This is more like a continuous or persistent bacteremia associated with relapsing disease. Malaria also is a classic example of relapsing disease associated with recurrent parasitemia.

Detection of intermittent bacteremia may require repeated blood cultures to find one or two positive. Bacteremia will usually be demonstrable 30 to 60 minutes before the temperature rises and before a chill. Prediction of the time of bacteremia is not always possible, but regularly spaced blood cultures throughout a 24-hour period or more, or cultures done as the temperature begins to rise are most likely to be productive.

The treatment of intermittent bacteremia, clearly, is treatment of the abscess or of the obstructed or specific infection. Demonstration of the bacteremia, however, may facilitate a specific microbial diagnosis and identify the treatment of choice.

Continuous Bacteremia

When each of several consecutive blood cultures are positive, the patient has continuous bacteremia, indicative usually of a serious infection. Intravascular infections are frequently responsible, but certain other types of infection also are characterized by continuous bacteremia. Typhoid, tularemia, brucellosis, plague, glanders, melioidosis, anthrax, and relapsing fever (*Streptobacillus moniliformis*), in addition to rat-bite fever (*Spirillum minus*), Weil's disease (*Leptospira icterohaemorrhagiae*), histoplasmosis, and several additional diseases, all are characterized by persistently positive blood cultures during early or active infection. Some, however, require special techniques for their detection.

Continuous bacteremia due to common pyogenic or nonpyogenic organisms, with or without a localized infection, is highly suggestive of intravascular disease, such as bacterial endocarditis, septic thrombophlebitis or infective endarteritis. The constant seeding of the blood with bacteria in these infections is attributable to their intravascular location. In bacterial endocarditis there are only minor variations in the number or organisms in the blood from time to time. When not all blood cultures are positive in these instances, the concentration of bacteria per ml. of blood and the volume of blood sampled for culture are probably small. It is important to emphasize, however, that intravascular infection can be associated with persistently negative blood cultures. This may be related to infection by organisms not readily grown in the usual culture media, to prior antibiotic therapy or for unexplained reasons. Because all blood cultures are usually positive in intravascular infection, if positive at all, more than three to five blood cultures from these patients are unnecessary. At times, bone marrow may be fruitfully cultured when blood cultures are negative. This has been particularly the case in typhoid, brucellosis, and histoplasmosis. Meningococci and rickettsiae can be identified in the cutaneous vascular lesions associated with infection by these organisms.

Falsely positive blood cultures are sometimes difficult to distinguish from transient or intermittent bacteremia. Certain bacteria are most often contaminants of blood cultures. These include *Bacillus subtilis*, some Corynebacteria, and *S. albus*. If identified in a single blood culture, no others having been taken, repeat cultures should be done, for these bacteria are occasionally pathogenic. If isolated from only one of several cultures in a patient having no evidence of infection, it may be designated a contaminant without further study. Virulent bacteria such as group A streptococci, pneumococci and meningococci, however, are always significant when isolated from a single blood culture and must be regarded seriously. Blood cultures, as with all other laboratory data, must be integrated, of course, with a thorough evaluation of the patient's problem.

Experimental data indicate that lumbar puncture, renal biopsy, and even intramuscular injections in individuals with bacteremia or viremia may result in localization of infection in the central nervous system, kidney, and muscle, respectively. In man, however, this occurrence is difficult to substantiate and has limited clinical importance.

The *reticuloendothial system,* including phagocytic cells of liver, spleen, and bone marrow, is largely responsible for removing microorganisms from the blood. Microbial specific serum antibody and the complement system may facilitate this clearance mechanism by opsonization of the infecting organisms, but are not always required for phagocytosis by the reticuloendothelial cells. Nonspecific serum factors adsorbing to or altering the surface of bacteria, however, probably contribute to phagocytosis of some microorganisms. The reticuloendothelial system has immense reserve capacity; and during terminal disease or massive bacteremia, organisms may be readily removed from the blood. Impaired reticulendothelial phagocytic function, therefore, must be rare.

Patients with *cirrhosis of the liver* occasionally may have transient, self-limited episodes of bacteremia with enteric organisms responsible for fever and chill. Cirrhosis predisposes patients to exaggerated pyrogenic and hypotensive responses to the endotoxin of gram-negative bacilli, but probably does not significantly impair reticuloendothelial phagocytic activity.

Splenectomy in children may be followed by increased frequency of pneumococcal disease with bacteremia possibly related to the resulting immunological impairment, but probably unrelated to removal of splenic phagocytic function.

The *clinical settings* commonly associated with bacteremia by organisms of moderate or low pathogenicity, such as the enteric, skin and upper respiratory tract indigenous microorganisms, are largely characterized by impaired immunological or granulocyte phagocytic activity.

Cardiovascular, cerebrovascular, hematopoietic and chronic respiratory diseases responsible for ischemia or vascular congestion, impaired cleansing of the respiratory tract, defective bladder emptying, and granulocytopenia, all are common disorders in which bacteremia occurs. Similarly, diabetes mellitus with peripheral vascular disease or acidosis, and uremic acidosis, resulting in defective granulocytic inflammation, also predispose to uncontrolled skin, respiratory, gastrointestinal and urinary tract infection leading to bacteremia. Necrotic tissue, as in exfoliative dermatitis and third-degree burns, producing avascularity and consequently impaired granulocyte inflammation, also are foci of infection leading to bacteremia. Foreign bodies, whether introduced accidentally or intentionally, as in using intravascular catheters, indwelling urethral catheters, or sutures and prostheses, predispose to uncontrolled focal infection and bacteremia, probably by interfering with phagocytic activity.

Immunological deficiency, as seen in congenital or acquired agammaglobulinemia, multiple myeloma and following use of immunosuppressive or corticosteroid drugs, for example, predispose to infection by microorganisms such as pneumococci, staphylococci and certain viral and other infections (Herpes zoster, cytomegalovirus, and pneumocystis, etc.), probably controlled by immune responsiveness. In contrast, infection by gram-negative bacilli, staphylococci, and candida are most frequent in patients with impaired granulocyte function, probably indicating the principle mechanism of host resistance controlling each microorganism's pathogenicity.

Gram-negative bacillemia usually arises from urinary tract infection. Staphylococcal and group A streptococcal bacteremia usually arise from skin infections. Infection of the respiratory tract is always the source of pneumococcal bacteremia. But gram-negative bacilli (Klebsiella, Pseudomonas) and gram-positive cocci (pneumococcus and staphylococcus) infecting the lung also may be responsible for bacteremia.

Because bacteremia by indigenous bacteria occurs largely in patients with impaired host resistance, more than one organism may produce infection simultaneously, and mixed bacteremia is not uncommon. Isolation of more than one organism from the blood, therefore, can be important and influence selection of antimicrobial therapy.

Bacteremic Shock

The association of circulatory collapse with severe infectious processes is well known. Early reports documented the occurrence of shock in the course of pneumococcal pneumonia, streptococcal and staphylococcal bacteremia. Subsequently, shock has been recognized in association with a wide variety of bacterial, fungal, viral, rickettsial and parasitic infections.

Currently, bacteremic shock is most commonly associated with gram-negative bacteremia. In about two-thirds of the cases, organisms such as *E. coli*, Klebsiella, Enterobacter, Proteus, and Pseudomonas are implicated. Other gram-negative bacteria such as the meningococcus, bacteroides, herellea, serratia, make up a variable percentage. Shock occurs in about 40 percent of gram-negative bacteremias. This syndrome is usually hospital acquired and is often directly related to some manipulative procedure such as catheterization or operation. The incidence of shock in gram-positive bacterial infections is not precisely known but probably amounts to more than five percent in infections due to pneumococcus, group A streptococcus and *Staphylococcus aureus*. While bacteremia can be demonstrated in most cases, occasionally blood cultures are negative. Transient or intermittent bacteremia not reflected by positive cultures may initiate shock.

The fundamental defect in shock is inadequacy of blood supply to vital tissues leading to cellular hypoxia and metabolic failure. Hemodynamic studies in patients have established that the pathophysiology leading to underperfusion may be cardiac failure, hypovolemia or pooling of blood in the periphery. Peripheral pooling of blood is not common, the usual hemodynamic abnormality being cardiac insufficiency frequently compounded by some degree of hypovolemia. Administration of gram-negative bacterial endotoxin to animals reproduces many of the features seen in shock occurring during gram-negative bacteremia in man. However, identical shock syndromes can be observed in patients infected with organisms devoid of endotoxin, such as gram-positive cocci and fungi. This suggests that the ways in which the cardiovascular system can react to bacteremia are relatively limited. Pharmacologic mediators such as kinins may participate in the pathogenesis of shock, but their importance is not clearly known.

Soon after the onset of bacteremic shock the cardiac index is often supranormal. Central venous pressure may be normal or elevated; hypotension and oliguria are present. Such patients are frequently hyperpneic; arterial blood gases at this stage reveal respiratory alkalosis, with pH of 7.45 or greater, diminished pCO_2 and bicarbonate. The total peripheral resistance is frequently diminished and the skin may be warm and dry. Simultaneous measurement of arterial and mixed venous pO_2 reveals a narrowed A-V oxygen difference. Oxygen transport to the tissues is inefficient when related to cardiac output, and overall oxygen consumption frequently declines. Despite the elevated cardiac index, the blood lactate level is increased. Such findings are consonant with a redistribution of blood within the vascular space characterized by A-V shunting, leading to hypoperfusion of vital tissues, increased anaerobic glycolysis and accumulation of blood lactate. Cellular metabolic failure with inability to utilize available oxygen, possibly related to bacterial toxins, may also be present.

In patients with shock complicating intra-abdominal infection, such as bowel infarction or peritonitis, hypovolemia is an added factor. Large amounts of fluid may be sequestered as inflammatory edema, intraluminal fluid or as free intraperitoneal fluid. Hemoconcentration is frequent. Such patients present with diminished central venous pressure and cardiac index. Total peripheral resistance is usually elevated. Respiratory alkalosis or compensated metabolic acidosis may be seen; blood lactate is elevated.

Aggressive therapy of patients with the previously described snydromes frequently reverses the shock process. With increasing duration or severity of septic shock, hemodynamic and metabolic parameters deteriorate further. Patients may pass from a high output, low resistance state to one characterized by falling cardiac index, increased total peripheral resistance and severe lactic acidosis. Whether all patients manifest these sequential changes is not clear. The rate of progression of such changes is highly variable from case to case. Certainly some patients seen apparently at an early time after inception of shock may already manifest the low output, metabolic acidosis syndrome. Once such a shock state has supervened, the prognosis for life is poor.

Other pathophysiologic processes which are common in bacteremic shock include disseminated intravascular coagulation, pulmonary insufficiency and renal failure.

Disseminated intravascular coagulation (DIC) probably occurs in all cases of bacteremic shock. DIC is thought to be initiated by endothelial or platelet damage from bacterial or other toxins resulting in activation of the intrinsic coagulation system. Whether or not DIC participates in the inception of shock or is a secondary feature is not clear. DIC results in formation of platelet and fibrin thrombi throughout the microvasculature and further reduces perfusion of vital organs. Thrombocytopenia, diminished factors II, V, VIII and fibrinogen and the appearance of fibrin split products in the serum are characteristic. Although coagulation factors are consumed by the process, overt bleeding apart from petechiae of skin and mucous membranes is unusual.

Arterial hypoxemia is observed in most patients even in the absence of recognized pulmonary disease. Oxygen exchange is inhibited and administration of increased inspired oxygen concentrations often fails to raise the arterial pO_2 to the expected value. Early in shock, major degrees of true pulmonary A-V shunting may cause hypoxemia. True shunting tends to decrease rapidly following resuscitative measures, to be replaced by ventilation-perfusion abnormalities secondary to atelectasis, pneumonia or pulmonary edema. Severe pulmonary edema may be observed and can progress to a fatal outcome even after the original hemodynamic abnormalities have been reversed. The mechanism of production of the "shock lung" syndrome is unknown. Factors such as capillary thrombosis from DIC, direct damage to capillaries by bacterial toxins or oxygen toxicity from prolonged exposure to high inspired oxygen concentrations may be implicated.

Oliguria and azotemia are usual in bacteremic shock. In most instances oliguria is secondary to renal vasoconstriction and diminished perfusion associated with hypotension. Gram-negative bacterial endotoxin also exerts a direct renal vasoconstrictor effect. The glomerular filtration rate is severely depressed. Continued hypotension leads to loss of renal concentrating ability secondary to renal tubular cell damage. Restoration of effective renal perfusion ordinarily results in increased urine output, but concentrating ability may be depressed for some time following clinical improvement. Rarely, partial or complete bilateral renal cortical necrosis occurs secondary to DIC.

Therapy of Bacteremic Shock

Prompt diagnosis and institution of effective therapy is critically important in saving life in bacteremic shock. This disorder should be suspected in any febrile patient with otherwise unexplained hypotension. Therapy is directed towards a) assuring a clear airway and efficient pulmonary gas exchange; b) restoring adequate blood perfusion of vital tissues; and c) eradication of the infectious process.

Certain measures are vital for correct management: hourly recording of central venous pressure, urine output, blood pressure, respiratory rate, pulse, rectal temperature. Arterial pH, pO_2, oxygen saturation, pCO_2 and bicarbonate should be measured frequently. Hematocrit, white blood cell count, serum creatinine and serum electrolytes should be monitored at least daily during the acute stage. Other parameters of great value but available usually only in specialized units include serial determinations of cardiac output, peripheral vascular resistance and blood lactate.

Pulmonary Gas Exchange. Once the diagnosis has been entertained, a clear airway and adequate alveolar ventilation must be established. Careful auscultation of chest, portable x-ray study and arterial blood gas determinations should be performed. Tracheobronchial aspiration is often necessary to remove secretions. Supplementary humidified oxygen should be supplied in view of the frequently observed arterial hypoxemia. Bronchoscopy and tracheobronchial lavage should be considered in the presence of atelectasis or mucous plugging of bronchi. Ventilatory failure may occur in the elderly or in patients recently subjected to thoracic or abdominal surgery. Inability of the patient to maintain a normal or lowered pCO_2, especially when associated with a low pO_2 (below 60 mm. Hg.), constitutes an indication for endotracheal intubation and respiratory assistance. In the severely ill shock patient ventilatory assistance materially dimishes work of respiration with its attendant demand for cardiac output and oxygen supply.

Fluid Replacement. The second major objective in therapy is to improve tissue perfusion, by ensuring adequate filling of the vascular space and improving cardiac performance. Adequate fluid replacement is best guided by serial central venous pressure (CVP) determinations. The CVP, normally 3 to 10 cm. H_2O, is a measure of the relationship between venous return and right ventricular pump capacity. Most patients do not have a primary volume deficit. Net vascular tone is usually decreased and the vascular space is expanded. CVP measurement in such patients may be normal or somewhat elevated due to a degree of myocardial insufficiency. Patients with intra-abdominal infection usually have major volume deficits. The CVP may be very low, normal or even elevated in the presence of myocardial insufficiency.

Valuable information is gained by observing the CVP response to rapid fluid infusions of 100 to 200 ml. over five-minute periods. Continuing low or normal CVP indicates cardiac competency and the need for further fluid. Patients with hematocrit below 40 percent should receive sufficient whole blood to replete the estimated deficit in red cell mass. Patients with normal red cell volume should receive either plasma, five percent albumin or isotonic saline. Excessive replacement of red cell mass should be avoided as this increases blood viscosity. In many patients, and particularly those with intra-abdominal infection, large amounts of fluid may be required to restore perfusion.

Correction of arterial pH towards normal in patients with lactic acidosis may be attempted with sodium bicarbonate infusions. Unless tissue perfusion and aerobic metabolism are restored, lactate will continue to accumulate.

Volume administration should be pushed until a good response is obtained, with rising systemic blood pressure, clearing mentation and increased urinary output (greater than 50 ml. per hour) or until the CVP becomes elevated. Aggressive fluid therapy given early may be sufficient to reverse the shock state.

Inotropic Agents. Patients with bacteremic shock suffer from variable degrees of impairment of myocardial contractility. Many will tolerate aggressive fluid therapy; the CVP may actually fall, indicating improved cardiac performance possibly secondary to increased coronary perfusion. In some patients following volume loading, body perfusion remains inadequate and the CVP rises to more than 15 cm. H_2O. Further fluid administration is dangerous and may precipitate pulmonary edema. Myocardial contractility in such patients may be improved by administration of isoproterenol. This agent augments cardiac rate and force of contraction by stimulating cardiac beta adrenergic receptors. In addition, stimulation of peripheral beta receptors induces vasodilation. Isoproterenol, 2.5 mg. in 500 ml. of 5 percent dextrose in water or isotonic saline should be infused at a rate of 1 ml. per minute. A favorable response is indicated by a decline in CVP to normal and increased urinary flow from oliguric levels to greater than 50 ml. per hour.

Should a good response not be obtained within 15 minutes of beginning the infusion, either the concentration of drug should be doubled or the infusion rate increased. Isoproterenol must be administered with caution and preferably under continuous electrocardiographic monitoring. Dangerous cardiac arrhythmias may be induced at rapid infusion rates, this being a particular hazard if ventricular rates consistently exceed 120 per minute. Most frequently though, the cardiac rate slows during favorable response to the drug. Therapy with isoproterenol should be continued for at least 24 hours after adequate body perfusion has been restored and the infectious process controlled. A dose adequate to maintain urine flow of at least 50 ml. per hour and systolic blood pressure of 90 mm. Hg should be employed.

Adrenal Corticosteroids. Although there is no controlled study available to establish their value in human bacteremic shock, the use of pharmacologic doses (20 to 40 mg./kg.) of steroid hormones, such as hydrocortisone, has become commonplace.

Other Measures. Failure to achieve a consistent elevation of cardiac index of more than 1 liter/min./M^2 with isoproterenol implies a poor prognosis. Should the CVP remain high and unresponsive to isoproterenol, a severe degree of myocardial insufficiency may be assumed, though cardiac tamponade or superior vena caval obstruction can produce this picture and should be excluded. Rapid digitalization of such patients may be beneficial.

Alpha adrenergic blockade with phenoxybenzamine combined with fluid loading remains largely an investigative procedure. Favorable results have been reported in some refractory shock patients but no general agreement exists as to whether mortality rates can be reduced. This form of therapy should be reserved for patients who do not respond to isoproterenol and fluid therapy. Because of a potent vasodilator effect, vascular volume may increase by up to 25 percent; large amounts of fluid should be administered. Improved tissue perfusion may follow, with a fall in CVP and increased urinary flow. Phenoxybenzamine exerts no inotropic effect on the heart. Occasionally the addition of 1-norepinehprine has been useful in increasing cardiac output in patients with established alpha blockade.

Heparin therapy to reverse the DIC syndrome has recently been evaluated. While coagulation parameters reverted towards normal in heparinized patients, their survival rate was apparently not improved. There exists no agreement as to whether all patients with bacteremic shock should receive heparin. Certainly patients with major hemorrhage attributed to DIC should receive adequate heparin therapy.

Antimicrobial Therapy in Bacteremia

The appropriate selection and administration of antimicrobial therapy is critical to the outcome of life-threatening bacteremia. Once recognized, an intensive effort should be devoted to 1) presumptive identification of the etiologic agent; 2) collection of appropriate specimens for precise identification and antimicrobial susceptibility testing of the infecting microorganism; and 3) prompt institution of antimicrobial therapy.

Presumptive Identification of the Etiologic Agent. A careful search for the source of bacteremia or for accessible, focal embolic lesions may provide useful clues to the identity of the infecting microorganism. Specimens should be obtained for gram-stain from each of the involved sites. If implicated, sputum, urine, aspirates of joint or cerebrospinal fluids, foreign bodies such as indwelling catheters, and infected material from abscesses or embolic cutaneous lesions, all should be examined. Stains performed by the gram method should always include appropriate material (such as scrapings of one's teeth) on the same slide to verify adequacy of the method.

Certain distinctive clinical and epidemiologic features of the patient's illness, as noted above, may provide useful clues to the diagnosis. In general, bacteremia arising from the urinary or gastrointestinal tracts is most likely due to gram-negative bacilli, while that originating in the skin or structures contiguous to the respiratory tract is more likely due to gram-positive pyogens.

Precise Identification and Antimicrobial Susceptibility Testing of the Infecting Microorganism. Cultures of blood and material from other sites involved in the infectious process should be obtained prior to the institution of antimicrobial therapy. Approximately three to five blood cultures should be taken. In constant bacteremia or emergencies they may be obtained in rapid succession. In intermittent bacteremia they should be drawn approximately one-half hour prior to a chill. If this is not possible, cultures may be spaced at regular intervals of no more than four to six hours. As soon as growth is detected, gram stains should be performed and subcultures should be made for antimicrobial susceptibility testing. Results of the gram stains and cultures should be reported immediately to the physician.

Selection of Antimicrobial Therapy. The general principles of drug selection and administration are outlined in the chapter on *Antimicrobial Therapy*. In patients with bacteremia, antimicrobial drugs must often be prescribed before the results of cultures and susceptibility tests are known. Use of extremely broad spectrum, multiple drug therapy should not substitute for a careful search for immediate clues to a presumptive identification of the infecting microorganism. More often than not, careful study of the patient will provide reliable information to assist in selection of specific therapy. In the vast majority of patients, distinction between gram-positive or gram-negative bacteremia is at least possible.

The general principles of drug selection and administration in bacteremia are as follows: 1) a single antimicrobial drug of known efficacy against the presumed etiologic agent(s) should be selected, if possible; 2) bactericidal drugs are preferable in most instances; 3) if more than one drug appears necessary, potentially antagonistic combinations should be avoided; 4) if the infection is severe, or threatens life, the drug should be administered intravenously; and 5) factors—such as abscess, obstruction, and foreign body—known to predispose to therapeutic unresponsiveness should be identified and eliminated whenever possible.

The antimicrobial susceptibilities of bacteria that frequently pose problems in drug selection are listed in Table 9.2. If presumptive identification of the infecting microorganism cannot be made, the following drugs are most useful in the indicated circumstances: 1) bacteremia due to unidentified gram-positive organisms—a penicillinase-resistant penicillin or cephalothin; 2) bacteremia due to unidentified gram-negative cocci—penicillin G; 3) bacteremia due to unidentified gram-negative bacilli—gentamicin, or in patients with profound renal impairment or leukopenia—carbenicillin; and 4) bacteremia of unknown etiology—cephalothin and gentamicin.

Since carbenicillin has little or no activity against strains of Klebsiella, gentamicin should be substituted when infection with this organism is suspected, even in patients with renal failure or leukopenia. Strains of enterococci and bacteroides may be resistant to each of the antimocrobial drugs listed above. Enterococcal bacteremia should be treated with large doses of ampicillin. Infection due to bacteroides may be suspected if 1) the source of the infection is in the bowel or female pelvis; 2) conditions at the site of infection favor anaerobiasis; 3) gas or putrid material is demonstrated in the tissues; 4) response to previous therapy with the

TABLE 9.2

*Antimicrobial susceptibilities of bacteria that frequently pose problems in drug selection**

Bacteria	Approximate number of strains tested	Antimicrobial agent and percentage of strains susceptible								
		Streptomycin	Chloramphenicol	Tetracycline	Penicillin	Ampicillin	Cephalothin	Kanamycin	Colistin or polymyxin B	Gentamicin
E. coli	3300	74	98	75	0.4	77	93	94	100	100
Klebsiella aerogenes	1600	80	92	76	0	7	95	85	99	100
Other Klebsiella	85	73	76	69	0	13	73	90	91	100
Enterobacter cloacae	420	84	91	75	0.3	15	8	90	98	100
Enterobacter aerogenes	350	78	92	73	1.	10	26	82	99	100
Proteus mirabilis	2010	92	92	6	3.	88	88	99	2	100
Other Proteus	25	91	78	29	0	35	39	100	17	96
Citrobacter	36	78	89	83	0	51	57	92	100	100
Providence	43	77	38	13	0	50	23	89	9	100
Serratia	130	46	72	14	0	14	4	85	28	100
Pseudomonas aeruginosa	1545	7	6	5	0	2	1	7	99	95
Herellea (*B. anitratum*)	93	79	44	82	4	42	16	92	97	100
Bacteroides fundiliformis	72	1	97	55	3	12	5	1	2	1
Other bacteroides	26	4	100	84	65	75	70	12	79	10
*Staphylococcus aureus***	1450	92	99	85	24	58	100	—	62	90
*Staphylococcus epidermidis***	1520	84	95	56	44	—	99	—	80	100
Enterococci	970	1	96	31	17	100	34	—	0	4

* Antimicrobial susceptibility tests performed on isolates from clinical specimens at the Shands Teaching Hospital, Gainesville, Florida, May 1970 to April 1971. Courtesy of Dr. Herman Baer.

** At least three-quarters of these isolates were also susceptible to erythromycin and lincomycin.

aminoglycosides has been poor; and 5) distinctive morphologic characteristics are noted on gram stain. Until laboratory tests confirm susceptibility of the bacteroides to less hazardous drugs, chloramphenicol should be administered.

SELECTED REFERENCES

Bennett, I. L. and Beeson, P. B.: Bacteremia: A consideration of some experimental and clinical aspects. Yale J. Biol. Med., *26*:241, 1954.

Cluff, L. E. and Reynolds, R. C., Page, D. L. and Breckenridge, J. L.: Staphylococcal bacteremia and altered host resistance. Ann. Int. Med. *69*:859, 1968.

Corrigan, J. J. Jr. and Jordan, C. M.: Heparin therapy in septicemia with disseminated intravascular coagulation: effect on mortality and on correction of hemostatic defects. N. Eng. J. Med., *283*:778, 1970.

Corrigan, J. J. Jr., Ray, W. L. and May, N.: Changes in the blood coagulation system associated with septicemia. N. Eng. J. Med., *279*:851, 1968.

Curtin, J. A., Petersdorf, R. G., Bennett, I. L. Jr.: Pseudomonas bacteremia: A review of 91 cases. Ann. Int. Med., *54*:1077, 1961.

DuPont, H. L. and Spink, W. W.: Infections due to gram-negative organisms: an analysis of 860 patients with bacteremia at the University of Minnesota Medical Center, 1958–1966. Medicine (Balt.) *48*:307, 1969.

Ebert, R. V. and Abernathy, R. S.: Septic shock. Fed. Proc., *20*:179, 1961 (Number 2, Part III).

Hardaway, R. M., James, P. M., Anderson, R. W., Bredenberg, C. E. and West, R. L.: Intensive study and treatment of shock in man. J.A.M.A., *199*:779, 1967.

Hodgin, U. G. and Sanford, J. P.: Gram-negative rod bacteremia: an analysis of 100 patients. Amer. J. Med., *39*:952, 1965.

Kardos, G. G.: Isoproterenol in the treatment of shock due to bacteremia with gram-negative pathogens. N. Eng. J. Med., *274*:868, 1966.

MacLean, L. D., Duff, J. H., Scott, H. M. and Peretz, D. I.: Treatment of shock in man based on hemodynamic diagnosis. Surg. Gynec. Obstet., *120*:1, 1965.

MacLean, L. D., Mulligan, W. G., McLean, A. P. H. and Duff, J. H.: Patterns of septic shock in man—a detailed study of 56 patients. Ann. Surg., *166*:543, 1967.

Martin, C. M., Cuomo, A. J., Geraghty, M. J., Zager, J. R. and Mandes, T. C.: Gram-negative rod bacteremia. J. Infect. Dis., *119*:506, 1969.

Mason, J. W., Kleeberg, U., Dolan, P. and Colman, R. W.: Plasma kallikrein and Hageman factor in gram-negative bacteremia. Ann. Intern. Med., *73*:545, 1970.

McCabe, W. R. and Jackson, G. G.: Gram-negative bacteremia. II. Clinical, laboratory and therapeutic observations. Arch. Intern. Med., *110*:856, 1962.

Robson, H. G. and Cluff, L. E.: Experimental pneumococcal and staphylococcal sepsis: effects of hydrocortisone and phenoxybenzamine upon mortality rates. J. Clin. Invest., *45*:1421, 1966.

Siegel, J. H. and Fabian, M.: Therapeutic advantages of an inotropic vasodilator in endotoxin shock. J.A.M.A., *200*:696, 1967.

Siegel, J. H., Greenspan, M. and Del Guercio, L. R. M.: Abnormal vascular tone, defective oxygen transport and myocardial failure in human septic shock. Ann. Surg., *165*: 504, 1967.

Strauch, M., McLaughlin, J. S., Mansberger, A., Young, J., Mendonca, P., Gray, K. and Cowley, R. A.: Effects of septic shock on renal function in humans. Ann. Surg., *165*:536, 1967.

Weil, M. H., Shubin, H. and Biddle, M.: Shock caused by gram-negative microorganisms: analysis of 169 cases. Ann. Intern. Med., *60*:384, 1964.

Weil, M. H., Shubin, H. and Rosoff, L.: Fluid repletion in circulatory shock: central venous pressure and other practical guides. J.A.M.A., *192*:668, 1965.

Weinstein, L. and Klainer, A. S.: Septic shock—pathogenesis and treatment. N. Eng. J. Med., *274*:950, 1966.

Wilson, R. E., Jablonski, D. V., and Thal, A. P.: The usage of dibenzyline in clinical shock. Surgery, *56*:172, 1964.

Chapter 10

HEMATOLOGICAL MANIFESTATIONS OF INFECTION

The interactions between microorganisms and the blood provide a fascinating array of clinical findings. In the following discussions three aspects are singled out for detailed analysis: the changes in hemostasis, the acceleration of red cell destruction, and the anemia of chronic infection. In each of these areas, the findings represent alterations in host systems which may be far removed from the specific site of infection. These changes may be the initial manifestation of infection or may be the deciding factor in the death of the patient. An understanding of these hematologic manifestations will enable us to more adequately help our patients with infection.

Anemia

The anemia found with infection usually is insidious in onset, moderate in severity, and obscure in origin. Should the infection be obvious, the physician may overlook the modestly reduced hemoglobin which rarely falls below nine gm percent. However, the appearance of an unexplained anemia may alert the physician to an otherwise occult infectious process such as bacterial endocarditis. Incomplete as our understanding of this association is, we can describe the features of the anemia sufficiently to provide a recognizable model. We shall explore the conditions in which it is found, discuss the clinical manifestations, differentiate it from similar anemias and describe appropriate management.

Infections which frequently lead to anemia are chronic and usually serious enough to produce other systemic findings such as fever, weight loss and leukocytosis. Lung abscess, osteomyelitis, endocarditis, and cholangitis are illustrative of these types of infection. Moreover, many chronic inflammatory diseases such as rheumatoid arthritis, ulcerative colitis, or disseminated neoplasia, all will produce an identical hematologic picture. This has been ably reviewed by Cartwright as the anemia of chronic disorders. Acute infections such as pneumococcal pneumonia, acute pyelonephritis, or rubella have a similar potential for producing anemia but usually resolve too rapidly for an appreciable drop in hemoglobin to be detected.

Upon close examination, the falling hemoglobin in infection is the result of a moderately accelerated hemolysis accentuated by an inadequate response from the erythroid bone marrow. Red cell survival studies typically show mean cell lifespan values of 30 to 90 days in contrast to the usual 120 days. The erythroid marrow normally can meet this stress by increasing its production of red cells. That it fails to do so under these circumstances is confirmed by a low reticulocyte count of less than 1.5 percent. Tests frequently helpful in detecting hemolysis, such as osmotic fragility and the Coombs' test, are normal. Products from inflamed tissue may possibly damage red cell membranes sufficiently to cause excessive removal of erythrocytes by the reticuloendothelial system. In fact, the cause for the hemolysis is unknown. Red cell morphology in most of these patients is entirely normal although occasional mild hypochromia and infrequent microcytosis may be found. The bone marrow is normal aside from granulocytic hyperplasia occurring in response to the need for more white cells.

Thus, the patient is anemic but red cell production fails to respond, raising the question as to whether the normal regulatory mechanism is operative. The rate of hemoglobin synthesis is largely controlled by the hormone erythropoietin which responds to the availability of oxygen in the kidney. One might anticipate that the serum erythropoietin levels in the anemia of infection might be low, thereby failing to accelerate hemoglobin synthesis. Animals with turpentine abscesses will respond with a reticulocytosis to injected erythropoietin, indicating marrow responsiveness in the presence of a sterile necrosis. But data in humans are scarce. Erythropoietin levels in the blood of patients with rheumatoid arthritis are generally lower than in patients with anemia of comparable severity from other causes. Significantly elevated erythropoietin levels, however, have been found in patients with infection when reticulocyte counts are low. This evidence suggests that the marrow responds less readily to the hormonal stimulus but that in most infections, the stimulus is sub-optimal.

In the anemia of infection, levels of serum iron are reduced. This decrease is frequently severe and mimics the levels seen in iron deficiency. The anemia in infection, however, does not respond to iron medication unless the patient is simultaneously iron deficient. A helpful datum in this

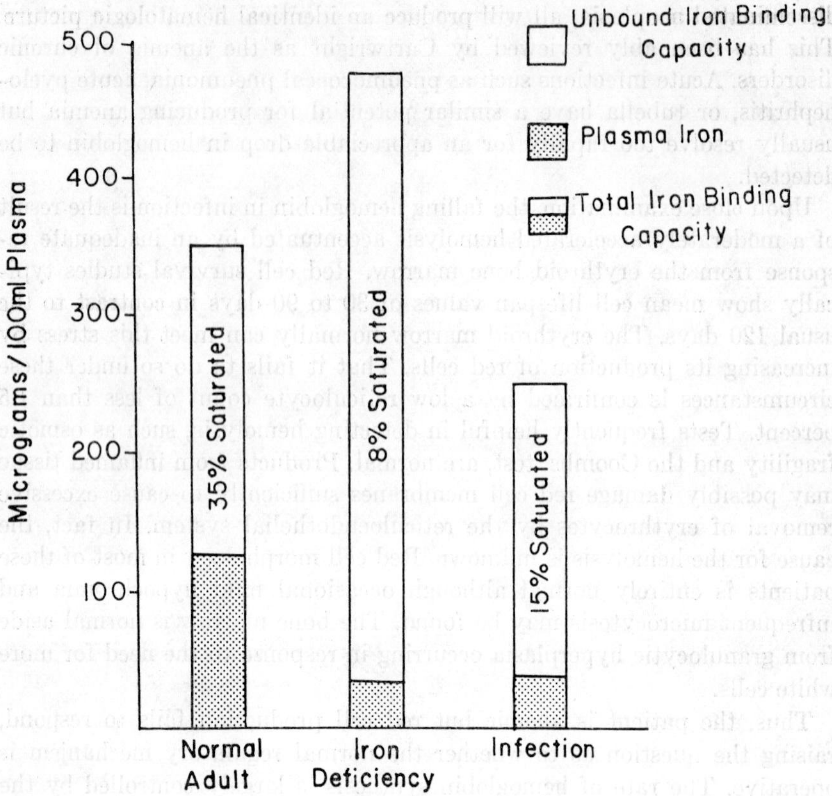

FIG. 10.1.

situation is the iron saturation of the serum iron binding protein (transferrin). Normally the saturation is 20 to 40 percent falling in iron deficiency to less than 15 percent. With infection, the transferrin level is normal or even diminished so that the saturation, despite a lowered serum iron, is usually 15 to 25 percent (Fig. 10.1). In patients with borderline values the finding of iron stores on bone marrow aspiration will help confirm the presence of body iron and implicate the infection as the basic disorder promoting the anemia (Fig. 10.2).

The concentration of iron in serum is regulated primarily by the reticuloendothelial (RE) cells and is derived from the continued breakdown of senescent red cells or from intra-cellular iron stores. With infection, the supply of senescent red cells is increased and therefore iron stores will be normal or increased. But the RE cell becomes miserly in its release of iron back into circulation. For example, animals with turpentine abscesses efficiently clear aged red cells from the circulation but the iron derived from these cells is slowly released to serum transferrin. Consequently, re-utilization of this iron for synthesis of hemoglobin is diminished. In contrast, iron bound to transferrin in vitro and infused directly into circulation is efficiently used for hemoglobin synthesis. This alteration in the RE handling of iron occurs promptly as serum iron concentration falls within six hours after the injection of endotoxin or within one day after tularemia infection.

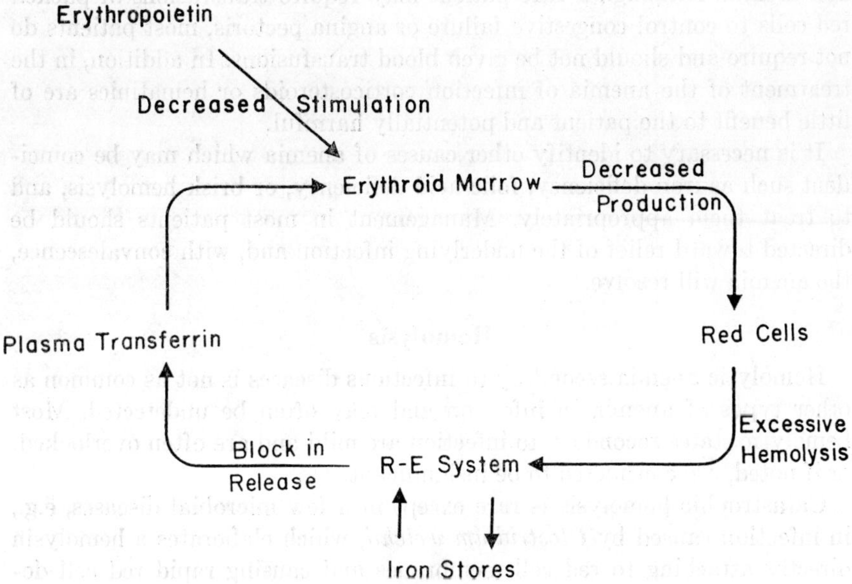

FIG. 10.2. Anemia of infection.

The bacteriostatic property of plasma is abolished when the transferrin is saturated with iron. The virulence of a number of pathogenic organisms is enhanced by an increased serum iron and the diminished release of iron from RE cells may have evolved to impede bacterial cell growth. Moreover, neutrophilic granulocytes have been shown to contain an iron-binding protein, lactoferrin, which is also found in the fluid of inflammatory exudates. In contrast to transferrin, its binding of iron remains stable down to pH 3; a pH found in inflamed tissues. The changes in iron transport during infection therefore may improve host resistance.

Metabolic changes during infection may retard red cell synthesis. Negative nitrogen balance, changes in amino acids, enhanced oxidation of succinate, elevated serum levels of copper and ceruloplasmin and increased activity of nicotinamide adenine dinucleotide glycohydrolase have been observed during infection. These changes serve to emphasize the need for better knowledge of the physiological and biochemical processes associated with infections.

Clinical Management of Anemia of Infection

Therapy of the anemia of infection in most patients is not only ineffective but unnecessary. Corticosteroids will reverse the lowered serum iron and improve the hemoglobin concentration in patients with rheumatoid arthritis, and similar effects may occur in infection. However, there is no evidence that a moderate fall in hemoglobin as seen in most infections is detrimental. Although a rare patient may require transfusions of packed red cells to control congestive failure or angina pectoris, most patients do not require and should not be given blood transfusions. In addition, in the treatment of the anemia of infection corticosteroids or hematinics are of little benefit to the patient and potentially harmful.

It is necessary to identify other causes of anemia which may be coincident such as iron deficiency, folic acid deficiency, or brisk hemolysis, and to treat them appropriately. Management in most patients should be directed toward relief of the underlying infection and, with convalescence, the anemia will resolve.

Hemolysis

Hemolytic anemia secondary to infectious diseases is not as common as other types of anemia in infection and may often be undetected. Most hemolytic states secondary to infection are mild and are often overlooked, or if noted, are considered to be insignificant.

Catastrophic hemolysis is rare except in a few microbial diseases, e.g., in infection caused by *Clostridium welchii*, which elaborates a hemolysin directly attaching to red cell membranes and causing rapid red cell destruction. A case of total hemolysis secondary to *Cl. welchii* infection has been documented in which the patient survived four or more hours after the hematocrit was found to be zero and the plasma had a burgundy wine color due to circulating free hemoglobin.

Other infectious organisms, such as *Bartonella bacilliformis* or malaria parasites, directly attack the red cell membrane, and erythrocyte destruction occurs in the spleen. The damaged red cells are unable to traverse the spleen more than a few times before lysing. Splenomegaly with hemolysis is generally the rule in these infectious diseases.

Viral Etiology

Viral infections have been associated with hemolytic anemia. In some cases this appears to be an immune hemolysis whereby cold agglutinins or other proteins or antibodies attach to the erythrocyte. In most instances the attachment of these agglutinins or proteins does not damage the red cell membrane, but when these enter the splenic circulation the protein is removed from the red cell membrane by the macrophages. In this process the red cell membrane is damaged and the life span of the erythrocytes is markedly decreased. Hemolytic anemia occurring during many viral diseases is unexplained. Viral hepatitis has recently been shown to cause hemolytic anemia, in some cases persisting for six months to a year after resolution of the liver disease. In these cases liver function returns to normal promptly, but the hemolytic anemia persists. Red cell survival in these patients, using autologous and homologous red cells labeled with Cr^{51}, reveals markedly shortened red cell survival, suggesting an extracellular hemolytic process. The osmotic fragility in these cases is also increased.

Microbial Etiology

Bacterial diseases causing hemolytic anemia often are associated with spherocytosis, increased osmotic fragility, and decreased red cell survival as measured by Cr^{51} labeling. The hemolysis in these cases is not usually attributable to immune mechanisms associated with positive Coombs' test and no hemolysins or agglutinins have been found.

Jandl has found hemolytic anemias in a variety of infectious diseases, including psittacosis, infectious hepatitis, malaria, miliary tuberculosis, and subacute bacterial endocarditis, as well as infectious mononucleosis. All of these patients had hemolysis with abnormal osmotic fragility and decreased red cell survival, but Coombs' test and other immunologic tests were negative. The spleens in these patients were enlarged. Infectious mononucleosis, however, also rarely causes immune hemolysis with a positive Coombs' test. An extremely severe hemolytic episode associated with infectious mononucleosis was reported by Mengel and associates in which megaloblastic arrest of the bone marrow occurred. This type of response is unusual and in most cases would not be expected, with the possible exception of hemolysis secondary to *Cl. welchii.*

Typhoid fever has been associated with hemolytic anemias which may persist after successful treatment of the infection. Corticosteroid treatment of the anemia can terminate the hemolytic episode, which has been shown to persist even after the bacteria have been destroyed with chloramphenicol. Because of this response, it has been suggested that reticuloendothelial hyperplasia plays an important role in the hemolysis.

Diagnosis of Hemolytic Anemia

It is only the rare infectious disease that will present with hemolysis severe enough to cause concern, but the diagnosis should be considered when the patient's hematocrit falls rapidly without blood loss, and when the hematocrit is 25 percent or less. An elevated reticulocyte count also may indicate hemolysis, but in severe or chronic infection the bone marrow is frequently suppressed, and the reticulocyte count will not be as high as is usual in hemolytic anemias. The peripheral blood smear in most instances will often reveal spherocytes. Splenomegaly may be found on examination by abdominal x-ray or by radioactive scan of the spleen. A positive Coombs' test can be helpful in making the diagnosis of immune hemolysis. Increased osmotic fragility of the red cells incubated in the test solution for 24 hours is usually found. In hemolytic anemia, however, all cells generally do not show increased osmotic fragility; the proportion of fragile erythrocytes may vary greatly. The survival of red cells labeled with Cr^{51} and radioactive scanning over the spleen to measure splenic sequestration of cells may document a hemolytic process.

In most instances it is not necessary or indicated to use all of these tests to demonstrate hemolytic anemia. Inspection of the peripheral blood smear, reticulocyte count, and osmotic red cell fragility usually will be sufficient. If further documentation is needed, the other tests can be used.

Management of Hemolytic Anemia

Therapy of the hemolytic anemia of infection is primarily treatment of the infection, if this is possible. In most cases this will terminate the hemolytic process and no further therapy is necessary. However, when the anemia is severe or the hematocrit is rapidly falling without bleeding, other measures must be instituted, including transfusion and administration of adrenal corticosteroids. When the hemolysis is severe or protracted and associated with a megaloblastic bone marrow arrest, folic acid may be indicated. It is important that these patients be followed, particularly since in some infections hemolytic anemia may persist for months.

Hemorrhagic Diatheses

Abnormalities of hemostasis may develop in association with infections either because of tissue injury produced by microorganisms, immunologic responses involving plasma coagulation factors and platelets, or because of the toxic effects of antibiotics and other drugs. Furthermore, underlying diseases, such as carcinoma, may also alter normal hemostasis and further complicate an already difficult diagnostic challenge. Since early recognition is essential for the successful treatment of most coagulation abnormalities associated with infection, seriously ill patients should be routinely screened for coagulation abnormalities.

Screening for Abnormal Blood Coagulation

Commonly acquired hemorrhagic disorders associated with infections include abnormalities of platelet function, thrombocytopenia, prothrombin deficiency, and disseminated intravascular coagulation (DIC). These abnormalities usually can be recognized by careful clinical observations and with relatively simple and commonly available laboratory tests.

Mucous membrane bleeding and petechiae suggest either thrombocytopenia or abnormalities of platelet function, while ecchymoses and large soft tissue hemorrhages are more commonly due to prothrombin deficiency. Since DIC leads to multifactorial deficiencies, including thrombocytopenia, patients with that complication may present with petechiae, large ecchymoses, and mucous membrane bleeding.

Though the above clinical points may be helpful, sorting out the specific deficiency (or deficiencies) which leads to bleeding is primarily a laboratory exercise. Thrombocytopenia may be suspected from initial inspection of the blood smear and confirmed by the platelet count. The presence of reduced platelets on the smear, some of which are macrothrombocytes, suggests that thrombocytopenia is due to increased peripheral destruction or consumption of platelets, and the platelet production is increased. Examination of the bone marrow will further substantiate increased platelet production if the number of megakaryocytes is normal or increased, while decreased megakaryocytes suggests failure of bone marrow and reduced platelet production.

Abnormal platelet function, which is commonly associated with uremia, liver failure, dysproteinemias, and therapy with drugs such as aspirin and antidepressants, should be suspected when there is mucous membrane bleeding associated with petechiae in the presence of a normal platelet count. Abnormal clot retraction at one hour (less than 15 percent retraction), prolongation of a well-done bleeding time, and abnormal prothrombin comsumption suggest impaired platelet function. Platelet adhesiveness to glass, aggregation with ADP or thrombin, and platelet Factor 3 assays provide more details of platelet function, but are unnecessary in the average clinical situation.

Demonstration of multiple coagulation factor deficiencies is necessary to confirm DIC; therefore, several screening tests are required. Macrothrombocytes on a thrombocytopenic blood smear with varying numbers of fragmented erythrocytes strongly suggests DIC. However, thrombocytopenia initially may not be present and fragmentation of erythrocytes often is minimal. Observation of whole blood coagulation and gross inspection of the resulting clot is essential. DIC is usually associated with a normal clotting time, but as the clot retracts to a small nubbin many of the erythrocytes fall out and the resulting contracted clot is small and soft, but does not lyse with further incubation at 37° C. This characteristic clot is often associated with reduced clottable fibrinogen (prolonged thrombin time), reduced Factors V and X (prolonged prothrombin time) and reduced Factor VIII (prolonged partial thromboplastin generation time). Early in the course of DIC all of the above tests may not be abnormal. Thus, each individual case requires careful initial and follow-up laboratory tests in conjunction with seasoned clinical judgment to diagnose this peculiar and poorly-understood syndrome.

Clinical Manifestations

Prothrombin Deficiency frequently occurs in association with infection following prolonged use of broad spectrum antibiotics which result in bowel sterilization. Similarly, antibiotics which alter intestinal absorption of fats, such as Neomycin, may lead to Vitamin K deficiency and the resultant deficiency of the Vitamin K dependent clotting factors. Cholangitis with common bile duct obstruction uniformly leads to malabsorption of Vitamin K and eventual prothrombin deficiency. Characteristically, prothrombin deficiency associated with these mechanisms promptly responds to parenteral Vitamin K therapy.

Abnormal Platelet Function. Mucous membrane and petechial bleeding associated with a normal platelet count strongly suggests abnormal platelet function. Because platelet membranes readily adsorb assorted materials and because platelet membranes are easily altered by certain drugs, abnormal platelet function of variable severity is extraordinarily common. Severe liver and renal failure are uniformly associated with abnormal platelet function because of the adsorption onto platelets of a variety of materials which accumulate in blood. However, acetylation of platelets resulting from the almost habitual use of aspirin for the relief of fever and other symptoms associated with infections is unquestionably the most common cause of abnormal platelet function though the abnormality is often of little or no clinical significance.

Thrombocytopenia and Disseminated Intravascular Coagulation. Bone marrow failure may occur as a result of toxicity from numerous drugs, especially chloramphenicol, but most thrombocytopenic bleeding associated with infection is due to increased peripheral consumption or destruction of platelets. Antiplatelet antibody may be synthesized in association with an immune reaction to drugs or microorganisms and typically occurs during convalescence (acute idiopathic thrombocytopenia of childhood). Abrupt onset of thrombocytopenic purpura without associated hemolysis, without other coagulation abnormalities and with normal numbers of bone marrow megakaryocytes, suggests immunologic thrombocytopenia.

Thrombocytopenia and the associated coagulopathy and hemorrhagic disorder, resulting from disseminated intravascular coagulation may occur during the early acute phase of any serious infection at the time of maximum tissue injury. Infected patients with DIC often present with hypotension since the tissue injury which initiates DIC may also lead to the synthesis of bradykinin, a potent vasodepressor. Infections occurring in patients with malignancies, chronic liver failure, extensive trauma, renal failure, cardiovascular surgery, and obstetrical complications frequently are associated with DIC.

Infections with gram-negative organisms (rods and cocci) account for most cases of DIC due to infections, but virtually every type of infection has been associated with this syndrome including viremia (purpura fulmanans of childhood), miliary tuberculosis, malaria, rickettsial and clostridial infections. Localized infection without bacteremia rarely is associated with DIC.

Treatment

Appropriate antibiotic treatment of the offending infection represents the most effective treatment of DIC due to infections. However, treatment of the associated hypotension with volume expanion (vasopressors are usually ineffective) and short term heparinization are important adjunctive measures. The effectiveness of therapy is best judged by following the platelet count and thrombin time (clottable fibrinogen), both of which should improve in 36 to 48 hours. Sequential improvement in quality and quantity of the well-contracted clot may be an equally reliable indication of response. Anticoagulant therapy should be continued three to four days after the infection is well-controlled and after the platelet count has returned to normal. Bacteroides infections require special mention since these organisms may produce heparinase leading to difficulties with heparin anticoagulation.

Though hypoprothrombinemia due to bowel sterilization or obstructive jaundice responds promptly to parenteral Vitamin K, one can prevent this coagulopathy by giving supplemental parenteral Vitamin K. It is suggested that patients who receive broad spectrum antibiotics for more than 14 days and those with obstructive jaundice for a similar period should receive Vitamin K therapy regardless of the prothrombin time.

Acquired thrombasthenia due to drug therapy may persist for several days after the offending drugs are discontinued. If significant hemorrhage is encountered or if surgery is planned, normal hemostasis can be achieved with platelet transfusions. However, abnormal platelet function associated with hepatic and renal failure cannot be specifically treated, and transfused fresh platelets rapidly acquire similar abnormalities rendering them ineffective in hemostasis. Platelet transfusions are of little or no value in the therapy of immunologic purpura because of rapid destruction by antibodies. However, adrenal steroids usually are dramatically effective. In all cases of immunologic purpura one should be highly suspicious of drug participation in the immuno process. Discontinuation of all nonessential drugs is of obvious importance.

SELECTED REFERENCES

Cartwright, G. E.: The anemia of chronic disorders. Sem. in Hemat., *3*:351, 1966.
Conrad, M. E.: "Persistent Haemolysis After Infectious Hepatitis" Gut, *10*:516, 1969.
Corrigan, J. J., Jr., Ray, W. L., and May, N.: Changes in the blood coagulation system associated with septicemia. N. Eng. J. Med., *279*:851, 1968.

Daykin, D.: The clinical challenge of disseminated intravascular coagulation. N. Eng. J. Med., *283*:636, 1970.

Dennis, L. H., Eichelberger, J. W., Inman, M. M., and Conrad, M. E.: Depletion of coagulation factors in drug-resistant plasmodium falciparum malaria. Blood, *29*:713, 1967.

Doan, H. M., Decker, C. L., and Baker, L. D.: Temporary survival in clostridial hemolysis with absence of circulating red cells. N. Eng. J. Med., *277*:700, 1967.

Freireich, Emil J., Miller, A., Emerson, Charles P., and Ross, Joseph F.: The effect of inflammation on the utilization of erythrocyte and transferrin bound radioiron for red cell production. Blood, *12*:972, 1957.

Giesner, B. M., Jenkins, S. R. Production of heparinase by bacteroides. J. Bact., *81*:595, 1961.

Gutinsky, A. and Van Dyke, D.: Normal response to erythropoietin or hypoxia in rats made anemic with turpentine abscess. Proc. Soc. Exp. Biol. Med., *112*:75, 1963.

Jandl, J. H., Jacob, H. S., and Daland, G. A.: Hypersplenism due to infection. N. Eng. J. Med., *264*:1063, 1961.

LoBuglio, A. F., Cotran, R. S., and Jandl, J. H.: Red cells coated with immunoglobulin G: Binding and sphering by mononuclear cells in man. Science, *158*:1582, 1967.

Martin, C. M., Jandl, J. H., and Finland, M.: Enhancement of acute bacterial infections in rats and mice by iron and their inhibition by human transferrin. J. Infect. Dis., *112*:158, 1963.

Mason, J. W., Keeberg, V., and Dolan, P.: Plasma kallikrein and Hageman factor in gram-negative bacteremia. Ann. Int. Med., *73*:545, 1970.

Masson, P. L., Heremans, J. F., and Schonne, E.: Lactoferrin, an iron-binding protein in neutrophilic leukocytes. J. Exp. Med., *130*:643, 1969.

Mengel, C. E., Wallace, A. G., and McDaniel, H. G.: Infectious mononucleosis, hemolysis and megaloblastic arrest. Arch. Int. Med., *114*:333, 1964.

McFadzean, H. J. S. and Choa, G. H. Haemolytic anaemia in typhoid fever. Brit. Med. J., *II*:360, 1953.

McKay, D. G., and Margaretten, W.: Disseminated intravascular coagulation in virus diseases. Arch. Int. Med. (Chicago), *120*:129, 1967.

Mowat, A. G., Hothersall, T. E., and Aitchison, W. R. C.: Nature of anemia in rheumatoid arthritis. Ann. Rheum. Dis., *28*:303, 1969.

Noyes, W. D.: Erythropoietin levels in the anemia of chronic disease. Clin. Res., *19*:75, 1971.

Rogers, D. E.: Sane thoughts about research in infectious disease. Clin. Res., *15*:154, 1967.

Shade, A. L. and Caroline, L.: An iron-binding experiment in human blood plasma. Science, *104*:340, 1946.

Ward, H. P., Gordon, B., and Pickett, J. C.: Serum levels of erythropoietin in rheumatoid arthritis. J. Lab. Clin. Med., *74*:93, 1969.

Ward, H. P., Kurnick, J. E. and Pisarczyk, M. J.: Serum level of erythropoietin in anemias associated with chronic infection, malignancy, and primary hematopoietic disease. J. Clin. Invest., *50*:332, 1971.

Chapter 11

FEVER

Fever is the clinical manifestation most often signalling the occurrence of an infectious disease, but occasionally may be absent, particularly when measured on only one occasion or sporadically. Determination of body temperature at regular intervals throughout 24-hour periods is necessary to detect some fevers. The pattern observed is often important diagnostically, and is useful in following the course of illness. The occurrence of fever and the febrile pattern can be altered by antipyretic drugs but at the risk of eliminating the value of fever as a diagnostic and prognostic indicator. Specific antimicrobial drug treatment also may profoundly alter the course of an infectious disease and correspondingly influence the fever pattern. Since treatment can result in abrupt or gradual termination of fever, awareness of the usual febrile course of an infectious disease after beginning antimicrobial treatment, therefore, should condition the physician's expectations and avoid confusion. It is as important today to know the usual course of treated disease, as it has always been to know the natural history of a disease (Chapt. 12).

Fever, obviously, is not a clinical manifestation exclusively seen in infectious diseases, and particularly when fever is prolonged and not associated with other significant findings may present a diagnostic dilemma. When fever persists for two weeks or more, therefore, the physician should appreciate the diagnostic possibilities and know the procedures necessary to identify the probable cause.

Fever may be the principal feature of illness, may be accompanied by other clinical manifestations or may be overshadowed by other features of illness. These other features or manifestations are often important diagnostically but also may be incidental. Fever frequently is accompanied by symptoms which occur with the physiological alterations responsible for the febrile reaction. Fever often is an "acute phase" reaction appearing as do changes in erythrocyte sedimentation rate, plasma fibrinogen, C-reactive protein and leucocytes, frequently occurring as a consequence of inflammation or tissue necrosis, irrespective of the cause.

The pathophysiology of fever now is fairly well understood. In addition, the pathogenesis of fever, particularly as it occurs in response to infection or allergic reactions, has been clarified. An appreciation of the pathophysiology and pathogensis of fever can assist in understanding the role of fever in disease.

In this Chapter, therefore, the pattern of the febrile response will be discussed, for it still represents the cardinal feature of infectious disease. The clinical manifestations often associated with fever and occasionally important diagnostically will be identified. The pathogenesis and pathophysiology of fever, as now understood, will be presented briefly. Finally, the dilemma of prolonged fever of unknown cause will be discussed, as identification of infection often provides the only basis for curative therapy.

Fever Patterns

Body temperature normally has a diurnal variation: higher in the late afternoon or early evening and lower in the early morning. Patients with febrile diseases generally have an exaggerated diurnal variation with the fever being most pronounced in the afternoon or evening. In some instances, this diurnal variation may be reversed, as in disseminated tuberculosis, or may be altered by administration of antipyretic drugs.

Depending upon the magnitude of the swing in the daily temperature, periodic return of temperature to normal and the recurrent or relapsing character of the fever, febrile patterns may be described as remittent, intermittent, sustained (continuous), or relapsing (recurrent) (Fig. 11.1 and Table 11.1). Erratic temperature elevations without some regularity and unaccompanied by corresponding tachycardia or other "acute phase" reactions also occur but often are factitious.

Intermittent fever, sometimes called hectic or septic fever, is characterized by widely varying temperature with high fever interrupted by return of temperature to normal usually during each 24-hour period. Pyogenic abscesses are most often responsible for this type of fever pattern, but the pattern also may occur in bacteremia with gram-negative bacilli as in urinary tract infection or pylephlebitis, disseminated tuberculosis and rarely malaria. Another common cause of this pattern is administration of salicylates to patients when their temperature exceeds a predetermined level, such as 104°F. Malaria caused by *Plasmodium vivax* often produces an intermittent fever with transient spikes in temperature occurring every other day, and when caused by *Plasmodium malariae* often produces temperature elevations every third day.

Remittent fever resembles intermittent fever, except that the tempera-

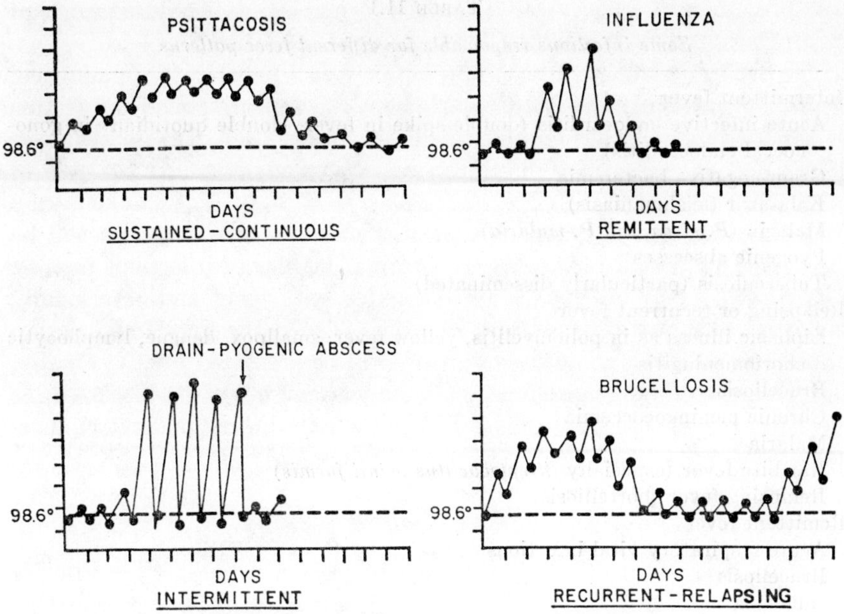

FIG. 11.1. Clinical examples of fever patterns.

ture does not become normal at any time and the swings in fever are less hectic or severe. This fever pattern is observed in patients with influenza, mycoplasma pneumonia, bacterial endocarditis, acute brucellosis, murine typhus and malaria caused by *Plasmodium falciparum*. Many non-infectious diseases produce similar fever patterns.

Sustained or continuous fever is characterized by a pattern with less marked swings in temperature than remittent fever, and usually a lower fever, but having minor diurnal variations. Pneumococcal pneumonia, group A streptococcal pharyngitis or cellulitis, typhoid and paratyphoid fever, many rickettsial infections and often meningitis produce this fever pattern in affected patients.

Relapsing or recurrent fever is characterized by several days of temperature elevation, either remittent, intermittent, or sustained, followed by several days of normal temperature, a pattern occasionally referred to as a Pel-Ebstein fever. Most often today, this febrile pattern is associated with lymphoma, but also is seen in patients with chronic meningococcemia, relapsing fever (*Spirillum minus* and *Streptobacillus moniliformis*), infective cholangitis and rarely malaria.

It is important to recognize that drug fever produced by hypersensitivity or allergy to an antimicrobial or other drug (Chapt. *29*) may result in prolongation or recurrence of fever in patients being treated for an infectious disease, may be unassociated with other allergic manifestations,

TABLE 11.1

Some infections responsible for different fever patterns

Intermittent fever
Acute infective endocarditis (double spike in fever—double quotidian—in gonococcal endocarditis)
Gram-negative bacteremia
Kala-azar (leishmaniasis)
Malaria (*P. vivax* and *P. malaria*)
Pyogenic abscesses
Tuberculosis (particularly disseminated)
Relapsing or recurrent fever
Biphasic illness as in poliomyelitis, yellow fever, smallpox, dengue, lymphocytic choriomeningitis
Brucellosis
Chronic meningococcemia
Malaria
Rat-bite fever (especially *Streptobacillus moniliformis*)
Relapsing fever (borrelliosis)
Remittent fever
Acute respiratory viral infections
Brucellosis
Influenza
Malaria (*P. falciparum*)
Tuberculosis
Typhoid fever
Sustained or continuous fever
Central nervous system infections
Brucellosis
Infective endocarditis
Pneumococcal pneumonia
Psittacosis
Rickettsial infection
Tularemia
Typhoid fever

and may complicate interpretation of the febrile course of the patient's illness.

Temperatures of 106°F or higher are rare in infectious diseases, and are more often attributable to heat stroke, hemorrhagic pancreatitis, intracerebral hemorrhage or other causes. Bacteremia caused by gram-negative bacilli, typhoid fever, malaria, disseminated tuberculosis, and meningoencephalitis may produce very high fevers, but rarely as high as 106°F. The rarity of such temperature elevations, except in unusual circumstances, militates against the use of antipyretics to prevent the hazards of hyperthermia in infection, except in the aged, very young, and those with cardiac decompensation.

Some microbial diseases are not ordinarily characterized by fever unless complicated, and these include tetanus, botulism, staphylococcal food poisoning, cholera, leprosy, most venereal diseases, some viral respiratory infections, and occasionally diphtheria. In addition, infection confined to mucous membranes or cutaneous surfaces, as in furunculosis, superficial mycotic infections, and acute or chronic bronchitis, often are unaccompanied by fever. Even infection confined to the lower urinary tract usually does not produce fever; and when fever occurs in these patients, it usually indicates pyelonephritis or extension of the infection, as in bacteremia following catheterization. Very young, very old, and debilitated persons are less likely to experience fever with any illness, than are other individuals.

Fever persisting for less than two weeks commonly is due to acute viral infections, particularly those responsible for respiratory disease, and including the myxoviruses, coronaviruses, reoviruses, adenoviruses, and picornaviruses. Many acute bacterial infections also cause fever of short duration, but may extend or produce chronic disease unless treated. The earlier antimicrobial treatment is initiated after onset of a bacterial infection, the more prompt is defervescence likely to be.

Clinical Manifestations Associated with Fever

Patients vary in the effect of fever upon their sense of well-being. Some have a vague sense of increased warmth, some experience considerable malaise and tiredness, some have headache or feel flushed, while others may feel quite normal. The severity of these symptoms associated with fever obviously is influenced by the severity of the disease, the type of infection, and the patient's sensitivity or awareness of illness (Chapt. 12).

Myalgia, arthralgia, anorexia, and impotence are also manifestations of fever in some patients, and may wax and wane with the severity of the febrile illness. Many patients with fever, particularly when caused by infection, experience a sensation of cold (*chillness*), and elect to use more clothing or prefer a higher than usual environmental temperature. This should not be confused with *chills* or *rigors* which may occur with intermittent fever, particularly associated with bacteremia, and often characterized by chattering of teeth and shaking (Table 11.2). Chills may be induced by administration of antipyretics to febrile patients; and when this happens, the symptom may erroneously suggest bacteremia or infections causing hectic or intermittent fever.

The respiratory and pulse rates are usually increased proportionally with the degree of temperature elevation. Typhoid fever and yellow fever are characteristically associated with relative bradycardia, but the heart rate also may not accelerate commensurate with fever in patients with cardiac decompensation, or may be increased excessively, for example, if the patient is anemic.

TABLE 11.2

Some infections responsible for chills

Group A streptococcal infection (cellulitis, erysipelas, puerperal sepsis)
Infective cholangitis
Infective endocarditis
Intermittent aspirin administration to febrile patients
Leptospirosis
Malaria
Osteomyelitis
Plague
Pneumococcal pneumonia
Pyelonephritis (acute)
Pyogenic abscesses (usually with bacteremia)
Rat-bite fever
Septic thrombophlebitis
Staphylococcal bacteremia
Tularemia
Typhus

Sweating usually accompanies fever, particularly during diurnal decline in temperature, and may result in dehydration, particularly in infants and children, causing considerable thirst, dryness of the mouth and other mucous membranes. If intravascular volume is decreased, and there is flushing with peripheral vasodilation or loss of vascular tone, postural hypotension may result. This can be disastrous in elderly patients by producing syncope.

Delirium or confusion frequently are the only manifestations associated with fever in elderly patients, but also may occur in others with particularly high fever who become dehydrated. Major motor seizures occur occasionally in infants or young children with high fever in the absence of central nervous system disease. Those children having convulsive seizures with fever, however, may be predisposed to development of convulsive disorders later in life.

"Fever blisters," occurring about the lips and nose and caused by *Herpesvirus hominus*, are particularly common only during certain infectious diseases, including meningococcal meningitis, pneumococcal pneumonia, salmonella infections other than typhoid fever and malaria. Fever alone cannot be responsible for activation of this herpetic infection as "fever blisters" would then be likely to occur with the same frequency in patients with all fevers, irrespective of the cause. Association of herpetic lesions with only certain infections suggests particular microbial factors may be involved. Even this seems less likely, however, when it is recognized that "fever blisters" are common in meningococcal meningitis but not in meningococcemia unassociated with meningitis.

TABLE 11.3
Causes of fever of unknown origin

	Petersdorf & Beeson*	Deal**
	1961 (%)	1971 (%)
Infections	36	35
Neoplasms	19	20
Connective-tissue diseases	15	15
Periodic fever	5	3
Others	18	7
Unknown	7	20

* Petersdorf, R. G. and Beeson, P. B.: Fever of unexplained origin: Report on 100 cases. Medicine, *40*:1–30, 1961.
** Deal, W. B.: Fever of unknown origin: an analysis of 34 patients. Postgrad. Med., *50*:182, 1971.

Prolonged Fever

Fever persisting for longer than two weeks without diagnostic findings is a perplexing problem. Infectious diseases account for about one-third of these problems, while the remainder are attributable to neoplasms, connective-tissue diseases, miscellaneous causes or remain undefined (Table 11.3). Detection in a patient of the cause of a prolonged, undiagnosed febrile illness ("fever or pyrexia of unknown origin") should be made by the use of diagnostic procedures selected rationally and in an orderly fashion.

Most patients with a prolonged, undiagnosed febrile illness have a normal total white blood cell count and urinalysis. Nevertheless, repeated observations are indicated as they may ultimately reveal evidence of a hematopoietic disorder or renal infection. Although the erythrocyte sedimentation rate (ESR) is a non-specific "acute phase reaction," as is fever, the presence of a normal ESR may indicate a factitious fever or plasma protein abnormality as in macroglobulinemia or multiple myeloma. When infection is responsible for the fever the ESR almost always will be rapid unless the patient has sickle cell disease or congestive cardiac failure.

Slight proteinuria is common with fever of any cause, but persistent moderate proteinuria may indicate infective endocarditis, perinephric abscess or chronic pyelonephritis, particularly if hematuria or pyuria also are present. Certainly, non-infectious causes also must be considered, including connective tissue disease such as lupus erythematosus, renal neoplasms, and vasculitis as seen with polyarteritis, Wegener's granulomatosis and necrotizing angiitis.

Serological tests with microbial antigens can be useful, particularly when selected to investigate a specific infectious disease. Commonly, physicians request "febrile agglutinins," not knowing what tests will be performed nor how reliable or useful they will be. Almost every investigation of large numbers of patients with prolonged undiagnosed fevers have failed to show these "febrile agglutinins" to be useful diagnostically, and most often they cause confusion rather than clarification. The infectious diseases to be most considered in these patients, for which serological tests may be useful, include leptospirosis, brucellosis, psittacosis-lymphogranuloma venereum, typhoid fever, and the systemic mycoses. If the epidemiological history suggests either of these as possible causes of the patient's illness, specific serological tests should be requested and done.

Bacteriological cultures of sputum, urine, blood, feces, and when indicated, cerebrospinal fluid should be done. If brucellosis is suspected as a cause of the patient's illness, special culture procedures will be required. If leptospirosis is considered, animal inoculations with urine or blood will be necessary. If meningococcemia is suspected, multiple blood cultures shculd be taken with special bacteriological techniques. Multiple blood cultures should be done, as bacteremia associated with meningococcemia or "hidden" abscesses may be positive only intermittently (Chapt. 9). The increasing recognition of infection by anaerobic bacteria, such as bacteroides, necessitates use of anaerobic procedures for cultures of blood, urine, pleural fluid and pus. The systemic mycoses, such as histoplasmosis, will require cultures for fungi, and bone marrow cultures may be useful in these circumstances as well as in brucellosis and disseminated tuberculosis.

Tuberculin skin testing should be done, preferably with a Tween 80 stabilized antigen. Other skin tests, such as with histoplasmin, coccidioidin or brucellergin, should not be done until after blood has been collected for serological study, as false positive serological titers may be induced by skin inoculation of the test antigens. A positive skin test to one of these antigens, however, may provide the signal for further diagnostic studies or eliminate some possibilities.

It is expected that routine chest x-ray will be performed. If a pulmonary or cardiac lesion is recognized, the necessary focus may be provided for further study. Otherwise, intravenous pyelography should be done to investigate a "silent" renal or urinary tract problem, and particularly to examine the possibility of renal tuberculosis and perinephric or psoas abscess. Barium contrast studies of the gastrointestinal tract may identify an abdominal mass indicative of abscess, neoplasia or a gastrointestinal lesion such as regional enteritis or colitis.

Studies carrying important risks, such as arteriography, lymphangiography or exploratory laporotomy should be performed only when symptoms or signs indicate their possible usefulness. Hepatic punch biopsy often is of importance when other studies are unrevealing. Caseous granulomata may indicate tuberculosis or histoplasmosis, and biopsy specimens always should be studied with microbiological stains. Non-caseating granulomata may be found in brucellosis, tularemia and Q fever, as well as in lymphoma and sarcoidosis. Hepatic and splenic radioactive scans may demonstrate hepatic abscess, splenomegaly or rarely splenic abscess.

Exploratory laporotomy as a final diagnostic maneuver should be considered, particularly if the patient has any evidence of intraabdominal disease manifested by abdominal pain, diarrhea, or hematochezia. When performed, liver biopsy, mesenteric lymph node biopsy, and complete examination of the gastrointestinal tract are required. Tissues biopsied or removed should be studied pathologically, examined and cultured for fungi and bacteria, including mycobacteria.

Therapeutic trials with antimicrobial drugs are rarely indicated in patients with prolonged undiagnosed fever unless there is some evidence directing the selection of a reasonably specific antimicrobial agent. Defervescence then is not always diagnostic but may occur coincidentally, and failure to defervesce does not exclude infection as a cause of the patient's illness. If a therapeutic trial is begun, however, it should be continued for the full course of treatment and not altered without new evidence.

Pathophysiology and Pathogenesis of Fever

Body temperature is maintained by a balance between heat production and heat loss. The thermoregulatory centers of the hypothalamus integrate heat production and dissipation by affecting metabolic activity and by influencing cutaneous circulation and sweating. Increased metabolism alone may increase body temperature very little, as indicated by the small elevations in temperature seen in hyperthyroidism and during exercise, as long as compensatory mechanisms of heat loss are intact. Excessive exercise may result in rise in temperature to a new level, and thyrotoxic crises may cause fever, but this is attributable to a diminution in compensatory heat loss as well as increased heat production.

Evaporation from the upper respiratory tract in man accounts for about 10 percent, and evaporation, radiation, and convection from the skin are responsible for the remaining 80 to 90 percent of total heat loss. Evaporation is the most effective mechanism of heat dissipation, but under normal conditions radiation is important in maintaining body temperature. Convection and radiation of heat are influenced by blood circulation through the skin. Peripheral vasoconstriction causes heat retention, and vasodilation causes heat loss. These vascular responses are controlled by local reactivity of blood vessels to environmental temperature, and by a central reflex mediated through proprioceptive nerve endings and the autonomic nervous system. Evaporation is influenced by sweating, but large amounts of moisture and heat may be vaporized by insensible perspiration. The degree of sweating, however, is determined by the autonomic nervous system, and influenced by the thermoregulatory centers of the hypothalamus.

With each degree (F) rise in body temperature above normal, there is an average increase of seven percent in metabolic activity. Therefore, irrespective of the cause of fever, metabolism is always increased. This change in metabolic rate in association with fever contributes to the increase in temperature but usually cannot be held directly responsible for it. It also contributes to the loss of weight often associated with febrile disease.

Fever, therefore, may be related to alterations in function of the thermoregulatory centers of the hypothalamus and to changes in peripheral blood vessel reactivity or circulation.

Chills or rigors are reflex phenomena attributable to cooling of the skin, either because of peripheral vasoconstriction or environmental temperature, stimulating the thermoregulatory centers to initiate muscular activity. Clinical and laboratory experimental studies reveal cooling of the skin followed by chill during malarial paroxysms. In addition, cooling the skin of normal persons to 31°C is associated with induction of a chill.

Most diseases associated with fever are characterized by tissue necrosis or inflammation, whether or not these are attributable to infection. Some microorganisms, particularly the gram-negative bacteria, however, possess a pyrogenic substance (endotoxin-lipopolysaccharide), which also may be responsible for febrile responses in certain circumstances. Many microorganisms, nevertheless, have no pyrogenic properties except as they may produce fever when responsible for an infectious disease. The fever of infection, therefore, cannot be attributable regularly to pyrogenic substances of the microorganisms.

Leucocytes and perhaps lymphoid cells, are the only cells of the body found to possess pyrogenic activity. Leucocytes elaborate a pyrogenic substance during phagocytosis, hypersensitivity reactions and upon stimulation by bacterial endotoxin. This leucocytic pyrogen appears to act directly upon the thermoregulatory centers of the hypothalamus to produce fever by decreasing heat loss and increasing heat production. This pyrogen is probably the common pathway in production of fever in diseases associated with inflammation and tissue necrosis, where leucocytic involvement usually is prominent.

Patients with agranulocytosis might be expected to experience less fever than those with normal leucocyte counts. Although diminution in febrile response can be detected in agranulocytic animals following injection of bacterial pyrogen, patients with agranulocytosis usually demonstrate what appears to be a normal febrile reaction to infection, possible because the marginal leucocyte pool and bone marrow stores are not often completely depleted.

Specific involvement of bacterial endotoxin in causing fever has been defined most precisely in acute transient bacteremia attributable to gram-negative bacilli, as may occur following urinary tract instrumentation or injection of solutions contaminated with endotoxin or bacteria. Circulating endotoxin has been transiently identified in the blood of such patients.

Summary

The pattern of fever demonstrated by recording body temperature at regular intervals provides important diagnostic and prognostic information. Although fever is an important and common but not invariable finding in infectious diseases, it also is a manifestation of other illnesses. Interpretation of the significance of fever in a patient, therefore, is best accomplished by understanding its clinical features providing diagnostic information, and appreciating the influence of therapeutic maneuvers upon its course and occurrence. The role of leucocytic pyrogen as a common pathway in the pathogenesis of fever due to infection and other causes has clinical implications and clarifies this important pathophysiologic process.

Prolonged undiagnosed fevers remain a diagnostic and therapeutic dilemma. The implication of infection as a cause of one-third of these clinical situations indicates the critical importance of searching for these diagnostic possibilities as they represent potentially treatable and curable illnesses, carrying a less ominous prognosis than might otherwise by expected.

No single chapter can identify all the important clinical or pathophysiologic aspects of fever, but the reader should recognize the reasons for detailed examination of fever patterns of patients, and become familiar with the diagnostic and prognostic features which can facilitate patient management. Treatment should never be directed solely to reduce the elevated temperature; fever alone is not a disease, and should be considered only as one important manifestation of illness.

SELECTED REFERENCES

Atkins, E.: Pathogenesis of fever. Physiol. Rev., *40*:580, 1960.

Bennett, I. L.: The significance of fever in infections. Yale J. Biol. Med., *26*:491, 1954.

Cluff, L. E. and Johnson, J. E.: Drug fever. In *Progress in Allergy*, ed. Kallos, P. and Waksman, B. H., Vol. VIII, p. 149. Karger, Basel/New York, 1964.

Deal, W. B.: Fever of unknown origin: An analysis of thirty-four patients. Postgrad. Med., *50*:182, 1971.

DuBois, E. F.: Fever and the regulation of body temperature. 1948, Charles C Thomas, Springfield, Ill.

DeBois, E. F. Why are fever temperatures over 106°F rare? Am. J. Med. Sci., *217*:361, 1949.

Kass, E. H. Is suppression of fever or hypothermia useful in experimental and clinical infectious diseases? J. Inf. Dis., *121*:81, 1970.

Petersdorf, R. G. and Bennett, J. I. L.: Factitious fever. Ann. Int. Med., *46*:1039, 1957.

Petersdorf, R. G. and Beeson, P. B.: Fever of unexplained origin: Report on 100 cases. Medicine, *40*:1, 1961.

Petersdorf, R. G. Fever of unknown origin. Ann. Int. Med., *70*:864, 1969.

Snell, E. S.: Hypersensitivity fever. Brit. J. Clin. Practice, *23*:73, 1969.

Wood, W. B., Jr. Studies on the cause of fever. N. Eng. J. Med., *258*:1023, 1958.

Chapter 12

RECOVERY FROM ACUTE INFECTION*

Infection, infectious disease, and illness are not synonymous. Infection, with few exceptions, indicates microbial replication and invasion. In some instances, infection is demonstrable only by evidence of the hosts' immunological response, as illustrated by a positive tuberculin test or positive specific serum antibody titer. At times replication may occur without microbial invasion, as in diphtheria. Infectious disease indicates the pathological or pathophysiological process resulting from infection and producing manifestations such as fever, leucocytosis, inflammation, or tissue necrosis. Not all patients with infection or an infectious disease are sick or ill. For example, tuberculosis of the lung may develop with x-ray and bacteriological findings, but the patient may feel well. Symptoms of illness associated with an infection may be clearly attributable to demonstrable disease, may be present before the disease becomes manifest, or persist after the infection has disappeared. The absence of demonstrable infection or disease, however, does not necessarily mean that symptoms of illness are unreal.

Attention will be focused upon recovery from infection (microbial replication and invasion), recovery from disease, and recovery from illness. In many instances these can be equated, but in other instances they cannot. Furthermore, the factors influencing and responsible for recovery from infection often differ from those responsible for recovery from disease and illness.

Recovery from Infection

The determinants of host resistance and susceptibility also affect recovery from infection. These include factors responsible for nonspecific and specific or acquired resistance. Diabetic acidosis, agranulocytosis, immunological deficiency, vascular insufficiency, and other diseases adversely affecting phagocytes or immune responsiveness, for example, not only predispose patients to infection by many different microorganisms, but

* "This paper was presented at the Eighth Annual Infectious Disease Symposium, Wilmington, Delaware and published in the November 1971 issue of the *Delaware Medical Journal*."

recovery occurs slowly if at all in these patients with infection unless the defect in resistance is corrected or the underlying disease is remedied. Once microbial replication begins and invasion takes place, mobilization of host resistance is essential to prevent progress and to initiate recovery from the infection.

Antimicrobial drugs certainly can terminate growth or kill microorganisms and contribute to recovery from infection. But if the microorganisms are not killed, host resistance is particularly important to prevent re-emergence of infection after discontinuing the antimicrobial drugs. Relapse after treatment of tularemia with tetracycline, relapses from bacterial endocarditis treated with "bacteriostatic" rather than bactericidal drugs, and re-emergent tuberculous infection treated for an inadequate period of time with INH or streptomycin, all are illustrative of dependency upon host resistance in recovery from infections treated with bacteriostatic drugs. Similarly, administration of tetracycline or chloramphenicol to patients incubating tularemia or Q Fever infection may prevent progression of the infection, but disease occurs when the antibiotic is discontinued.

Termination of microbial replication, therefore, is not always synonymous with cessation of infection. *Persistence of infection* without progressive microbial replication or further invasion is a problem in chronic infections such as tuberculosis, syphilis, malaria, brucellosis, histoplasmosis, and *Herpes simplex* infection, for example. These persistent infections may be the source of relapsing or advancing disease when natural resistance declines. Many of these persistent infections are associated with intracellular parasitism, and some are associated with appearance of atypical bacterial forms, protoplasts, spheroplasts, or L-forms. The mechanisms responsible for microbial persistence are not known, but these infections are becoming increasingly important in aged persons, and other patients with impaired resistance to infection. Unfortunately, some bacteria assume atypical form or become protoplasts, with defective or absent cell walls, under the influence of antimicrobial drugs, particularly penicillin, which act by interfering with cell wall synthesis. Microbial persistence is an interesting and important problem associated with the use of antibiotics. Attenuated or altered microorganisms may persist in tissues after infection, to re-emerge later as sources of progressive disease. Recovery from infection, therefore, implies eradication or elimination of the infecting microorganism and its variants and not only cessation of microbial replication.

Recovery from Disease

The pathological processes set in motion by different infections do not evolve, progress, or resolve in the same way. The pathological or pathophysiological events associated with infectious diseases do not disappear during recovery in the same way or at the same rate. For example, fever may disappear long before elimination of the microorganism or resolution of the pathological lesion. The pathological lesion may subside before the affected patient's weight returns to normal. The patient may continue to feel ill after all objective manifestations of the disease have disappeared.

Traditionally, it is considered wise to know the natural history of a disease to enable prognostication and to temper expectations during the course of disease. As the course of many infectious diseases can now be influenced by antimicrobial drug therapy, however, it is equally important to know the course of treated infection. Figure 12.1, for example, illustrates the type of defervescence ordinarily expected following administration of an effective antibiotic to patients with typhoid fever, pneumococcal pneumonia, meningococcemia and meningococcal meningitis. Rarely will patients with typhoid fever become afebrile in less than 3 to 5 days, while patients with pneumococcal pneumonia may be afebrile in less than 12 to 24 hours.

Defervescence in patients with meningococcemia is ordinarily much more rapid than in patients with meningococcal meningitis, illustrating

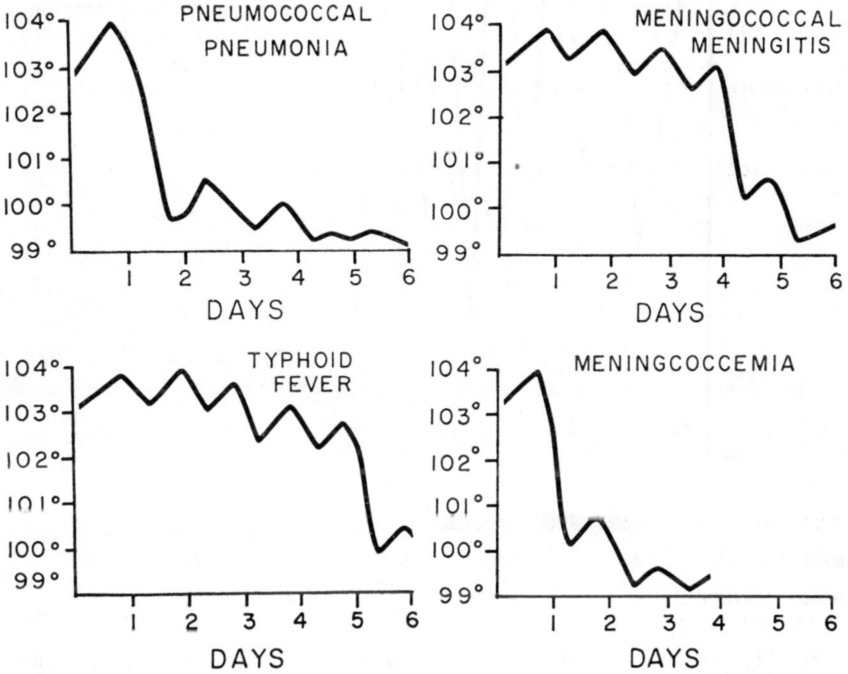

FIG. 12.1. Variable but usually expected defervescence following specific antimicrobial therapy of different infectious diseases.

that localized suppuration impedes the rapidity of response after beginning treatment. The reasons for this variability in recovery from treated infection are not well understood. At times, it is related to chronicity or intracellular parasitism characteristic of the infection. Most important, however, recovery occurs slowly if at all following initiation of antibiotic treatment if an obstructed or undrained abscess is present (Fig. 12.2). Similarly, infection involving a foreign body may persist or recur despite drug administration. Drainage of the abscess and removal of the foreign body will have more effect upon recovery than administration of antibiotics. Rarely, is the ineffectiveness of antimicrobial treatment in these cir-

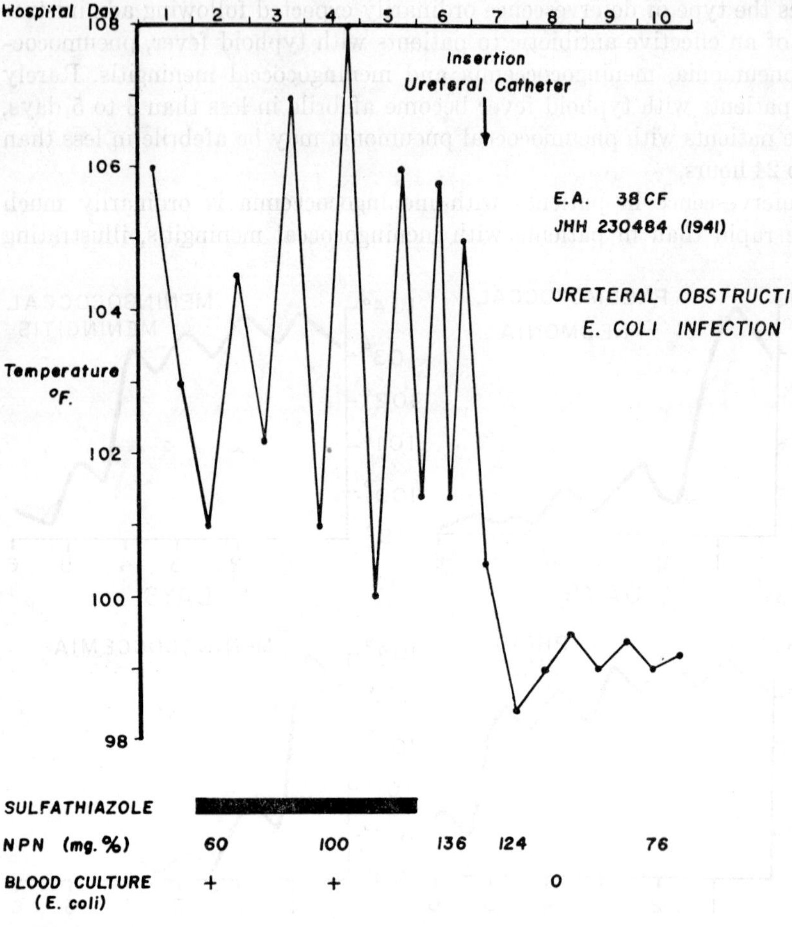

Fig. 12.2. Removal of obstruction to drainage essential to recovery from an infectious disease. Diabetic patient with *E. coli* urinary tract infection, obstructed ureter and bacteremia.

cumstances attributable to failure of drug penetration into the site of infection.

The rate of defervescence also may vary significantly in patients treated for the same type of infectious disease. Figure 12.3 illustrates the four principle patterns of defervescence in patients with pneumococcal pneumonia. Defervescence in 12 to 24 hours, 2 to 3 days or after 4 to 5 days is observed in about one-third of patients, respectively. A few patients may defervesce promptly but have recrudescence of fever after 5 to 10 days. This recrudescent fever may be caused by a pyogenic complication of the infection, such as pyoarthritis or empyema, but this rarely occurs if the complication was not present when penicillin therapy was begun. In most instances, such recurrent fever is attributable to drug fever.

The reasons for the other variable patterns of defervescence often are not apparent. The speed of defervescence, however, is related to the duration of disease before beginning antibiotic therapy. There is an almost direct relationship between the duration of disease prior to administering antibiotics and the days required for the patient to become afebrile. Awareness of this variability, conditions the physician's expectations, avoids unnecessary concern, reduces the dilemma associated with changes

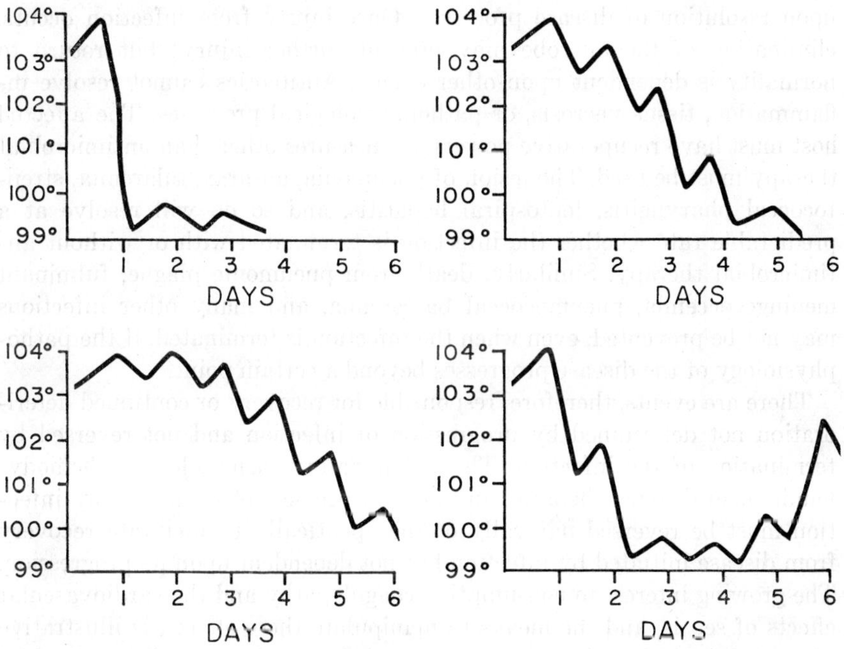

FIG. 12.3. Variability in defervescence in uncomplicated pneumococcal pneumonia treated with penicillin.

in sputum bacteriology, and eliminates unjustifiable alterations in antibiotic therapy. The patient who has had pneumonia for four days before starting penicillin follows the usual pattern of recovery if he continues to have fever on the second or third day of therapy.

Unfortunately, antibiotic administration may initiate recovery from one manifestation of an infectious disease without altering another and without eliminating the infection. For example, streptococcal pharyngitis and its suppurative complications may resolve after sulfonamide or tetracycline therapy, but the streptococcus may persist in the pharynx and rheumatic fever may supervene. On the other hand, penicillin therapy may provide no other benefit to the course of the pharyngitis or its suppurative complications, but can eradicate the streptococcus and prevent rheumatic fever.

Unfortunately, antibiotic treatment of the patient with an infectious disease may delay as well as facilitate recovery. Large doses of antibiotics may alter the normal balance between bacteria of skin and mucous membranes allowing resistant microorganisms to replicate and superinfect. In addition, antimicrobial drugs can produce adverse pharmacologic or allergic reactions. Diseases caused by these drugs frequently are responsible for delayed recovery from infectious diseases.

Antimicrobial drugs can eradicate microorganisms but have no effect upon resolution of disease processes. Once injury from infection occurs, elimination of the microbe may prevent further injury; but return to normality is dependent upon other events. Antibiotics cannot resolve inflammation, tissue necrosis, or pathophysiological processes. The affected host must have recuperative powers, or measures other than antimicrobial therapy must be used. The lesion of pneumonia, anthrax, tularemia, streptococcal pharyngitis, leptospiral hepatitis, and so on will resolve at a predictable rate whether the infection is terminated with or without antimicrobial therapy. Similarly, death from pneumonic plague, fulminant meningococcemia, pneumococcal bacteremia, and many other infections may not be prevented, even when the infection is terminated, if the pathophysiology of the disease progresses beyond a certain point.

There are events, therefore, responsible for recovery or continued deterioration not determined by progression of infection and not reversed by termination of the infection. The inflammatory, hematological, hemodynamic, neural, renal, hepatic, and other processes set in motion by infection must be reversed naturally or therapeutically to facilitate recovery from disease initiated by infection but not dependent upon its progression. The growing interest in consumptive coagulopathy and the cardiovascular effects of sepsis, and the means to manipulate these effects, is illustrative of our appreciation that the disease of infection is more than microbial replication and invasion.

Recovery from Illness

Premonitions of being sick, variability in severity of illness, and differing speeds of returning to normal health occur in patients with an infectious disease. Often this is related to the intensity of infection, the severity of the disease and rate of resolution of the pathological process. Certainly, the patient developing cirrhosis of the liver as a result of hepatitis often will continue to feel ill, and patients developing influenzal pneumonia might remain ill longer than patients who have uncomplicated influenza. Even with these differences, however, there is great variation in the speed of convalescence from illness among patients with disease of similar severity.

Patients with uncomplicated influenza may return to a feeling of good health within seven days, but some may continue to feel ill for three weeks or more. Brucellosis often has been held responsible for chronic ill health after recovery from the acute disease. Patients recovering from infectious mononucleosis and malaria have had lingering disability after manifestations of disease have subsided. All infections and many other diseases probably are associated with delayed recovery to normal health in some patients.

Prior to the influenza pandemic of 1957, we began to examine the reasons for delayed recovery from illness associated with this disease. Approximately 600 employed, active individuals under continuing care in one clinic were evaluated clinically and psychologically several weeks before appearance of influenza. The Asian strain of influenza virus responsible for this pandemic had not previously affected the population, and negative specific serological titers to the viral antigen were found uniformly. Vaccine available prior to the appearance of the influenza outbreak was generally of little value and had no effect upon rates of influenzal infection. About 26 of the individuals came to the clinic during the outbreak with disease typical of influenza and from whom virus was isolated or at least a four-fold rise in specific serum antibody titer was observed.

These individuals were followed to evaluate their disease and symptoms of illness. About one-half of the patients were free of symptoms within seven days, while most of the other half still felt ill at three weeks. There was a distinct grouping of the patients and only two individuals had illness persisting for an intermediate period of time. The ages of the two groups were similar; no underlying or associated diseases differentiated them; the height and duration of fever in the two groups were the same; disease complications (pneumonitis and otitis media) occurred rarely and with the same frequency in patients of each group; the immune response as measured by elevation in serum antibody titer was the same in each group. There were, in essence, no clinical or laboratory changes which explained the delay or speed of recovery in the individuals.

The psychological data from each person in the study prior to the influenza outbreak was obtained by the Minnesota Multiphasic Personality Inventory, the Cornell Medical Index, and a social questionnaire. This data was analyzed and interpreted before the outbreak of influenza and independent of the clinical study. Characterization of the patients identified as having influenza, using the data collected before the pandemic, revealed that almost all patients recovering slowly from their illness had a "depressive propensity." With a high degree of accuracy, it would have been possible to predict before the outbreak which persons would have lingering illness following the infection.

The major persisting symptoms in patients recovering slowly from influenza were tiredness, weakness, insomnia, headache, anorexia, and feeling "blue." Myalgia, arthralgia, malaise, and anorexia were common symptoms during the acute disease. The protracted illness merged imperceptibly with the symptoms of the acute illness.

It might be concluded that the delay in recovery from illness was attributable to the "depression propensity" and that the symptoms were interpreted by the patient as related to the influenza. Certainly, the "depression-proneness" was identified before the acute infection, and the persistent symptoms were those usually associated with depression. On the other hand, the persisting symptoms could be attributable to subtle manifestations of disease undetected by the evaluation methods.

Influenzal illness was reported by 12 percent of all patients identified as being "depression-prone," but only by 3 percent of all other individuals. This suggested the possibility that the former group might be more susceptible to influenzal infection.

Serological examinations obtained before and after the epidemic in the "depression-prone" and other individuals, however, revealed an infection rate in the "depression-prone" group of about 40 percent, and about 34 percent in all others. The difference between these rates of infection was not statistically significant, indicating that susceptibility to infection was not different in the two groups. These observations suggested that the disease in "depression-prone" persons might be more severe when infection occurs, but the clinical observations of the two groups of patients presenting with influenzal illness did not show any differences in severity of their disease. The possibility developed that the "depression-prone" individuals were more likely than others to report sickness when infected, indicating a heightened awareness of disease.

Several additional observations have further suggested the heightened awareness by "depression-prone" individuals of the presence of disease. The questionnaires completed before the epidemic showed an increased awareness by these persons of disease in distant family members; previous visits to the clinic for common problems (diarrhea, constipation, common cold, etc.) were more common; and previous complaints about reactions to vaccination were more frequent. A subsequent prospective study of reactions to vaccination in the two groups confirmed their increased reporting or awareness of adverse vaccine reactions but no measurable differences in the objective manifestations of vaccine reactions in the "depression-prone" persons contrasted with other individuals.

The sum and substance of these studies, therefore, support the conclusion that persons identified as "depression-prone" have no increased susceptibility to infection, no increased severity of infectious disease, delayed recovery from symptoms of illness, and a heightened awareness of disease in themselves and others. This increased awareness might be equated to an enhanced reactivity to disease. It probably is not appropriate to imply that this is entirely caused by psychological determinants. It seems equally possible that the so called "depression-proneness" is only another manifestation of enhanced physiological responsiveness. Conceivably, future studies will reveal a biological difference between these groups of individuals manifested by varied physiological reactivity of a different responsiveness to stimuli. Perhaps, the difference between these groups of persons may be reflected in variable effects of pharmacologically active drugs.

Weakness and tiredness are the most common persistent symptoms in persons recovering slowly from influenza. Myalgia and weakness are major manifestations of the acute disease. Possibly, the persistent symptoms are the expression of gradually resolving neuromuscular disease common in all patients with influenza, but appreciated only by those with an increased awareness of the presence of disease. Other studies are required to clarify these and other questions.

Summary

Infection is defined as microbial replication and invasion of a host. Infectious disease is defined as the pathological and pathophysiological processes caused by infection. Illness is defined as the symptoms appreciated by the infected individual. Infection can occur without detectable disease and disease may persist or resolve long after infection has been eliminated. At times infection may persist without progression of disease, and there are instances where persistence of infection may lead to delayed consequences, either by emergent infectious diseases or by late non-infectious sequelae. Treatment of infection is important in control of infectious disease, but once the pathological or physiological processes set in motion by infection develop, elimination of the microorganism may not be accompanied by enhanced recovery.

There is considerable variability in recovery of patients following antimicrobial drug treatment of an infection. Awareness of this variability between infectious diseases is essential to avoid confusion in interpreting microbiological, serological, and clinical findings, and to prevent unneces sary changes in antimicrobial drug therapy.

Patients vary in their speed of recovery from an infectious disease. Often this is related to complications or severity of the process. Often, however, persistent symptoms of ill health are not explainable in this way. There is a relationship between awareness and reporting of disease by individuals, "depression-proneness," and speed of recovery from illness. Conceivably, this could be related to variable reactivity to different endogenous and exogenous stimuli.

SELECTED REFERENCES

Overholt, E. L., *et al.*: An analysis of 42 cases of laboratory acquired tularemia. Treatment with broad spectrum antibiotics. Am. J. Med., *30:*785, 1961.

McCrumb, R. F., Jr., Snyder, M. J., and Woodward, T. E.: Studies on human infection with pasteurella tularensis: Comparison of streptomycin and chloramphenicol in the prophylaxis of clinical disease. J. A. Am. Physicians, *70:*74, 1957.

Tigertt, W. D. and Benenson, A. S.: Studies on Q fever in man. J. A. Am. Physicians, *69:*98, 1956.

McDermott, W.: Microbial persistence. Yale J. Biol. Med., *30:*257, 1959.

Sanders, E. and Cluff, L. E.: Antimicrobial drugs: Mechanisms of action and factors influencing their action in antimicrobial therapy. ed. Kagan, B. M., 1970, W. B. Sanders Co., Philadelphia.

Cluff, L. E. and Johnson, J. E., III: Drug fever. Prog. in Allergy, *VIII:*149, 1964.

Imboden, J. B., Canter, A., and Cluff, L. E.: Convalescence from influenza. Arch. Int. Med., *108:*393, 1961.

Cluff, L. E., *et al.*: Brucellosis II: Medical aspects of delayed convalescence. Arch. Int. Med., *103:*398, 1959.

Tumulty, P. A., Nichols, E., Singlwald, M., and Lidz, T.: An investigation of the effects of recurrent malaria. Medicine, *25:*17, 1946.

Greenfield, N., Roessler, R., and Crosby, A. J.: Ego strength and length of recovery from infectious mononucleosis. J. Nerv. Ment. Dis., *128:*125, 1959.

Imboden, J. B., Canter, A., and Cluff, L. E.: Symptomatic recovery from medical disorders. J.A.M.A., *178:*1182, 1961.

Cluff, L. E., Canter, A., and Imboden, J. B.: Asian influenza infection, disease and psychological factors. Arch. Int. Med., *117:*159, 1966.

Imboden, J. B., Canter, A., and Cluff, L. E.: Separation experiences and health records in a group of normal adults. Psychosom. Med., *25:*433, 1963.

Canter, A., Imboden, J. B., and Cluff, L. E.: The frequency of physical illness as a function of prior psychological vuluneraibility and contemporary stress. Psychosom. Med., *28:*344, 1966.

SECTION
THREE

SPECIFIC INFECTIOUS DISEASES

Chapter 13

INTRODUCTION

Infectious diseases usually are distinguishable from each other clinically as well as microbiologically. Isolation and identification of a pathogen is most definitive, but the clinical manifestations of many infectious diseases, if properly identified and analyzed, also enable a reasonably precise diagnosis before microbiological evidence becomes available. Initiation of the appropriate treatment usually is necessary before definitive microbiological data are obtained, and arriving at a reasonably certain clinical impression is required if treatment is to be rational. Knowing the manifestations which are characteristic of different infections, therefore, is essential. Dependence upon randomly chosen laboratory procedures such as "febrile agglutinins" or "routine" cultures are as often useless as they may be misleading. Selection of those procedures most likely to assist in differentiation or identification of particular infections also is dependent upon a carefully derived clinical impression.

Patients suspected of having an infectious disease do not present with a label indicating they have tuberculosis, klebsiella lung abscess or coccidioidomycosis. It is the physician's responsibility and burden to identify the probable possibilities and to initiate those studies most likely to reveal the precise microbiological cause of the patient's illness.

Infectious diseases are most often discussed by considering the few or many clinical syndromes attributed to specific microorganisms. Although this is the simplest method of covering the subject, this is not the method the physician must employ in defining a patient's disease. Patients present with fever or no fever, chills or no chills, chronic or acute illness, regional or systemic manifestations. The first step for the physician is to determine if the patient does or does not have an infection. If infection seems possible, he must then identify the particular features of the illness in each patient which can assist in deciding what type of infection may be present, e.g., is it pyogenic, acute or chronic, epidemic or sporadic, related to environmental exposure or animal contact, or involve a particular organ or system. If the patient's disease dominantly affects lung, kidney, central nervous system, or other organs, for example, certain microbial causes become more important than others.

Although the host's reactions to infection are not infinite, each infecting microorganism often produces characteristic manifestations. The features of disease may be extraordinarily diverse or uniform, depending upon the infecting microorganism. Tuberculosis, for example, has protean manifestations, may affect virtually every organ or system, and can mimic many other diseases. Nevertheless, tuberculosis affecting one organ produces features often differentiating it from other infections of the same organ. In contrast, influenza predominantly affects the respiratory tract, and the clinical syndrome produced, although varying, is much more uniform than respiratory infection caused by the staphylococcus, streptococcus or tubercle bacillus. Awareness of the variety of clinical syndromes produced by some microorganisms, and the uniformity of syndromes produced by others, therefore, assists in recognizing or excluding them in particular patients.

Localization of the manifestations of disease to a particular region facilitates recognition and interpretation of the infectious process. At times, however, localized infections may not produce similarly localized manifestations of disease, and expression of the infection may be at a distant site or characterized only by non-specific manifestations such as fever, generalized myalgia, tiredness, weakness, weight loss, fatiguability, anemia and impotence. Manifestations distant to the primary site of infection, however, often are characteristic of particular infections, e.g., the rash of scarlet fever associated with group A streptococcal infection of the throat, or the embolic features of infective endocarditis. When only non-specific manifestations of illness are present, however, certain features such as chill may suggest a hidden pyogenic infection or abscess, and chronicity will exclude the acute viral infections and be more indicative of a chronic infection such as tuberculosis, histoplasmosis, or infective endocarditis. This form of differentiation requires a knowledge of infectious diseases but, most importantly, necessitates a rational, logical approach and ability to examine all possibilities.

The chapters included in this section are not meant to be comprehensive. Rather, they have been selected for one or more reasons. *First,* they represent specific microbial infections illustrating differing syndromes or features of (1) an acute pyogenic infection, (2) a chronic graunlomatous, occasionally necrotizing and often intracellular infection, (3) an acute infection with a predominant organ involved, and (4) an acute infection producing late non-infectious sequelae. *Second,* they represent a variety of differing infections affecting a single organ or system. *Third,* they represent localized infection producing predominantly distant manifestations of disease. From this selection, hopefully, the reader will appreciate the ways in which infectious diseases occur and will gain an approach to an organizational perspective. *Fourth,* the diseases covered represent exceedingly important hospital infections or are major epidemiological problems.

Chapter 14

PNEUMONIA

Pneumonia represents inflammation of the lung parenchyma produced by microbial infection. Localized symptoms including cough, pleuritic pain, and sometimes dyspnea are usually prominent, and physical findings of pulmonary consolidation are detectable. Systemic manifestations characteristically include fever, chills, prostration, and at times cyanosis or jaundice. Considerable variability in symptoms is noted, however, depending upon the etiologic agent as well as the age and clinical status of the patient. Viral pneumonias, for example, often produce few if any physical findings, and confirmation of pulmonary involvement depends upon chest x-ray.

The diagnosis of pneumonia must be considered in any patient presenting with fever and a pulmonary infiltrate. Although such findings are highly suggestive of pneumonia, non-infectious processes may also produce these changes. For example, pulmonary infarction, various granulomatous diseases, atelectasis secondary to bronchial obstruction, and inhalation of toxic or irritating substances, all may lead to pulmonary infiltration or consolidation in association with fever.

Variability of Clinical Findings with Etiologic Agent

The most common cause of bacterial pneumonia in essentially healthy persons is the pneumococcus (*Diplococcus pneumoniae*), a microorganism frequently found in the upper respiratory tracts of normal individuals. Other bacterial organisms which less commonly cause pneumonia are *Staphylococcus aureus,* Group A beta-hemolytic streptococcus, *Klebsiella pneumoniae* (Friedlander's bacillus) and *Hemophilus influenzae.* Other gram-negative organisms including *Escherichia coli, Pseudomonas aeruginosa* and Proteus species are increasingly being implicated. The clinical syndromes produced by infection with these organisms may be quite similar, the definitive diagnosis depending upon isolation and identification of the organism from the sputum. Nevertheless, certain features are characteristic of particular infections and may strongly suggest the etiologic agent. Thus, pneumococcal pneumonia typically is explosive in onset, heralded by a single shaking chill, and (depending on the time of institution of appropriate therapy) associated with massive lung involvement, a short course, abrupt termination and relatively rapid resolution of the infiltrative process.

Staphylococcal pneumonia most often occurs in individuals with significant impairment of resistance to infection: following influenza, and in debilitated states. In contrast to the single shaking chill and sustained fever typical of pneumococcal pneumonia, staphylococcal pneumonia is usually associated with multiple chills and often a hectic fever. Staphylococcal pneumonia is a necrotizing process and often leads to abscess formation. Particularly, pneumatocoeles and pyopneumothorax may develop in children.

Pneumonia due to the hemolytic streptococcus (now rare) may also follow influenza and be associated with hectic fever and multiple chills. It is almost never seen, however, as a sequel to scarlet fever or streptococcal pharyngitis. Rapid accumulation of relatively thin serous or serosanguinous, non-clotting pleural fluid is characteristic. The nature of the pleural fluid is related to the elaboration of streptococcal enzymes which lyse fibrin and leukocytes.

Klebsiella (Friedlander's) pneumonia is a necrotizing process in which abscesses tend to occur and in which the sputum tends to be quite viscid, mucoid or "stringy" and often grossly bloody. Alcoholics and patients with uncontrolled diabetes are especially susceptible.

Recently other gram-negative baccilli have been increasingly recognized as important causes of pneumonia. The organisms responsible include *Escherichia coli*, pseudomonas species, proteus, bacteroides, and *Serratia marcescens*. Pneumonia produced by these organisms almost always occurs in patients with serious underlying diseases including chronic lung disease, renal disease, and diabetic ketoacidosis, and in patients whose resistance has been further impaired by treatment with corticosteroids, or immunosuppressive agents. Inhalation therapy may play a significant role in transmission of these organisms.

Pneumonia due to *Hemophilus influenzae* is much more common in children under the age of two years, since older children and adults usually possess significant immunity to this organism. Very rarely in adults a syndrome indistinguishable from pneumococcal pneumonia may be due to *H. influenzae*.

Clinically mycoplasmal, viral and rickettsial infections usually develop more insidiously than the common bacterial pneumonias. Symptoms may be less severe, the temperature lower, and leucocytosis slight or absent. A hacking cough is characteristic of mycoplasmal and some viral pneumonias, and sputum production is usually minimal or absent. Specific etiologic causes of this "atypical pneumonia syndrome," formerly grouped in a single catch-all category, are now being identified.

An important determinant of the occurrence of a particular type of pneumonia is the setting in which it occurs. In the case of the indigenous bacteria, age, senility, alcoholism, preceding influenza or other viral infections and carriage rate are significant factors. Infections with these organisms, including the pneumococcus, occur sporadically. In pneumonias due to organisms with primary virulence such as tularemia, plague or anthrax, an exposure history is a significant clue; and they tend to occur in clusters and at particular times of the year or in particular geographic areas.

Pathogenesis

Pneumococcal pneumonia is the classic prototype from which our knowledge of the pathogenesis of pneumonia has evolved. Pneumococci may be carried in the upper respiratory tracts of normal individuals, involving from about 5 percent up to as high as 60 percent of the population depending upon the season and particular community. Insight into the epidemiology of the pneumococcal carrier state has been gained by utilizing serological typing of the more than 82 specific serotypes now known.

Identification of serotype depends upon the unique capsular polysaccharide produced by each of these potentially virulent types. It is the capsule which is responsible for virulence since the polysaccharide is anti-phagocytic and resists engulfment by leukocytes. Accordingly, type-specific antibodies, which usually appear between the 5th and 10th day of infection, opsonize (or "coat") the capsule and facilitate phagocytosis by neutrophiles and the mononuclear phagocytic system. Fixation of complement during the antibody-antigen reaction leads to the generation of activated complement components which in turn further contribute to the effectiveness of phagocytosis.

Fortunately, phagocytosis may proceed, although less efficiently, in non-immune individuals with the help of normally present polyspecific heat-labile opsonins and through the mechanism of "surface phagocytosis" by which leukocytes entrap encapsulated bacteria against cell surfaces and in fibrin clots.

By means of serotyping it has been shown that about 75 percent of adult cases of pneumonia are due to 9 pneumococcal serotypes (1, 3, 4, 5, 7, 8, 12, 14 and 19). In childhood pneumonia, types 1, 6, 14 and 19 predominate. The higher-numbered types which rarely produce disease account for much of the carriage by normal individuals while the more virulent lower-numbered types are not often associated with high carriage rates. Exceptions may occur in closed communities such as hospitals or custodial institutions.

Sporadic occurrences of pneumococcal pneumonia are related to conditions under which carriage of the few pathogenic types increases: crowding of people into confined spaces, and the season of the year. Viral respiratory infections, most common in winter and early spring, facilitate aspiration of infected secretions as do other factors which similarly interfere with pulmonary clearance mechanisms such as alcoholic intoxication and anesthesia. Normal carriers actually are more important in the transmission of highly virulent pneumococcal types than are patients with pneumonia.

Following lodgment of pneumococci in pulmonary alveoli, there is an outpouring of edema fluid which may facilitate intralobar spread of organisms to other alveoli (via the pores of Cohn). Polymorphonuclear leukocytic accumulation ensues, leading to consolidation of the lobe or segment. In the outer zone of the actively spreading lesion, edema and hemorrhage are prominent, leading to characterization of these areas as "red hepatization." To the older central parts of the lesion the term "grey hepatization" is applied. Spread *between* lobes may occur via the bronchi under the influence of respiration, coughing, and gravity. In addition to typical lobar" consolidation, the pneumococcus may also produce a more diffuse patchy distribution of lesions termed "bronchopneumonia."

An interesting and important feature of pneumococcal pneumonia is its tendency to undergo complete resolution without residual damage to lung parenchyma. In contrast, organisms such as staphylococci and klebsiellae produce necrosis of alveolar septal walls with significant parenchymal tissue destruction leading to cavitation, abscess formation and fibrosis. (The type III pneumococcus, which has a particularly thick capsule, may also occasionally produce abscess formation.)

The mechanism by which the pneumococcus actually produces inflammation remains poorly understood. Although the organisms elaborate a spreading factor and an hemolysin (pneumolysin), the capsule, which through its anti-phagocytic properties determines virulence, is itself nontoxic. In fact, no pneumococcal tissue-damaging toxin has been identified. By contrast staphylococci elaborate several toxins capable of producing tissue damage. Toxic factors which produce tissue necrosis have also been identified for other organisms including pseudomonas.

Along with the pneumococcus, other common bacteria such as staphylococci, streptococci and *Hemophilus influenzae* also may be found in the upper respiratory tracts of normal persons. Respiratory carriage of gram-negative bacilli is particularly likely to occur in hospitalized patients. As with the pneumococcus, infection with the other common bacteria is facilitated by aspiration of bacteria-laden secretions and is particularly likely to occur when local or systemic defense mechanisms are significantly impaired.

Additional predisposing conditions include chronic bronchopulmonary disease, cerebrovascular accidents, and convulsive disorders. Pneumonia may also develop by the direct extension of infection from adjacent sites, as from a subdiaphragmatic abscess or through the blood stream from a distant focus of infection.

In contrast to the indigenous bacteria which produce infection primarily when resistance is lowered, other bacteria appear to possess primary virulence for man and produce infection whenever a sufficient dose of organisms reaches the lung. This occurs principally by inhalation of microbial aerosols. Such is the case with *F. tularensis*, *B. anthracis*, *Pasteurella pestis* ("pneumonic" plague), and *M. tuberculosis*. Other microorganisms producing disease principally through inhalation include *Mycoplasma pneumoniae* (a major cause of "primary atypical" pneumonia), rickettsiae (Q fever), bedsoniae (psittacosis), viruses (adenovirus and others) as well as fungi (coccidioidomycosis and histoplasmosis). An epidemiologic history of exposure to an infected person or environment is therefore of considerable importance in establishing the correct diagnosis in these disorders.

Clinical Presentation

Modes of Presentation

The patient with pneumococcal pneumonia typically has noted symptoms of an upper respiratory infection for several days when he abruptly develops a single shaking chill followed by a rapid rise in temperature to 103 to 105°, pleuritic chest pain and cough productive of a "rusty" (muco-purulent, slightly blood tinged) sputum. Tachypnea, slight cyanosis and increasing chest pain are common, and the patient appears acutely ill. Pleuritic pain is often the predominant complaint and myalgia and headache are relatively less prominant or severe. Physical examination reveals restricted chest movement on the involved side, crackling inspiratory rales and variable evidence of consolidation. A pleural friction rub is sometimes noted. Particularly in early pneumonia the symptoms may be prominent at a time when x-ray findings are minimal. The following day after rehydration of the patient, typical radiological consolidation may be evident. Suppression of breath sounds and decreased sputum production may be noted in patients with mucous plugging of the bronchi.

The classical presentation is unmistakable, but it is important to realize that many patients do not present in this way. Especially in elderly, alcoholic or debilitated patients, symptoms may be much less dramatic or completely overshadowed by systemic symptoms of prostration, extra-pulmonary signs or mental disturbance. Elderly patients, for example, may be afebrile, but show severe prostration, confusion, or even evidence of psychosis. Patients with underlying heart disease may present with congestive failure and pulmonary edema as the major manifestations. At times, patients with evidence of infection elsewhere in the body—such as pyarthrosis, hypopyon, meningitis and endocarditis—are found to have underlying pneumonia as the source of metastatic infection.

Pneumonia in an alcoholic patient is usually accompanied by marked prostration and often delirium. Involvement of upper lobes and upper segments of lower lobes occurs as a result of the aspiration of secretions by the supine patient in a comatose or semi-conscious state. In addition to the pneumococcus, Klebsiella is a relatively frequent cause of serious and life-threatening pneumonia in alcoholics. Infection in such patients tends to be overwhelming and is often associated initially with a diminished host response as indicated by a normal or low white blood count and little or no fever.

Epileptic patients similarly are susceptible to aspiration of bacteria-laden secretions or carious teeth during seizures, and fever in the post-ictal state is often overlooked or ascribed to the convulsive episode.

In patients with chronic bronchopulmonary disease, such as chronic bronchitis or bronchiectasis, who frequently have cough and bouts of purulent sputum production, recognition of early pneumonia may be difficult. Symptoms may not be strikingly different from the patient's usual complaints. In patients with chronic bronchitis on tetracycline or other broad-spectrum antibiotic prophylaxis, the development of pneumonia must suggest the possibility of a drug-resistant etiologic agent such as the staphylococcus. Fortunately, such superinfection has been uncommon in patients on the usual prophylactic doses of broad spectrum antibiotics.

An important group of patients are those whose pneumonia develops distal to an area of bronchial narrowing or obstruction. Recognition of such patients is important since possible causes of such obstruction include neoplasm, tuberculosis or a foreign body, all of which have important therapeutic implications. Bronchostenosis should be suspected in patients with recurrent episodes of pneumonia, especially when in the same area, and in patients with slow resolution of pneumonia. Early bronchoscopy may be helpful both diagnostically and therapeutically by facilitating drainage. After the acute phase, bronchographic studies may be useful. Cytopathologic studies of bronchial secretions are also indicated although sometimes difficult to interpret in the presence of acute infection.

Generalized Manifestations

Fever

Fever is an almost constant feature of pneumonia, and its onset usually parallels the appearance of clinical symptoms. Fever in pneumococcal and staphylococcal pneumonia appears suddenly and rapidly reaches levels of 103 to 106°. Usually it is sustained or mildly remittent, although occasionally in staphylococcal and Klebsiella pneumonia, there may be wide swings in temperature resulting in a hectic fever pattern. The rapidity of rise and degree of elevation tends to be less in the pneumonias of slow onset. In general, however, the febrile pattern alone is not particularly helpful in identifying the cause of the infection.

Characteristically, marked prostration accompanies the fever. In tuberculosis, however, the patient may feel surprisingly well despite high fever. Response of fever to therapy may be quite dramatic, as in the case of pneumococcal pneumonia treated soon after onset, in which temperature often returns to normal within a few hours after institution of penicillin treatment. The rapidity of defervescence in fact directly correlates with the time which elapses before treatment is started. The patient with tuberculous pneumonia, however, may remain febrile for a week or longer after starting treatment. Persistence of fever despite adequate antibiotic therapy may be due to bronchial obstruction with inadequate expectoration of purulent material from the bronchial tree. In such cases, institution of adequate drainage usually results in dramatic cessation of fever. Recurrence of fever during the course of treatment of pneumonia may signify a complication such as empyema or dissemination of the infection with resultant endocarditis, meningitis, or other pyogenic lesions. In pneumococcal pneumonia treated with penicillin, however, recurrence of fever after the first few days is now more likely to represent drug fever, a manifestation of hypersensitivity to penicillin.

Pulse

In most common pneumonias, pulse rate is elevated in parallel with the fever. However, in tularemia, psittacosis, and mycoplasmal pneumonia relative bradycardia is often found. Peripheral vascular collapse which may complicate pulmonary infection, particularly during bacteremia, may result in a rapid thready pulse becoming faint as the blood pressure falls.

Chills

Pneumococcal pneumonia characteristically begins with a single vigorous shaking chill or rigor at the onset. This may be followed be emesis. A series of chills occurring late in the course of the infection is distinctly unusual, but may indicate dissemination of infection. Multiple chills with associated hectic fever are more typical of acute staphylococcal pneumonia. Chills are less common in tularemia and tuberculosis, and distinctly uncommon in non-bacterial pneumonias. A most important cause of chills is the haphazard administration of antipyretics to febrile patients, resulting in wide swings in temperature with accompanying rigors. Such treatment usually *increases* the patient's discomfort. If antipyretics are administered they should be given in small frequent doses on a regular schedule.

Skin and Mucous Membrane Findings

Mild *jaundice* is common in pneumococcal pneumonia as a result primarily of suppression of hepatic function. Severe bilirubinemia, however, is a poor prognostic sign and indicates overwhelming infection or severe liver disease. Mild elevation of serum bilirubin is also commonly seen with pulmonary infarction, and may confuse the diagnosis. *Herpes simplex* (fever blisters), particularly on the lips and in the mouth, are common in pneumococcal pneumonia but unusual in viral pneumonias and tuberculosis. *Erythema nodosum* is particularly frequent in coccidioidomycosis, and somewhat less commonly seen in histoplasmosis and tuberculosis. *Petechial lesions* occur with rickettsial infections, with the exception of Q fever. The cutaneous lesions of varicella when associated with a pulmonary infiltrate suggest varicella pneumonia, which may be quite severe, particularly during pregnancy. Cyanosis indicates severe or diffuse pulmonary involvement or associated disorders such as congestive heart failure.

Systemic Complications

Ileus or gastric dilatation may occur in the severely ill patient, and peripheral vascular collapse or shock may ensue in the course of the infection. Congestive heart failure may supervene when there is underlying cardiac disease. Such complications require immediate management. Confusion, delirium, or toxic psychosis may be observed in pneumonia. Alcoholics may develop delirium tremens and are often severely dehydrated.

Pneumonia during epidemics of influenza is often severe and may represent either primary influenzal pneumonitis characterized by cyanosis, tachypnea, and diffuse bilateral patchy infiltrates, or superimposed staphylococcal or other bacterial pneumonia which is more likely to be lobar in distribution. Primary influenzal pneumonia is particularly likely to occur in elderly patients with underlying cardiac or pulmonary disease.

Local Manifestations

Cough

Cough, though not invariably present, is a very common manifestation of pulmonary infection. In pneumococcal pneumonia, it is more likely to appear after the onset of the chills. In contrast to the bacterial pneumonias, in which cough is usually productive of purulent sputum, with or without blood, cough in viral pneumonias is more often nonproductive and "brassy." Purulent sputum, however, may be noted in the later stages of viral pneumonia.

Sputum

Sputum in pneumococcal pneumonia frequently has a "rusty" appearance, indicating a serosanguinous exudation into the area of infection at the alveolar level so that the blood is fairly evenly distributed throughout the sputum specimen. In staphylococcal pneumonia, which is usually productive of a bright yellow purulent sputum, there occasionally may be blood streaking as well. The sputum in Klebsiella pneumonia is characteristically extremely thick, stringy, viscid and often quite bloody. In tuberculosis, the sputum often has a salty taste to the patient.

Chest Pain

In pneumococcal pneumonia the patient usually experiences a severe stabbing pain in the chest appearing with the onset of the chill and fever. The pain is accentuated by deep respiration, and the patient may obtain relief by lying on the affected side. The pattern of breathing tends to be rapid and shallow since shorter chest excursion results in less pain. Viral pneumonias are less likely to have a pleuritic component, but it should be noted that pleuritic-type pain is common in infections due to Coxsackie virus (pleurodynia). Involvement of lung parenchyma is uncommon in this infection. Other conditions with pleuritic pain which must be differentiated from pneumonia are pulmonary infarction, acute costochondritis and rib fracture. In the latter two instances localized tenderness is present.

Character of Respiration

Dyspnea, tachypnea, and cyanosis may accompany the diffuse pneumonitis of influenza or varicella, or multilobe involvement in pneumococcal pneumonia.

Physical Findings in the Chest

Typically, lobar pulmonary consolidation can be detected by physical examination, which reveals an area of percussion dullness, tubular breath sounds and fine crackling rales. Physical findings of consolidation, however, are not always demonstrable even though pneumonia is found on chest x-ray. In addition to classic lobar involvement, pneumococcal pneumonia may also produce a diffuse patchy process (bronchopneumonia). Viral pneumonias often show fairly widespread pulmonary involvement on chest x-ray despite few if any physical findings. Presence of a friction rub synchronous with respiration indicates involvement of the pleura. Deviation of the trachea toward the involved side may signal atelectasis, but when the deviation is away from the involved side, pleural effusion or empyema is usually present. Fixation of the mediastinum by previous inflammatory processes such as tuberculosis may limit such deviations. Lung abscesses are more difficult to demonstrate by physical examination, although an area of amphoric breathing may be present. Splinting of respiration is often present especially when there is pleural involvement. A respiratory lag may be noted on the involved side. Chronic pulmonary disease may obscure the findings of acute pneumonia, and fever, dullness and auscultatory manifestations may be atypical.

Resolution of Pneumonia

Pneumococcal pneumonia characteristically resolves rapidly with complete disappearance of the pulmonary lesion. Occasionally in pneumonia due to the type 3 pneumococcus pulmonary abscesses may develop. Staphylococcal and Klebsiella pneumonias are more likely to result in chronic abscesses.

Complications

Pleuritis with serous effusion occurs in about 10 percent of pneumococcal pneumonia cases, but empyema is now rare and is unlikely to develop after adequate penicillin therapy has been instituted. Stiff neck and headache may signal the appearance of meningitis. Endocarditis and meningitis may occur together as complications of pneumococcal pneumonia and may be indicated by the occurrence of repeated chills. Pyogenic pericarditis may ensue by direct extension. Other possible extrapulmonary complications include pyogenic arthritis and peritonitis. Metastatic abscesses are more likely to occur in overwhelming staphylococcal pneumonia.

Laboratory Findings

White Blood Count

Bacterial pneumonias usually produce leukocytosis in the range of 15,000 to 40,000 white cells per mm^3 with a preponderance of young neutrophiles. Occasionally, a patient with pneumococcal pneumonia may present with leukopenia, indicating a particularly severe or fulminating infection. This is more likely to occur in alcoholics or aged patients and reflects suboptimal host response to infection. Viral, rickettsial and tuberculous pneumonias may be associated either with a normal white blood count or an initial leukopenia followed by leukocytosis in the second week of infection. Eosinophilic pneumonitis (Loeffler's syndrome), in which evanescent fleeting pulmonary infiltrates occur, is associated with a very high level of blood eosinophiles. Monocytosis or a myelocytic leukemoid reaction may occasionally be seen in tuberculosis.

The *erythrocyte sedimentation rate* is usually increased following the onset of infection. This finding is non-specific, however, and has little diagnostic value. Failure of elevation of the sedimentation rate despite the presence of significant infection occurs in abnormal red cell states such as sickle cell anemia and in congestive heart failure.

As a rule, *anemia* does not result from acute infections. In chronic infections, however, moderate suppression of marrow activity may occur with consequent normochromic normocytic anemia. Rarely in staphylococcal infection anemia may result from the production of a hemolytic toxin. In primary atypical pneumonia due to the *Mycoplasma pneumoniae*, cold agglutinins commonly appear in the serum during convalescence and may possibly be associated with a hemolytic anemia.

Proteinuria, microscopic hematuria, and pyuria occur frequently in pneumonia, but in most instances are mild in degree and rapidly reversible.

Examination of the Sputum

Gram stain of the sputum is a valuable tool in diagnosis before beginning treatment but may occasionally be misleading. It is important that the specimen examined represent a true sample of sputum rather than salivary or other secretions. When a valid specimen is properly gram-stained, the etiologic agent usually appears as the predominant organism on the smear. Thus, in pneumococcal pneumonia, myriads of typical lancet shaped gram-positive diplococci can usually be seen both intra- and extracellularly. The type-specific polysaccharide capsule is usually not evident unless the *quellung* reaction is performed with appropriate antisera. It is of particular importance to be alert for the presence of staphylococci or of gram-negative encapsulated rods typical of Klebsiella (Friedlander's bacillus). In varicella pneumonia microscopic examination of tracheal aspirates may reveal characteristic intracytoplasmic inclusion bodies.

It is essential that culture of the sputum be carried out to confirm the diagnostic impression of the gram stain. Both aerobic and anaerobic cultures should be prepared, and when indicated appropriate media should be inoculated for culture of fungi and tubercle bacilli.

Mycoplasma pneumoniae and viruses require more complex techniques which are not usually available in routine bacteriological laboratories.

Blood Cultures

Cultures of blood obtained during the acute illness are often of value in confirming the bacteriologic diagnosis. About 30 percent of patients with pneumococcal pneumonia will be found to have bacteremia, usually found when one or two blood cultures are taken before beginning treatment.

Bacteremia is very commonly found during staphylococcal pneumonia but is rare with Klebsiella pneumonia. Blood cultures are usually negative in mycoplasma, tularemia, and rickettsial pneumonia.

Dysproteinemia, particularly in multiple myeloma and hypogammaglobulinemia, may be found in patients with recurrent pneumococcal pneumonia.

Radiological Findings

X-ray examination of the chest is of great importance in the diagnosis of pneumonia since, as indicated, some forms of fairly extensive pulmonary involvement produce few if any physical findings. Pneumococcal pneumonia may occur in any lobe of the lung, but most often produces consolidation of the right lower lobe. When the upper lobes or apical segments are involved, atelectasis is more likely to develop, and produce delayed resolution. In children, pneumococcal pneumonia is often diffuse or patchy (bronchopneumonia) and may involve several lobes. Abscesses or cavities are rarely seen in pneumococcal infection but are common in staphylococcal and Friedlander's pneumonia. The aspiration of vomitus or other foreign material may result in "aspiration pneumonia." The right lower and the right middle lobes are most frequently involved. Cavitation and subsequent calcification is characteristic of tuberculosis, but may be seen in mycotic infections as well. Actinomycosis is particularly likely to result in sinus tract or fistula formation. Tularemia pneumonia is usually associated with mediastinal lymph node enlargement. The pulmonary lesion of anthrax is primarily hemorrhagic mediastinal lymphadenopathy.

Mycoplasma and adenovirus pneumonia usually produce patchy or confluent lobular densities confined to part of one lobe, and air bronchograms are often seen. In contrast, widespread lobular consolidations or reticular infiltrations throughout *both* lungs are characteristic of other severe viral pneumonias produced by varicella, herpes, variola and cytomegalovirus. Primary influenza pneumonia may appear as either localized or diffuse bronchopneumonia but in association with rheumatic heart disease may produce a perihilar "butterfly" pattern.

Management

Antibiotic Therapy

Two principal questions should be answered before treatment of pneumonia is begun: Is the infection acute or chronic? What is the probable infecting microorganism? Staphylococcal, Klebsiella and pneumococcal pneumonia, as well as viral, rickettsial and mycoplasmal pneumonias are usually acute in onset, and the patient will be seen by the physician within a few days of the start of illness. Tuberculosis and mycotic infections of the lung also may appear to be acute in onset but the patient usually gives evidence of chronic disease, including weight loss, fatiguability, malaise and pulmonary symptoms. The distinction between acute and chronic pulmonary infection, therefore, is usually not difficult, even when a patient with chronic pulmonary disease such as emphysema or bronchiectasis develops acute pneumonia. The identification of *probable* infecting microorganism depends, however, on a careful appraisal of manifestations of illness and epidemiological considerations as well as a gram stain of sputum. The gram stain for example may be an important guide in distinguishing coccal from bacillary pneumonia. Since it is difficult to differentiate mycoplasmal from viral pneumonias, it is probably desirable to treat "primary atypical pneumonias" as though due to mycoplasma.

Choice of Antibiotic

The outcome of acute pneumonia is strongly influenced by the selection of the correct antibiotic. The drug of choice in pneumococcal pneumonia is penicillin, in a dose of 600,000 to 1.2 million units per day intramuscularly. Oral penicillin has been used effectively, but its absorption from the gastrointestinal tract is less predictable, particularly in acutely ill patients. In the presence of peripheral vascular collapse, penicillin should be administered intravenously because of the danger of impaired absorption from intramuscular sites. There is no evidence that larger doses of penicillin are of value in pneumococcal pneumonia. Broad spectrum antibiotics including the tetracyclines, cephalosporins as well as erythromycin are also generally effective and may be used, for example, in patients allergic to penicillin. Treatment should continue until the patient has been afebrile for two to three days. In uncomplicated pneumococcal pneumonia with a resolving x-ray infiltrate, it is not necessary to continue treatment until x-ray resolution is complete.

Staphylococcal pneumonia is potentially a more serious disease. Since up to a third of staphylococcal infections acquired outside of hospitals now are resistant to penicillin as are the majority of hospital acquired staphylococcal infections, the initial drug of choice is a penicillinase-resistant penicillin such as methicillin or oxacillin (in a total daily dose of four to six grams parenterally). If bacteriological studies indicate that the staphylococcus is sensitive to penicillin G, it is reasonable to substitute this less expensive and highly effective drug in a dose of 4 to 6 million units a day. Treatment of staphylococcal pneumonia should be continued for a minimum course of four weeks in most instances.

Klebsiella pneumonia in most cases may be effectively treated with gentamicin or cephalothin. Other potentially effective agents include kanamycin, chloramphenicol and colistimethate. In seriously ill patients it is customary to employ combination therapy, such as cephalothin plus gentamicin. Treatment should be continued until evidence of progressive resolution of the pulmonary lesion is obtained. Treatment of other gram-negative bacillary pneumonias pending antimicrobial susceptibility studies requires knowledge of the antibiotic sensitivity pattern in the particular hospital or community. (See Chapt. 27.)

Mycoplasma pneumonia is preferably treated with tetracycline or erythromycin for two to three weeks.

When culture data become available, it may be necessary for the physician to change his diagnosis and alter the therapeutic regimen accordingly. After beginning antibiotic treatment, however, the nasopharyngeal and sputum bacteriology will almost invariably be altered, commonly with the appearance of gram negative bacilli. This change in flora after beginning treatment should not be used as a criterion for a change in drug treatment unless evidence of superinfection with worsening of the patient's condition is evident.

SELECTED REFERENCES

Austrian, C. R. and Austrian, R.: Pneumococcal pneumonia (lobar pneumonia) in: *Tice's Practice of Medicine*, Hagerstown, Md., W. F. Prior Co., Inc, 1959. Vol. 1, p. 1.

Austrian, R. and Gold, J.: Pneumococcal bacteremia with especial reference to bacteremic pneumococcal pneumonia. Ann. Int. Med., *60*:759, 1964.

Fisher, A. M., Trevor, R., Curtin, J. A., Schultze, G., and Miller, D. F.: Staphylococcal pneumonia: A review of 21 cases in adults. N. Eng. J. Med., *258*:919, 1958.

Forsythe, B. R. and Chanock, R. M.: Mycoplasma pneumonia. Ann. Rev. of Med., *17*:371, 1966.

Heffron, R.: Pneumonia with special reference to pneumococcus lobar pneumonia. New York, The Commonwealth Fund, 1939.

Manfredi, F., Daly, W. J., and Behnke, R. H.: Clinical observations of acute Friedlander pneumonia. Ann. Int. Med., *58*:642, 1963.

Pierce, A. K., Sanford, J. P., Thomas, G. D., and Leonard, J. S.: Long-term evaluation of decontamination of inhalation-therapy equipment and occurrence of necrotizing pneumonia. N. Eng. J. Med., *282*:528, 1970.

Shulman, J. A., Phillips, L. A., and Petersdorf, R. G.: Errors and hazards in the diagnosis and treatment of bacterial pneumonias. Ann. Int. Med., *62*:41, 1965.

Tillitson, J. R. and Lerner, A. M.: Pneumonias caused by gram-negative bacilli. Medicine, *45*:65, 1966.

Triebwasser, J. H., Harris, R. E., Bryant, R. E., and Rhoades, E. R.: Varicella pneumonia in adults. Medicine, *46*:409, 1967.

Wood, W. B., Jr.: Studies on the cellular immunology of acute bacterial infections. The Harvey Lectures, Series *47*: 72–98, 1951–52.

Wood, W. B., Jr.: Studies on the mechanism of recovery in pneumococcal pneumonia. I. The action of type specific antibody upon the pulmonary lesion of experimental pneumonia. J. Exp. Med., *73*:201, 1941.

Chapter 15

INFLUENZA

Introduction

Influenza is the principal remaining infectious disease which has defied measures to prevent its becoming pandemic. This is attributable to at least three factors: 1) variable antigenicity among viral strains responsible for pandemics: 2) difficulty in preparation of effective vaccines for mass immunization of non-immune populations at risk of infection by a viral strain to which there has been no prior exposure: and 3) unavailability of a chemotherapeutic agent which will reliably and safely prevent or treat infection. Control of pandemic influenza and its devastating effects probably will be dependent upon development of an immunogenic agent with broad specificity or improvement of present methods for production of new vaccines for mass immunization.

Endemic and epidemic influenza usually are caused by infection of non-immune persons previously escaping, or with waning immunity following infection by pandemic or well established influenza viruses.

Influenzal infection may produce no apparent illness, mild febrile respiratory symptoms, or severe potentially fatal disease with pneumonia. During a pandemic, many more persons will demonstrate infection by rises in specific serum antibody titer than will be recognized as having influenzal disease. Persons dying with influenza most often have some associated disease exaggerating the severity of their infection.

Transmission of influenza virus from one person to another is by close contact or droplet. In small particle aerosols (droplet nuclei) the virus does not long retain its viability or virulence. Outbreaks of the infection, as expected, therefore, occur most prominently among persons in close contact, as during winter months, in schools, or in other crowded conditions.

There are no completely satisfactory therapeutic measures which will terminate or eliminate influenzal infection. Symptomatic management and treatment of complications are the principal measures which can be employed to help the affected individual.

Historical Perspective

Pandemics and epidemics of respiratory diseases like influenza have been recorded for over 400 years. The catastrophic and mysterious periodicity, as well as the relationship to climatic conditions, of these out breaks led to naming the disease "influenza," meaning influence of heavenly bodies or of cold. The first well-studied pandemic of influenza occurred in 1889–1892, when the spread of influenza was shown not to be in the direction of prevailing winds, and bacteriological studies erroneously related the infection to *Hemophilus influenzae*. The major thrust of this pandemic, as with others, was followed by lesser outbreaks in waves over the following few years. Many pandemics of influenza have begun in the far East, in Russia, Japan, and China. A major pandemic towards the conclusion of World War I resulted in over 10,000,000 deaths during one year.

A virus responsible for influenza was identified first in 1933 by infection of ferrets. The virus isolated than was called influenza A, but subsequently other related strains of virus have been characterized as responsible for pandemic, epidemic, and endemic infection. The three principle antigenically distinguishable variants of type A influenza virus thus far identified have been designated A_0, A_1, and A_2. More recently a Hong Kong variant also has been recognized. Each of these subtypes have been responsible for pandemics in the past 25 years; one in 1946–47, and the others in 1956–57 and 1967–68.

Cultivation of influenza virus in embryonated eggs in 1940 resulted in further characterization of the agent and led to development of a vaccine. This was immediately followed by demonstration of erythrocyte agglutination by influenza virus, providing a tool accelerating virological research and useful for assaying serum antibody and virus.

Epidemiology

The likelihood of influenzal infection is related to the degree of acquired immunity, risk of exposure to an infected person, and virulence of the virus. Infection usually induces an antibody response demonstrable in respiratory secretions and in serum, but levels of antibody decline after several weeks and within one year may be undetectable. Reinfection with the same influenza virus strain can occur in those with waning immunity, but may induce an accelerated immune response. Declining individual, group or population immunity probably is responsible for the periodicity of influenza epidemics. Epidemics of influenza A, for example, may occur every two to three years among persons in communities with declining immunity acquired during a previous outbreak. All communities are not on the same cycle, however, and epidemics of influenza A are usually reported in different communities annually. Such epidemics usually begin in the winter months in north temperate zones and persist for only about one month. These epidemics have a low mortality rate, and persistence of immunity in some members of the community prevents the devastating events seen more often during pandemics caused by an antigenically new viral strain.

Pandemics of influenza are caused by virulent viral strains antigenically dissimilar from strains previously responsible for infection, and therefore affecting a non-immune population. Appearance of such an influenza virus characteristically is followed by spread throughout the world, sequentially affecting one country after another over several months, and such pandemics have arisen about every 10 to 12 years. Most recorded pandemics have first begun in Asia, but the reasons for this are completely unknown. The origin of the new viral strains is unknown. The impact of these pandemics is great, resulting in massive numbers of sick, temporarily disabled individuals, and usually high mortality rates particularly in the old, the very young, and those with chronic respiratory or cardiovascular disease.

Endemic influenza probably occurs continually in all populations, resulting in sporadic respiratory disease in individuals not protected by immunity acquired during epidemic cycles. Identification of the influenza virus in such sporadic cases is not usually done, however, and the presence of influenza during the intervals between epidemics is poorly defined.

The risk of developing influenza also is importantly related to crowding and close contact of groups of individuals. The congregation of individuals together in heated buildings during cold weather probably is responsible for the relationship of epidemics to winter months. Control of epidemics, therefore, should include restriction of group aggregates. The airborne or droplet transmission of influenza has resulted in use of face masks during epidemics and pandemics, but the usefulness of this measure in preventing naturally occurring infection is not proven; although if worn whenever there is person-to-person contact, an effective mask should prevent acquisition of the virus.

The incubation period of influenza is 24 to 48 hours; the illness begins abruptly and persists for less than 7 days if uncomplicated. During pandemics, however, more than 30 percent of the population may be infected while only 5 percent of the population will report being sick. It is probable that the infected but asymptomatic person is a source of infection for others as is the ill person. Any protective device or measure, therefore, must include not only protection from those who are sick but from asymptomatic individuals as well.

Influenza is caused by an RNA virus having two virus coded protein antigens on its surface—hemagglutinin and neuraminidase. The hemagglutinin is responsible for virus attachment to cells, and the enzyme neuraminidase facilitates release of newly formed virus particles from infected cells. These proteins are antigenic, and antibody to both may be necessary for development of acquired immunity.

A nucleoprotein antigen of influenza virus enables separation of strains into three main types—A, B, and C. Type A viruses are the most important and are the only ones isolated during pandemics. Type B is a rare cause of epidemics and infection with this type is uncommon. An outbreak of infection by type C virus has been described but also is a rare cause of epidemic disease. Antigenic variants of type B virus, based on differences in surface or envelope antigens, have been identified but significant antigenic variation among type C strains are not known.

The three principal subtypes of influenza A virus have a common nucleoprotein antigen but dissimilar envelope (hemagglutinin) antigens. These variants of type A virus, as mentioned, have been responsible for major pandemics in the past 30 years. They may represent viral mutations, emergence of a latent virus or perhaps transmission of a strain from an animal reservoir. Influenza A viruses probably do not have the capacity for infinite antigenic changes.

The subtypes of type A identified in the past several years may have been responsible for infection long before, as older persons in some populations have been found to have low titer serum antibody directed against surface antigens of these type A variant viruses. Conceivably, the viruses could remain latent for years and emerge for unexplained reasons as causes of major outbreaks. Latency of a influenza virus has been described in swine, the disease appearing only after pulmonary infection of these animals with a pathogenic bacterium or lung parasite. In addition, the virus may assert its pathogenicity only after exposure of the animal with latent infection to cold. The observation that animals may be infected by influenza viruses antigenically like those causing disease in man suggests either that viral strains causing outbreaks of infection in man may be transmitted from animals or the infection of man may be transmitted to animals. There is experimental evidence demonstrating simultaneous infection with two different strains of virus resulting in hybrid viruses deriving genetic information and antigenic features of the two parent strains. This recombination may account for emergence of different strains but its importance as a cause of outbreaks of infection has not been shown.

Pathogenesis

Necrosis or denudation of the ciliated epithelium of the respiratory tract is the primary lesion of influenza. The trachea is most severely affected, but the upper respiratory tract also may be involved. Re-epithelization begins after the third day of infection with appearance of epithelium simulating metaplasia. Ciliated cells appear after two weeks, and there are then no residial lesions in uncomplicated influenza.

Involvement of the lung parenchyma by influenza virus (primary influenzal pneumonia) produces thickening of the alveolar septa with hyaline membranes lining alveolar ducts and alveoli. The alveoli contain edema fluid with fibrin and some monouclear and neutrophilic cellular exudation. Focal hemorrhage and inflammation may occur in the submucosa of the trachea, bronchi, and bronchioles.

Lymphocytopenia is common early in the disease but may be followed by leucocytosis of mild degree with neutrophilia. The fever of infection may be attributable to pyrogenic activity of the virus and to its effect upon phagocytic cells releasing endogenous pyrogen. Acute phase reactions such as the erythrocyte sedimentation rate may be increased. When pneumonia develops, there frequently are impairments of pulmonary function. Otherwise, no pathological, physiological, or biochemical changes explain the manifestations of influenza infection. Viremia is not known to occur in influenza, but the intense myalgia and the neurological manifestations are indicative of a systemic illness.

Recovery from influenza is not related to appearance of serum or local antibody. The infection does induce the elaboration of interferon, a relatively non-specific antiviral substance, from infected cells preventing further viral synthesis. Interferon, therefore, may be primarily responsible for termination of the infection, by interfering with the combination of viral messenger RNA with cellular ribosomes in forming functional polysomes on which viral proteins are synthesized.

Clinical Manifestations

Asymptomatic infection is the most common form of influenza. The majority of persons who become sick experience an acute febrile illness with myalgia, frontal or orbital headache, dry harassing cough, and substernal aching. Rhinitis and pharyngitis, common manifestations of rhinovirus and adenovirus infection, are uncommon in influenza. Diarrhea and vomiting are not characteristic of influenza, and the phrase "intestinal flu" is inaccurate, often indicating enterovirus infection. Conjunctival injection and scattered rales or rhonchi in the chest, even without abnormal x-ray findings, often are observed in influenza.

The fever of influenza is sustained but is lower in the morning and higher in the evening. Sweating at night may be intense, particularly if aspirin is given at bedtime. Aspirin also will cause prompt defervescence in most patients and relieve much of the discomfort of illness. If given irregularly, however, the patient may experience chills with defervescence, and sweating may lead to prostration and dehydration. Aspirin, therefore, may improve the patient's state of well being, cause defervescence, but also may produce adverse consequences. Generally, the fever persists for only three to four days unless there are complications such as pneumonia or sinusitis. Weakness, fatiguability, anorexia, and malaise, however, will disappear within one week or persist for three weeks or more. When uncomplicated, delay in recovery from these symptoms is seen mostly in patients who are more aware of illness, frequently report minor complaints to physicians and have a "depressive propensity" even though otherwise emotionally and functionally normal and in absence of evidence for persistence of infection. (See Chapt. 12.)

Complications

Influenza virus pneumonia is a devastating form of the disease, usually fatal, and develops rapidly after onset of infection, producing dry harassing cough, dyspnea, diffuse pulmonary infiltrative involvement by x-ray, cyanosis, and hypoxemia. Many patients developing influenza pneumonia have valvular heart disease or, less commonly, pre-existing lung disease or pregnancy. The manifestations of pneumonia may be confused with pulmonary congestion and heart failure, but the central venous pressure and blood volume are normal in influenzal pneumonia.

Bacterial pneumonia may occur as a complication three days or more after onset of influenza and is characterized by deteriorating clinical status and beginning purulent productive cough. Pulmonary findings by x-ray are those of consolidation and confluent pneumonitis rather than diffuse pulmonary infiltrate. Hypoxemia may be less evident and cyanosis may not be present. Many patients developing these complications are elderly, pregnant, or have pre-existing chronic pulmonary disease and, less commonly, valvular heart disease.

Young children with influenza may develop obstructive laryngotracheitis, and have difficulty in clearing the respiratory tract of tracheal secretions. Encephalitis, polyneuritis, radiculitis, Guillain-Barre syndrome and myocarditis are less common complications of influenza and usually resolve without residual abnormalities. A form of Parkinsonism has been suggested as a complication of influenza, particularly following the 1918–1919 World War I pandemic.

Management

Symptomatic care is all that can be done to treat patients with uncomplicated influenza. The fever can be reduced with antipyretics, such as aspirin. For adults, 0.6 gm. aspirin every 4 hours will suffice. If aspirin is given, it should be taken regularly and not prescribed only when the temperature exceeds a specified level. The latter often results in marked swings of temperature, with intense sweating and chills, which may exhaust the patient and cause dehydration. Aspirin also is effective in relieving headache, myalgia, and malaise, but the patient may then engage in excessive activity and possibly prolong his illness. Bed rest ordinarily need not be prescribed, for the patient will voluntarily restrict his activities unless his sense of well being is improved with aspirin. The patient should be advised, therefore, that despite symptomatic improvement following aspirin administration, he should restrict his activities. This is particularly a problem in children.

Patients having cough without sputum production and associated substernal aching with tracheitis may be given codeine as a cough suppressant. Occasionally, inhalation of steam will also produce significant relief of cough and the tracheitis. If the cough is productive of much sputum, codeine should not be used, or given with caution, and steam inhalation is preferred. The principle pathological lesion of influenza is denudation of the respiratory tract epithelium, particularly of the trachea, and this is responsible for the cough, substernal discomfort and predisposition to bacterial superinfection. The steam inhalation keeps the trachea moist and this may be the mechanism whereby it is effective.

The management of influenza virus pneumonia is directed largely towards alleviation of hypoxemia by oxygen administration. Antimicrobial therapy is required if bacterial pneumonia supervenes but administration of antibiotics, otherwise, will not reduce the likelihood of bacterial pneumonia and will increase the probability of infection by antibiotic-resistant bacteria. Staphylococci are important in causing bacterial pneumonia in patients with influenza, and if gram stain of sputum reveals pus cells and clusters of gram-positive cocci, a penicillinase-resistant antibiotic such as methicillin, oxacillin, cloxacillin, or cephalothin should be used until further bacteriological data are available. If pus cells and gram-negative bacilli are seen in sputum, initial treatment with ampicillin for *Hemophilus influenzae* infection should be used as this organism also is an important cause of bacterial pneumonia in patients with influenza. Other bacteria may cause pneumonia in patients with influenza and the information in Chapter 14 will be helpful in recognizing these and guiding the appropriate treatment.

Most patients with influenza recover without complication; and unless complicated, these patients should not be hospitalized. They can be cared for at home, and there is a risk of superinfection in the hospital with antibiotic resistant microorganisms.

Corticosteroids have been used to treat influenza viral pneumonia but without proven benefit.

Prevention

Inactivated influenza virus vaccines have been used for many years, and their effectiveness has been demonstrated in prevention of infection by corresponding infecting viruses when the quantity of viral antigen in the vaccine is adequate. Vaccination one to two months before an expected epidemic is recommended, followed by a booster dose prior to the outbreak. As mentioned before, mass production of vaccine to newly appearing viruses has not provided enough vaccine of sufficient antigen concentration to significantly affect pandemics. This is the most important unresolved problem in prevention of influenza. Recognition of antigenic overlap between influenza type A viruses and possible utilization of neuraminidase as a common antigenic vaccine may lead to better means for control of these problems in the future.

Influenza infection largely, if not exclusively, involves the respiratory mucous membranes. Furthermore, there is not a precise relationship between immunity to influenza and serum antibody. Recent observations suggest that locally secretory antibody may be more important in immunity to infection of mucous membranes. The induction of local antibody production in the respiratory tract by topical application of vaccine may prove to be an important adjunct in prevention of influenza. (See Chapt. 4.)

Amantadine hydrochloride given prior to infection with influenza A virus decreases the rate of infection, as determined by the absence of antibody rise to viral antigens. The drug has the disadvantage of having little or no value in treatment of established infection or control of the disease once it develops. Amantadine may be given to adults in doses of 200 mg. daily. To prevent influenza, treatment must be started as soon as possible after exposure and continued for at least 10 days or up to 30 days in patients with repeated and unknown exposures. There is no evidence indicating efficacy of amantadine in other respiratory viral illnesses, or influenza B or C infection.

SELECTED REFERENCES

Chanock, R. M., Smith, C. B., Friedewald, W. T., Parrott, R. H., Kapikian, A. Z., and Gharpure, M. A.: Resistance to parainfluenza and respiratory syncytial virus infection-implications for effective immunization and preliminary study of attenuated strain of respiratory syncytial virus. In: *First International Conference on Vaccines Against Viral and Rickettsial Diseases of Man.* Sci. Publ. No. 147 PAHO, pp. 53–61 (Pan-Amer. San. Bur., Washington, 1967).

Davenport, F. M., Minuse, E., Hennessey, A. V., and Francis, T., Jr.: Interpretations of influenza antibody patterns in man. Bull. W.H.O., *41*:453, 1969.

Fazekas de St. Groth, S. and Donnelley, M.: Studies in experimental epidemiology of influenza. IV. The protective value of active immunization. Aust. J. Exp. Biol. Med., *28*:61, 1950.

Fedson, D. S.: Characteristics of serum antibody response to infection and vaccination. Ann. Intern. Med., *71*:386, 1969.

Francis, T., Jr.: The inactivation of epidemic influenza by nasal secretions of human individuals. Science, *90*:198, 1940.

Fukumi, H.: Summary report on the Asian influenza epidemic in Japan, 1957. Bull W.H.O., *20*:187, 1959.

Jordan, W. S., Jr.: The mechanism of spread of Asian influenza. Amer. Rev. Resp. Dis., *83*:29 (NO.2), 1960.

Kasel, J. A., Fulk, R. V., and Couch, R. B.: Antigenic relationship between the equine and the Hong Kong human variant of influenza type A virus. J. Immunol.,

Kilbourne, E. D., Christenson, W. N., and Sande, M.: Antibody response in man to influenza virus neuraminidase following influenza. J. Virol., *2*:761, 1968.

102:530, 1969.

Kilbourne, E. D., Laver, W. G., Schulman, J. L., and Webster, R. G.: Antiviral activity of antiserum specific for an influenza virus neuraminidase. J. Virol., *2*:281, 1968.

Kilbourne, E. D.: Recombination of influenza A viruses of human and animal origin. Science, *160*:74, 1968.

Louria, D. B., Blumenfeld, H. J., Ellis, J. T., Kilbourne, E. D., and Rogers, D. E.: Studies on influenza in the pandemic of 1957–1958. II. Pulmonary complications of influenza. J. Clin. Invest., *38*:213, 1959.

Masurel, N.: Relation between Hong Kong virus and former human A isolate and the A/Equi/2 virus in human sera collected before 1957. Lancet *1*:907, 1969.

Mills, J. and Chanock, R. M.: Temperature-sensitive mutants of influenza virus. 1. Behavior in tissue culture and in experimental animals. J. Infect. Dis., *123*:145, 1971.

Mulder, J., and Masurel, N.: Pre-epidemic antibody against the 1957 strain of Asiatic influenza in the serum of older persons living in The Netherlands. Lancet, *1*:810, 1958.

Pereira, H. G., Tumova, B., and Webster, R. G.: Antigenic relationship between influenza A. viruses of human and avian origins. Nature, *215*:982, 1967.

Schulman, J. L. and Kilbourne, E. D.: Airborne transmission of influenza virus infection in mice. Nature, *195*:1129, 1962.

Seto, J. T. and Roth, R.: Functional significance of sialidase during influenza virus multiplication. Virology, *30*:731, 1966.

Smith, C. B., Purcell, R. H., Bellanti, J. A., and Chanock, R. M.: Protective effect of antibody to parainfluenza type 1 virus. N. Eng. J. Med., *275*:1145, 1966.

Stuart-Harris, C. H.: Twenty years of influenza epidemics. Amer. Rev. Resp. Dis., *83*, No. *2*:54, 1960.

Tumova, B. and Easterday, B. C.: Relationship of envelope antigens of animal influenza viruses to human A influenza strains isolated in the years 1957–1968. Bull. W.H.O., *41*:429, 1969.

Waldman, R. H., Bond, J. O., Levitt, L. P., Hartwig, E. C., Prather, E. C., Baratta, R. L., Neill, J. S., and Small, P. A., Jr.: An evaluation of influenza immunization. Bull. W.H.O., *41*:543, 1969.

Waldman, R. H., Mann, J. J., and Small, P. A., Jr.: Immunization against influenza. J.A.M.A., *207*:520, 1969.

Woodall, J., Rowson, K. E. K., and McDonald, J. C.: Age and Asian influenza, 1957. Brit. Med. J., *2*:1316, 1958.

Chapter 16

TUBERCULOSIS

Introduction

Tuberculosis is caused by *Mycobacterium tuberculosis*, a slowly multiplying, non-motile bacillus which is an obligate aerobe. It is acid-fast on Kinyoun stain and produces few if any toxins harmful to the human body. Because it multiplies best in a high oxygen environment, the predominant infection caused by this organism is most often found in the lung. Tissue damage occurs because of the delayed cellular hypersensitivity reaction induced when infection occurs. Although methods for control of this disease are known to be effective, it remains a quantitatively important worldwide health problem, particularly in the underdeveloped countries.

Transmission and Pathogenesis

Exposure of the previously uninfected individual to a patient with tuberculosis may result in contagion of the disease. That this new infection will be acquired by the respiratory route seems certain, but the exact way in which transmission occurs has taken many years to delineate. Contagion begins with the tuberculous patient, whose pulmonary infection is manifested by cough. Coughing expulses droplets, most of which travel two to three feet before falling to the floor or impinging upon another person or piece of furniture. It is not these droplets, however, that are inspired by the susceptible individual. Some droplets promptly evaporate, leaving particulate matter which contains tubercle organisms. These "droplet nuclei" can persist in the air of a closed room for many hours. Their size is correct for inhalation and, therefore, they have been strongly implicated as the vehicles which carry acid-fast organisms to the susceptible individual. The droplet nucleus is inhaled and it carries the infectious mycobacteria into the alveoli.

When such droplet nuclei are inhaled, they may go to any area of the lung. Since ventilation is greater in the lung bases, preferential deposition occurs there. The organisms may multiply in these areas, unmolested by body defenses until delayed hypersensitivity is evoked. The latter is manifested by a conversion to positive of the tuberculin skin test (PPD) and may take four to five weeks after infection. During this time it is thought that dissemination of some organisms occurs through the blood stream. In the vast majority of patients, the disseminated organisms are destroyed by body defenses everywhere except in the apex of the lung. Presumably, the higher oxygen tension in this area favors their growth. In rare instances organisms may also remain viable in the kidneys, adrenals, bones, or any other organ. None of these necessarily causes symptomatic disease. The apical focus (or other foci if present) may become walled off, the primary focus healed, and the only remnant of infection may be the positive skin test, a primary complex and a Simon focus at the apex. These foci may all be microscopic and, indeed, this is probably what happens in the usual tuberculin skin test conversion.

Alternatively, primary tuberculous infection may lead to an area of infiltration in the lungs or pleura, plus mediastinal adenopathy. Clinical primary tuberculosis, however, occurs in the minority of infected persons. In even fewer persons does the dissemination lead to post-primary miliary, meningeal, renal, or other extra-pulmonary disease.

Usually, there is a lack of clinical disease of any kind with PPD skin test conversion. Today, positivity of the PPD is thought to signify *living organisms* somewhere in the body. The bulk of evidence would suggest that such organisms are located in the apical areas of the lung, but are temporarily non-invasive. Studies have shown that these organisms may escape their confinement at any time during the life of the individual and cause clinical disease. The case rate per 100,000 persons per year for PPD positive individuals with no other added risk factors is 70 as opposed to 2/100,000 for tuberculin negative patients. When the apical lesions become clinical disease, they produce the classic apical cavity tuberculosis which therefore is properly termed re-exacerbation of endogenous tuberculosis rather than exogenous re-infection. This "unitary concept" of the pathogenesis of all types of tuberculosis from a single, often long-past, infection recently has been popularized.

Isolation Procedures

Isolation procedures should obviously bear relation to the mechanism of spread. Since fomites are not thought to be instrumental in spreading tuberculosis, it makes little sense to wear gown, cap, and gloves when entering the room of a patient with tuberculosis. Similarly, it makes little sense to handle in any special way every piece of equipment brought into such a room. What should be handled carefully is the air in the room. One can decrease the number of sputum particles entering the air by placing a mask on the patient. This is, in practice, difficult to maintain at all times, since patients must eat and generally do not like to wear masks constantly. Obviously, a corollary to this method is to instruct the patient in the proper way to cough, which is into something rather than directly into the air of the room.

Assuming that droplet nuclei cannot be completely prevented from entering the air by mask and cough instruction, elimination of these nuclei from the air must be accomplished. Good room ventilation, with rapid turn-over of the air and no recirculation into the room, is effective in eliminating organism-containing droplet nuclei. The addition of ultra-violet light to the ventilation duct also will kill the organisms as they pass through. Lastly, the job of prevention of contagion has been made immensely easier by the observation that drug-treated individuals place organisms into the air which are less capable of transmitting infection. Therefore, a tuberculous patient, on chemotherapy, may cough living organisms into the air; however, they are unlikely to cause disease, even if inhaled by a susceptible person. This point will be covered in more detail later, but it is the key to handling tuberculosis today.

Epidemiology

The intermediate PPD skin test containing five tuberculin units (TU) of purified protein derivative has been the epidemiologic tool used in most studies. There are three general categories of reaction that can occur. Positivity generally connotes an area of skin induration of greater than 10 mm. in largest diameter at 48 hours. A positive test certainly means some past exposure to *Mycobacterium tuberculosis*. In the absence of clinical and x-ray activity at the time of the test, a positive PPD is now thought to reflect living organisms, usually in the apex of the lung. A negative test is present when the area of induration is less than 5 mm. in greatest diameter. Negativity connotes no previous infection with *Mycobacterium tuberculosis*. Intermediate degrees of induration (5–9 mm.) often reflect previous infection with an atypical Mycobacterium, predominantly group III (Battey). If dual, simultaneous testing is done with PPD-S (5 TU PPD) and PPD-B (5 TU-Battey) in patients with intermediate reactions, often the specific skin test for the atypical mycobacterial infection will show a greater degree of induration than that for *Mycobacterium tuberculosis*.

The risk of acquiring tuberculous disease appears to depend directly upon the reactivity of the PPD. Risk, however, also depends upon whether there is exposure to exogenous infection as well. For instance, the population with a negative PPD has a low incidence of acquiring tuberculosis because exposure is infrequent today. The same persons, if exposed to a case of active tuberculosis, would be most likely to acquire the infection. On the other hand, an individual with a positive PPD is unlikely to be reinfected if exposed to an individual with active tuberculosis. However, re-exacerbation of endogenous tuberculosis is likely. The individual with intermediate sensitivity to PPD and a PPD-B skin test greater than PPD-S may be most protected against infection, and there is little likelihood of exacerbation of infection by atypical mycobacteria. There is evidence that past infection with an atypical organism may protect against exogenous infection with *Mycobacterium tuberculosis*. Therefore, the likelihood of future tuberculosis in individuals with intermediate sensitivity to PPD is lower than in other persons.

Host Factors

The probability of developing active tuberculous disease varies even among normal individuals. Individual variability in cell-mediated delayed hypersensitivity and immunity are probably related to the development of clinical disease. The tools with which to study these immunologic phenomena have been recently developed and they will likely shed light on the following important questions: 1) Why does one patient develop primary tuberculosis and another only convert his PPD skin test in the face of an apparently equal challenge with the inhaled tubercle organism? 2) Why does the apical living organism cause re-exacerbation tuberculosis at a specific time in life?

Certain host factors have been implicated in producing a predisposition toward clinical tuberculosis. Alcoholism has been shown to alter red cell, platelet and leukocyte function and is also a frequent underlying host factor in the patient with tuberculosis. Poor nutrition, debilitating disease and subtotal gastrectomy may also predispose toward re-exacerbation tuberculosis by as yet unknown mechanisms. The Negro, while more likely to be exposed to infection because of socioeconomic factors, also may develop more advanced disease. Diabetes and steroid therapy depress leukocyte migration and delayed hypersensitivity, respectively, and both have been associated with a relatively high frequency of clinical tuberculosis. Reticuloendothelial malignancies similarly depress cellular immunity and are associated with tuberculosis.

An additional host characteristic related to clinical tuberculous disease is a history of previous clinical tuberculosis. Untreated, healed infection, particularly when associated with a radiologic pulmonary scar, is highly correlated with the future development of disease. Presumably these old, healed but non-drug-treated lesions harbor significant quantities of viable organisms which may re-exacerbate still again in the lifetime of the individual.

Prevention

Based upon these observations, recommendations for the prevention of tuberculosis can now be discussed rationally. If a positive PPD connotes infection by viable mycobacteria, the increased incidence of future tuberculosis in this group probably could be prevented by treatment with isonicotinic hydrazide (INH). Controlled studies with one-half of the population taking INH and one-half taking a placebo have shown a decreased rate of tuberculous disease during the year of drug therapy and a continued decrease in incidence during the following 10 years. The reduction in incidence was greatest in the patients who were judged more reliable in taking their drugs. These findings might justify treating all patients having a positive PPD with a year of INH at a dose of 300 mgm./day. The magnitude of such an undertaking, however, has led to recommendations for treating only those persons with positive PPD most likely to develop tuberculous disease, including the following and those identified in Table 16.1:

1. Persons with a past history of tuberculosis who received inadequate or no drug therapy.
2. Persons with radiologic evidence of healed tuberculosis, a positive PPD and negative sputum.
3. Persons with a positive PPD receiving prolonged corticosteroid therapy.
4. Persons with gastrectomy and positive PPD.

TABLE 16.1

*Relative risks of developing active tuberculosis**

New Active Case Rate per 100,000

All U.S.A. 1965	25
Tuberculin negative:	
non contact	2
close contact	500
Tuberculin positive:	
Males over 45	250
Grade school children	300
High school children	650
Hospital admissions	450
"Inactive" TB	900
Abnormal x-ray	2,000
Gastrectomy	2,000
Household contacts	3,500
Recent converters	3,500
Other contacts	700
No added risk	70

From multiple sources, particularly studies by USPHS and the Danish Tuberculosis Index.

* From Green, Robert A. *Clinical Patterns of Pulmonary Tuberculosis* in *Rational Therapy and Control of Tuberculosis*, edited by Johnson, Joseph E. III, University of Florida Press, Gainesville, Florida.

5. Persons with reticuloendothelial disease, such as leukemia or Hodgkin's disease.

6. Persons with diabetes mellitus and positive PPD.

7. Pregnant women with a positive PPD (chemoprophylaxis to be started in the last trimester and continued for a year).

8. Persons in close contact with an active case of tuberculosis if the PPD is positive. Negative contacts should be retested at three month intervals and treated if the PPD becomes positive.

9. Persons with a recent conversion of PPD from negative to positive.

10. Persons under age 20 with a positive PPD.

Individuals with a negative PPD generally can be considered to be not infected, and the development of tuberculosis depends entirely upon exposure to persons with active disease. In the United States today the overall risk of exposure is low; therefore, no prophylactic treatment is needed. In areas of higher exposure, however, prophylaxis may be desirable for some persons with negative PPD. For the individual with a negative PPD and a high risk of exposure, periodic skin testing with PPD and prompt treatment with INH upon conversion to positive has proven to be successful in preventing clinical tuberculosis. If periodic skin testing is not possible, persons at great risk probably should be vaccinated with BCG.

Clinical Spectrum

Tuberculosis is a protean disease, and description of all its possible manifestations is impractical here. Several selected, relevant clinical problems will be discussed with emphasis on practical management.

Primary Tuberculosis

Development of tuberculous disease soon after first exposure (primary tuberculosis) is uncommon. When disease occurs it differs from exacerbating or late emergent tuberculosis. Primary tuberculosis occurs most often in the younger age groups and frequently in children. There is a predilection to involvement of mid and basilar lung fields where a small parenchymal infiltrate may develop. The disease may progress to involve the mediastinal or hilar lymph nodes, causing them to enlarge. This combination of a peripheral pulmonary infiltrate and enlarged nodes in the areas of drainage is called the *primary pulmonary complex*. If a primary infection has been massive, or if the patient is debilitated, disease may involve larger areas of lung parenchyma, producing pneumonia, but cavitation is rare. Most often primary tuberculosis does not proceed farther than the involvement of the lung and the regional lymph nodes. Spontaneous healing may proceed to calcification of both the parenchymal lung lesion and the involved nodes. This type of healing produces the *calcified primary complex* consisting of an isolated calcified pulmonary nodule (Ghon focus) and a cluster of calcium deposits in the hilar nodes. Drug treatment accelerates such healing and is quite effective in this type of tuberculosis.

Pleural Effusion

Occasionally the primary infiltrate involves the pleural surface, causing an acute or chronic pleurisy with effusion. On thoracentesis, the fluid will often be exudative (SG > 1.015, Protein > 3.5 gm%, LDH > 500 u (Berger-Broida method)), clear or cloudy yellow in color, with varying numbers of cells which are mainly mononuclear, but are occasionally polymorphonuclear leukocytes. The definitive diagnosis of tuberculous effusion is made by a smear or culture of the fluid in only 25 to 50 percent of the cases. Sputum smear or culture for acid-fast organisms will be positive in only 10 to 15 percent of cases. Pleural biopsy with either a Cope or Abrams needle will increase the diagnostic yield considerably. Histological examination of a biopsy specimen will reveal granulomata with or without stainable acid-fast organisms in 63 to 71 percent of cases, thus allowing early definitive diagnosis. Culture of a biopsy specimen will grow acid-fast organisms in 55 to 76 percent of cases. By combining all the mentioned procedures, between 80 to 95 percent of tuberculous effusions can be diagnosed without surgical intervention. In the remaining patients, the American Thoracic Society recommends either empiric treatment with antituberculous drugs or open surgical pleural biopsy.

This remaining undiagnosed group, of course, presents to the physician as the combination of a positive PPD skin test and an undiagnosed pleural effusion. Every patient with this combination does not have tuberculosis, and empiric therapy with antituberculous drugs would not always be indicated. In this author's opinion, when confronted by a patient with this problem, the probabilities must be weighed before coming to a decision on empiric antituberculous therapy versus thoracotomy for pleural biopsy. In the younger patient (i.e., under 40 years) the likelihood of bronchogenic, or other types of carcinoma involving the pleura is lower. Perhaps in this type patient, empiric treatment for tuberculosis could be carried out. In the older patient with a long smoking history, bronchogenic carcinoma is more likely and perhaps open pleural biopsy should be performed.

Cavitary Tuberculosis

As mentioned earlier, any part of the body may be asymptomatically seeded at the time of the primary infection. The apical regions of the lung are most commonly the site of persistence of living tubercle organisms. They are also the most common site of breakdown and re-exacerbation tuberculosis. This form of pulmonary tuberculosis is that which is more familiar to the practicing internist. Cavitary disease is common, as is the clinical picture of hemoptysis, weight loss, and night sweats.

The extent of disease is classified according to the following scheme taken from the National Tuberculosis and Respiratory Disease Association booklet on diagnostic standards and classification of tuberculosis.

Minimal lesions include those of slight to moderate density *without* demonstrable cavitation. The total extent, regardless of distribution, should not exceed the volume of the lung on one side, which is above the second chondrosternal junction and the body of the 5th thoracic vertebrae.

Moderately advanced lesions may be present in one or both lungs. Their total extent should not exceed the following limits: lesions of slight to moderate density which do not exceed the volume of one lungfield in extent; dense and confluent lesions comprising a volume no greater than one third of a lungfield; total diameter of cavitation less than four cm.

Far advanced: describes lesions more extensive than moderately advanced.

Disseminated Tuberculosis

Virtually any organ of the body can be involved with tuberculosis. Miliary tuberculosis probably involves all organs of the body. It may occur in the immediate post-primary period if massive numbers of organisms invade the blood stream from the primary focus. In adults, however, miliary spread occurs from breakdown and dissemination of the apical focus; from a distant seeded focus, particularly urogenital; or from a caseous mediastinal node. These may rupture into the blood stream either directly or via the lymphatics. The syndrome, sometimes abrupt in onset, probably reflects a single dissemination; therefore, the miliary lesions seen on x-ray are all the same size and age. Patients with miliary tuberculosis are often quite ill, debilitated, wasted, and frequently have meningitis as well. Miliary lesions on chest x-ray, associated with choroidal tubercles seen on fundoscopic examination are quite suggestive, but are not diagnostic, of miliary tuberculosis.

Sputum smear is infrequently diagnostic, and sputum culture requires a prolonged wait for definitive diagnosis. Since delay in diagnosis of both miliary and meningeal tuberculosis can be extremely dangerous, emphasis should be placed on early lumbar puncture and liver biopsy if these diseases are considered. In the presence of meningitis the former will show elevated cerebrospinal fluid (CSF) pressure, increased cell count (usually lymphs, but polys may be present early), elevated protein, and decreased CSF sugar. Acid-fast bacilli may be seen in 30 percent on stain of the pellicle that forms if the CSF is left to stand. These organisms can be cultured in 60 percent. Liver biopsy in miliary tuberculosis usually reveals granulomata and allows early presumptive diagnosis and drug therapy.

Other Forms of Tuberculosis

Tuberculous pericarditis is thought to occur after a tuberculous mediastinal node erodes and ruptures into the pericardium. The signs and symptoms are those of pericarditis of any etiology. The PPD is positive and the pericardial fluid will grow acid-fast organisms in 50 percent of the cases. In those cases where culture is negative, considerable difficulty is encountered in making a definitive diagnosis. Early pericardiectomy for both diagnosis and therapy is occasionally necessary. Triple drug therapy plus steroids have been recommended both for treating acute pericarditis and in the hope of preventing the complication of constrictive pericarditis.

Tuberculosis of the peritoneum, kidney, adrenal, or bone may result from deposition of organisms at the time of the primary infection with late re-exacerbation. Tuberculous peritonitis leads to a syndrome characterized by fever, ascites, weight loss, abdominal pain, and night sweats. A positive PPD plus exudative peritoneal fluid is suggestive, but a peritoneal biopsy with a Cope or Abrams needle may be diagnostic. Often laparotomy is necessary to establish a diagnosis. Once therapy is begun, the prognosis in tuberculous peritonitis is quite good.

Renal tuberculosis is often asymptomatic, presenting as a mild backache plus sterile pyuria or hematuria. The predominant symptoms may be secondary to involvement of the urinary bladder by infection carried from the kidney through the ureter. Therefore, cystitis with urinary frequency and dysuria is common. Intravenous pyelogram (IVP) may reveal distortion of the calyceal system or ureteral stricture. When early morning or 24-hour urine collections are cultured for acid-fast organisms, the diagnostic yield is high. Treatment with antituberculous chemotherapy has been quite successful, making the need for surgical intervention rare.

Skin Testing in Active Tuberculosis

In all forms of tuberculosis, the PPD skin test is expected to be positive. Unfortunately, in almost every form of tuberculosis there is a small percentage of patients who, with proven active tuberculosis, will not react positively to tuberculin. The reasons for the negative PPD in various situations are manifold. They generally divide into spurious negative and real negative skin tests.

The reasons for spurious negatives begin with the obvious causes, such as the use of outdated PPD solutions, reading of the skin test at the wrong time, and subcutaneous instead of intradermal placement. Additionally, there is the not so obvious problem of leak of PPD solution back along the needle as the attempt is made to inject intradermally. This problem has been frequently encountered by the author and leaves one unsure of how much purified protein derivative has been injected and how much has leaked out.

A skin test plagued by any of the aforementioned problems should obviously be repeated. However, in practice, it is often read as a negative PPD. A spurious problem which is even more subtle relates to the observation that conventional PPD may adsorb to glass either in the ampule or in the syringe. This may lead to no problem if the diluent is added, the resulting solution is promptly drawn up and immediately injected. Studies, however, have shown a fairly rapid drop off of radioactively labeled PPD in solution over several hours. In the first day after mixing, up to 60 percent of the purified protein derivative may adsorb to the glass of the ampule. Therefore, if this solution were subsequently used, less PPD than expected would be injected and more frequent negative tests would occur. The addition of tween-80 to the solution will stabilize it and prevent the adsorption to glass. Such stabilized PPD is now available commercially (Panray Division, Ormont Drug and Chemical Co., Inc., Englewood, N. J. 07631) and studies have begun to show its clinical superiority.

Even if the test is performed perfectly, and tween-stabilized solutions are used, a percentage of patients with culture-proven tuberculosis will have negative skin tests to intermediate PPD. These remaining negative reactors will often be anergic because of severe overwhelming disease which depresses delayed hypersensitivity. In addition, older individuals will presumably have decreased delayed hypersensitivity and, consequently, a higher frequency of negative skin test. Anergy due to disease of the lymphoreticular system, or due to corticosteroid therapy, may also prevent the positive PPD. In a tuberculous military population—young persons with disease of limited extent—the PPD skin test should virtually always be positive if properly done. In old, debilitated, sick patients in the general hospital, the PPD may be negative in the face of clinical tuberculosis for the reasons mentioned.

Therapy

Chemotherapy

The treatment of tuberculosis has become infinitely easier since the introduction of effective, relatively non-toxic, antituberculous chemotherapy. New drugs continue to be introduced which will soon make even the tuberculosis caused by primary drug resistant organisms amenable to chemotherapy. Table 16.2 is a brief compilation of the major first line antituberculous agents available today. Second line drugs will be listed only. Their usefulness is limited to the disease caused by organisms resistant to the primary drugs, and their pharmacology can be found in standard texts.

With this available array of drugs, it is often difficult for the non-expert to figure out how many drugs to give. One reads of one drug for prophylaxis, two-, three-, and four-drug regimens for disease, and often no single rationale is evident among the recommendations from various experts. One method of integrating the rationale for therapy in all forms of tuberculosis has been presented by Johnston and Hopewell, and alluded to by Fox. This reasoning has appealed to this author and will be presented here, although it is not completely accepted by all experts in this field.

The rationale essentially states that the greater the number of organisms present in a lesion, the more drugs should be given. If one accepts the thesis that mutation to drug resistance does not occur *because* drugs are given, the addition of INH to the milieu in which the acid-fast organism is growing will not *cause* an organism to mutate. In other words, if 1,000 sensitive organisms are present in a lesion and INH is administered, it will kill all 1,000 organisms. The emergence of drug resistance occurs when one of the original organisms was resistant to INH and the drug killed all the others and allowed that single resistant organism to overgrow. The reason for using more than one drug then would be to kill the single organism originally resistant to INH.

It seems reasonable, if the above is true, that the likelihood for one, two, or three organisms to be resistant to INH would be directly related to the numbers of organisms present in the lesion. In patients with PPD skin test conversion and no visible pulmonary lesion, very few organisms are present. The chance of one of these being resistant to INH is low. Therefore, one can treat with INH alone. In cavitary lesions the population of acid-fast organisms may reach or exceed 100,000,000. Therefore three drugs would be appropriate treatment since a possibility exists that one of these organisms might be resistant to one or even two drugs. Lesions in between these two extremes might require only two-drug therapy. The more extensive the disease, the larger the number of bacilli; and the larger the number of bacilli, the greater the chance that a significant number of drug resistant organisms may be present.

Such reasoning might also be extended to include the different phases of treatment in an inividual patient. Early in treatment, more organisms are likely to be present in a lesion than after months of drug therapy have been administered. Consequently, triple-drug therapy for six weeks to three months has been advocated until the bacillary population has been reduced. Presumably, both completely sensitive and single drug resistant organisms would be eradicated at the same rate. Late in treatment, when smaller populations of bacilli exist, two drugs could be used and, perhaps after six months to one year, small enough numbers of viable organisms would be left to allow the administration of only one drug for the remainder of treatment. Such a regimen has been described by Wallace Fox and has appealed to this author because of its inherent logic and apparent effectiveness.

TABLE 16.2

Drug	Dose	Toxic effects	Allergic manifestations	Usefulness	Availability	Precautions and problems
Isoniazid (INH)	Adults: 3–5 mg/kg/d. Usually 300 mgm/day. Children: 10–20 mgm/kg/d. Not over 400 mgm/d.	Peripheral neuritis (0.3%). Rare neural toxicity. Rare hepatitis. Asymptomatic transaminase elevation (?10%)	0.1% incidence Skin rashes Fever Arthralgias Malaise	Best drug currently available for both treatment and prophylaxis. Orally administered.	Inexpensive. Commercially available. Often available through local Health Dept.	Pyridoxine given if dose greater than 5 mg/kg. Otherwise not necessary. Relatively nontoxic but very effective drug.
Ethambutal	15 mgm/kg/day	Retrobulbar neuritis, with central scotomato and loss of green perception if dose higher than recommended is given.	Rare skin rash	Probably second drug of choice today. Has replaced PASA in many areas. Never used alone to treat TB, always is accompanied by INH. Orally administered.	Relatively inexpensive. Available commercially. Often available through Health Dept.	Base-line and monthly visual acuity tests recommended but at proper dose, ophthalmic changes are rare.
PASA	200 mgm/kg/day. Usually 9–12 gm/day	10% incidence of GI distress. 0.1% goitrogenic. G-6-P.D. anemia	7.2% incidence Fever Rash Hepatitis (0.2%) Myalgia Arthralgia	Prior to ethambutal, was 2nd drug of choice. Numerous large pills and consequent stomach upset often led patient to skip this drug. Never should be used alone to treat TB. Good as companion drug to INH. Orally administered.	Inexpensive. Commercially available. Numerous preparations varied to help overcome gastric toxicity. Often available through Health Dept.	Always given with meals. May be given with antacids. May start with small dose and gradually increase to adequate levels.
Streptomycin	Adults: 15 mgm/kg/d. Usually 1 gm/d for 60–90 d, then 1 gm biweekly. Children: 20–40 mgm/kg/d. Not over 1 gm/d.	Vestibular dysfunction, vertigo, dizziness, nausea. (10–15% of patients receiving daily treatment for 2–3 mo). Rare renal injury. Rare peripheral neuropathy. Pain at injection site.	5.8% incidence Skin rash Fever (rare) Lymphadenopathy (rare) Blood dyscrasia (rare) Anaphylaxis (rare)	Injectable drug. Less useful in outpatient treatment. After initial daily course, biweekly treatment o.k. on OPD basis. Never should be used alone. Usually used as 3rd drug in triple therapy.	Commercially available.	Routine audiometry and BUN. Observation for signs of vestibular or auditory dysfunction.

Rifampin	Adult: 600 mgm/d.	Icterus with SGOT elevation. Transient leukopenia. Red-orange pigmenturia. G.I. upset—nausea and diarrhea.	Skin rash (rare)	Orally administered. Seems as effective as INH.	Recently released on market in U.S. Used extensively in Europe.	Appears to be relatively non-toxic, effective drug. Its place in therapy remains to be seen. Perhaps would be best to reserve this drug and PASA for treatment of tuberculosis resistant to INH, Streptomycin and Ethambutal.

Second Line Drugs: 1 Pyrizinamide, 2. Viomycin, 3. Kanamycin, 4. Capreomycin, 5. Cycloserine, 6. Ethionamide.

Corticosteroid Therapy

In the last 15 years, corticosteroid therapy has acquired a place in the treatment of certain types of tuberculous infection. Certainly, steroids should *never* be used alone, but rather in conjunction with effective antituberculous drug therapy. Those situations in which steroids have been found useful include the following:

(1) In extremely ill, toxic patients, the administration of corticosteroids will often improve the general clinical condition. This abrupt improvement may allow the patient to survive long enough for antituberculous drug therapy to act on the tuberculosis itself. The corticosteroids apparently make the patient better in some non-specific way, but do not affect the basic tuberculous infection.

(2) Proven tuberculous pleural effusions usually resolve under chemotherapy with or without complete drainage by thoracentesis. Occasionally, such an effusion will persist or reaccumulate over a period of months despite adequate antituberculous chemotherapy. In this situation, corticosteroid administration will often hasten resorption of the fluid.

(3) As mentioned above, uncontrolled studies have implied that concomitant corticosteroid therapy, early in the management of tuberculous pericarditis, may suppress inflammation and enhance reabsorption of the pericardial fluid. This author's limited personal experience would support this contention. Whether this early therapy will prevent later constrictive pericarditis is not known.

(4) Tuberculous meningitis has often been treated with supplemental steroids in order to prevent subsequent fibrosis at the base of the brain. Presumably, such treatment would decrease the incidence of post-inflammatory hydrocephalus. Recent controlled studies indicated that acute treatment with steroids (and antituberculous drugs) led to a more rapid fall in CSF pressure, less frequent herniation of the brain, increased survival, and more frequent return of cell counts, protein, and glucose to normal. The conclusion was that steroids were clearly indicated in the treatment of cerebral edema associated with the meningitis. Although the numbers were small, and the increased survival was therefore not statistically significant, the steroid-treated group had a 45 percent survival and the control 25 percent.

(5) Controlled studies have implied that primary tuberculosis in children, complicated by endobronchial disease, will resolve more quickly if treated with corticosteroids. The more usual primary tuberculosis without endobronchial manifestations will resolve promptly with antituberculous chemotherapy, and does not require the addition of steroid treatment.

Early Reversal of Infectiousness

As mentioned earlier, the observation that adequate drug therapy reduced the infectiousness of the tubercle organisms has revolutionized current ideas, both concerning isolation techniques and the length of hospitalization. In a study designed to assess the efficiency of ultraviolet light as a decontaminant, Riley *et al*, constructed a ventilation system that allowed all the air from the rooms of selected patients with tuberculosis to pass through guinea pig chambers. The subsequent rates of PPD conversion and clinical tuberculosis in the pigs were used as a measure of the infectiousness of those particular patients, as well as a measure of the beneficial effects of irradiation of the ventilation system. In this study, it was noticed that the air from the rooms of drug-treated, sputum-positive patients produced a markedly decreased incidence of guinea pig infections. It was stated by these authors that this was "highly suggestive evidence that drug therapy produces a prompt and striking reduction in infectiousness when the organisms were susceptible to the drug which is administered." Unfortunately, the promptness of this phenomenon was not then, and to date, still has not been quantitated.

Subsequent to this suggestive work, epidemiologic evidence has accumulated to strongly support the suggestion of reduced infectiousness due to drug therapy. Several studies have compared the incidence of PPD conversions among exposed hospital personnel in the pre-chemotherapy as opposed to the post-chemotherapy era. The conversion rate during nursing school training was noted to have fallen from 66 percent in the years 1948 to 1951 to 3.5 percent between 1959–1964. Similarly, the conversion rate in VA hospital personnel had fallen to 2.3 percent for the year 1963. This phenomenon was attributed to both the use of drug therapy and better understanding of isolation techniques.

Additional, strongly supportive, data has been reported from India where large numbers of tuberculosis patients were randomly allocated to either in-hospital or home treatment programs. Both groups received INH and PAS; both did equally well in arresting the tuberculous infection. Follow-up studies were performed to assess the incidence of tuberculosis in the close family contacts of the two groups. It was found that *no added risk* of infection in contacts occurred as a result of the outpatient treatment for the entire course of chemotherapy. The incidence of active tuberculosis was no greater in the contacts of patients treated at home than in the contacts of patients treated in the sanitorium, either in the first year or over the subsequent four years. The major risk to the contacts of both groups resulted from exposure of the patient *prior to diagnosis*.

Based upon such data, in various parts of the United States, the sanitoria have been closed and outpatient treatment of tuberculosis has been instituted. As a result, numerous patients are treated at home who would have previously been considered to be infectious on the basis of positive sputum cultures or smears. The fact that new case rates of tuberculosis continue to decline in these areas lends further support to the contention that such drug-treated patients are at least relatively non-infectious. Current thinking would suggest, therefore, that indications for long term hospitalization would be based on severe, debilitating, clinical disease or unreliability on the part of the patient in taking drug therapy. Unfortunately, tuberculosis often occurs in unreliable patients and the latter indication warrants many prolonged hospitalizations.

The unsolved question, however, relates to the duration of drug therapy necessary to reduce infectiousness. A rule of thumb used at this author's hospital is to isolate the tuberculous patient for one to two weeks and to discharge him to home care when clinical manifestations allow and when reliability is assured. Fortunately, primary multiple drug resistance is rare and such drug resistant organisms appear to be less infectious than the usual *Mycobacterium tuberculosis*. Hopefully, further research will elucidate the exact timing, incidence, and predictability of this early reversal of infectiousness.

Summary

Spread of tuberculosis from person to person occurs by inhalation of organisms contained in droplet nuclei. The resultant primary infection and the subsequent re-exacerbation of disease can be logically explained by the "unitary concept" of the pathogenesis of tuberculosis. Proper isolation techniques should be related to the proposed method of contagion. Proper control measures should be related to the pathogensis of active disease and to the probability, in given population groups, of the occurrence of primary or re-exacerbation type of disease. Selected aspects of the clinical spectrum of tuberculosis are presented with emphasis on practical means of diagnosis and treatment. A brief listing of available chemotherapeutic agents and a rationale for drug therapy are discussed. The indications for concomitant corticosteroid therapy are enumerated and the current theory of early reversal of infectiousness with adequate drug therapy is presented.

SELECTED REFERENCES

Chemoprophylaxis for the Prevention of Tuberculosis. A Report of the Ad Hoc Committee on Chemoprophylaxis. Am. Rev. Resp. Dis., *96*:558, 1967.

Comstock, G. W. and Webster, R. G.: Tuberculosis studies in Muscogee County, Georgia. VII. A twenty-year evaluation of BCG vaccination in a school population. Am. Rev. Resp. Dis., *100*:839, 1969.

Dawson, J. J. Y., Devadatta, S., Fox, W., *et al.*: A 5-year-study of patients with pulmonary tuberculosis in a concurrent comparison of home and sanatorium treatment for one year with isoniazid plus PAS. Bull. Wld. Health Org., *34*:533, 1966.

Diagnostic Standards and Classification of Tuberculosis. National Tuberculosis and Respiratory Disease Association, New York, 1969.

Fox, W.: The John Barnwell Lecture. Changing concepts in the chemotherapy of pulmonary tuberculosis. Am. Rev. Resp. Dis., *97*:767, 1968.

Horne, N. W.: A critical evaluation of corticosteroids in tuberculosis. Adv. Tuberc. Res., *15*:1, 1966.

Infectiousness of Tuberculosis. A Report of the NTA Ad Hoc Committee on Treatment of TB Patients in General Hospitals. Am. Rev. Resp. Dis., *96*:836, 1967.

Johnson, J. E., III.: *Rational Therapy and Control of Tuberculosis,* Univ. of Fla. Press, Gainesville, Florida, 1970.

Johnson, J. R., Turk, T. L. and MacDonald, F. M.: Corticosteroids in pulmonary tuberculosis. III. Indications. Am. Rev. Resp. Dis., *96*:62, 1967.

Johnston, R. F. and Hopewell, P. C.: Chemotherapy of pulmonary tuberculosis. Ann. Int. Med., *70*:359, 1969.

Kamat, S. R., Dawson, J. J. Y., Devadatta, S., *et al.*: A controlled study of the influence of segregation of tuberculous patients for one year on the attack rate of tuberculosis in a 5-year period in close family contacts in South India. Bull. Wld. Health Org., *34*:517, 1966.

Kent, D. C. and Schwartz, R.: Active pulmonary tuberculosis with negative tuberculin skin reactions. Am. Rev. Resp. Dis., *95*:411, 1967.

Landi, S., Held, H. R., Harschild, A. H. W. and Hilscheimer, R.: Absorption of tuberculin PPD to glass and plastic surfaces. Bull. Wld. Health. Org., *35*:593, 1966.

Lattimer, J. K.: Renal tuberculosis. N. Eng. J. Med., *273*:208, 1965.

Levine, H., Metzger, W., Lacere, D. and Kay, L.: Diagnosis of tuberculous pleurisy by culture of pleural biopsy specimen. Arch. Int. Med., *126*:269, 1970.

Levine, I.: Tuberculosis risk in students of nursing. Arch. Int. Med., *121*:545, 1968.

O'Grady, F. and Riley, R. L.: Experimental airborne tuberculosis. Adv. Tuberc. Res., *12*:150, 1963.

O'Toole, R. D., Thornton, G. F., Mukhergee, M. K. and Nath, R. L.: Dexamethasone in tuberculous meningitis. Relationship of cerebrospinal fluid effects to therapeutic efficiency. Ann. Int. Med., *70*:39, 1969.

Palmer, C. E. and Edwards, L. B.: Identifying the tuberculous infected. J.A.M.A., *205*:167, 1968.

Riley, R. L.: Airborne pulmonary tuberculosis. Bacteriol. Rev., *25*:243, 1961.

Riley, R. L.: Apical localization of pulmonary tuberculosis. Bull. Johns Hop. Hosp., *106*:232, 1960.

Riley, R. L., Mills, C. C., O'Grady, F., *et al.*: Infectiousness of air from a tuberculosis ward. Ultraviolet irradiation of infected air: comparative infectiousness of different patients. Am. Rev. Resp. Dis., *85*:511, 1962.

Riley, R. L.: The hazard is relative. Am. Rev. Resp. Dis., *96*:623, 1967.

Rooney, J. J., Crocco, J. A. and Lyons, H. A.: Tuberculous pericarditis. Ann. Int. Med., *72*:73, 1970.

Scharer, L. and McClement, J. H.: Isolation of tubercle bacilli from needle biopsy specimens of parietal pleura. Am. Rev. Resp. Dis., *97*:466, 1968.

Singh, M. M., Bhargava, A. N. and Jain, K. P.: Tuberculous peritonitis, an evaluation of pathogenetic mechanisms, diagnostic procedures and therapeutic measures. N. Eng. J. Med., *281*:1091, 1969.

Smith, D. T.: Diagnostic and prognostic significance of the quantitative tuberculin tests. The influence of subclinical infections with atypical mycobacteria. Ann. Int. Med., *67*:919, 1967.

Stead, W. W.: Pathogenesis of a first episode of chronic pulmonary tuberculosis in man: Recrudescence of residuals of the primary infection or exogenous reinfection? Am. Rev. Resp. Dis., *95*:729, 1966.

Stead, W. W.: Pathogenesis of the sporadic case of tuberculosis. N. Eng. J. Med., *277*:1008, 1967.

Therapy of Pleural Effusion. A Statement by the Committee on Therapy. Am. Rev. Resp. Dis., *97*:479, 1968.

Zuck, M. B. and Fulkerson, L. L.: Clinical reliability of stabilized and nonstabilized tuberculin PPD. Am. Rev. Resp. Dis., *102*:91, 1970.

Chapter 17

HISTOPLASMOSIS

Histoplasmosis is a common infectious, non-contagious disease caused by *Histoplasma capsulatum*, a dimorphic fungus with nearly world-wide distribution. In humans the fungus is intracellular, parasitizes the reticuloendothelial cells, and may involve any organ of the body singly or in multiples, giving rise to a variety of manifestations of illness.

In 1905 Samuel Darling, two years after graduation from medical school and while serving as a pathologist in the Canal Zone, described the first three human infections of histoplasmosis. Since the fungus resembles a large encapsulated plasmodium engulfed by histiocytes, he mistook it for a protozoan and named it *Histoplasma capsulatum*. Darling actually believed he had found a variety of Kala-azar.

Histoplasmosis remained an autopsy curiosity until 1934 when Dodd and Tompkins made the first antemortem diagnosis. The fungus was recovered from this patient and used by DeMonbreun to study its characteristics in culture and animal infections.

Christie and Petersen in 1945 used a culture filtrate of the fungus (histoplasmin) to skin test 181 children in an orphanage outside of Nashville. Seventy-four percent of these children demonstrated a positive skin reaction. These investigators suggested that histoplasmosis was responsible for the many individuals with pulmonary calcifications and negative tuberculin tests and postulated that the disease was commonly a mild or asymptomatic infection.

Palmer skin tested 10,000 nursing students with histoplasmin and demonstrated the high incidence of endemic infection among residents in the Mississippi River valley and east central United States regions. In addition, she incriminated histoplasmosis as the commonest cause of pulmonary calcification in the United States.

Today there are an estimated 30 million individuals in the United States with positive skin reactions to histoplasmin. Another 500,000 develop this immunological marker of presumed infection each year.

Morphology and Pathogenesis

H. capsulatum is a dimorphic fungus growing as a mold in its natural soil habitat but changing to a yeast when infecting an animal or human. In soil the growth of the fungus is sparse. It reproduces by two types of spores. The spherical conidia (spores) are 2 to 4 μ in diameter and when inhaled by man easily reach the alveoli. The macroconidia are 8 to 14 μ in diameter. The spores are not airborne for any appreciable distance. The yeast phase seen in human infection is similar to any other budding yeast. If cultures are maintained at 37°C, the yeast form persists while cultures of *H. capsulatum* at ambient temperature characteristically grow as a mold.

Like most fungal infections there is little understanding of the pathogenicity of *H. capsulatum.* It does not elaborate any known toxin. It is never part of the normal flora of the human body. Man and animals are infected through the inhalation of spores from an environmental source. Contagion is unknown. The manifestations of human infection appear to be related to the quantity of infectious material inhaled by the infected person and his state of health at the time of exposure.

The mouse is peculiarly susceptible to experimental infection by *H. capsulatum.* Either a single macroconidium or a few yeast cells injected intraperitoneally will infect the mouse. Although only a few organisms are required to infect a mouse, it requires more than a million yeast delivered intravenously to kill a mouse. The mouse serves as an excellent laboratory vehicle to isolate the fungus from soil samples.

H. capsulatum infection stimulates antibody formation in man and animals. Although these immunological reactions are helpful in diagnosis, there are no proven relationships between any antibody formation and host resistance.

Pathology

Virtually all the early patients diagnosed as having histoplasmosis represented disseminated disease. This was uniformly fatal and the early pathology reports of this illness focused on this form of the infection. By means of biopsies and cultures the illness is now recognized antemortem. Actually, lung resections of solitary nodules now yield the greatest source of tissue specimens with *H. capsulatum.*

In disseminated disease the organism is contained within the reticuloendothelial system. Histiocytes which engulf the fungi are increased individually in size and in total numbers. This accounts for the characteristic enlargement of the lymph nodes, liver and spleen seen in this illness. Since reticuloendothelial cells are present in reasonable numbers in the mucous membranes of the mouth and intestinal tract, enlargement and multiplication of these cells occurs, and ulceration may take place. Caseous necrosis, particularly in the adrenal glands, may develop. The organisms do collect anywhere in the human body and account for such rare manifestations of illness as cerebral abscesses, mediastinitis and endocarditis. Some heart valve lesions have suggested in pathological specimens a transitional form of the fungus with well developed hyphae in evidence along with budding yeasts.

Within the histiocyte, *H. capsulatum* is a small oval body between 1 and 4 μ in diameter. The fungus appears to have a rigid wall and in the process of tissue fixation, the protoplasm retracts from the wall and gives the false appearance of a capsule. It was this pseudo capsule that mislead Darling in his original description of the disease and accounts for the incorrect designation of *H. capsulatum*. The fungus is easily seen with ordinary hematoxylin and eosin stain. Although it may be confused with leishmania or toxoplasma, this difficulty is resolved by the use of special fungal stains.

For years pathologists have reported some resected lung tissue as morphologically compatible with tuberculosis but with no mycobacterium demonstrated. Unquestionably many of these specimens represented lung tissue infected with *H. capsulatum*. Typically the lung presents a histologic pattern of epithelioid cell granulomas sometimes including Langhan's giant cells. Necrosis and calcification of the central portion of the lesions occur while fibrosis is characteristic of the periphery. If the lung lesions are large, cavitation takes place.

The solitary nodule resulting from *H. capsulatum* at times is pathologically obscure. In size the lesion may vary from less than a cm. to 4–5 cm. in diameter. The lesion may show little more than a fibrotic surface enclosing some caseous and calcific material. Usually hematoxylin and eosin staining does not demonstrate any fungi. Fungi are sometimes seen, not always clearly, with special fungal stains such as the Gridley or periodic acid Schiff reaction. There are no histiocytes in these lesions as they presumably have degenerated. These old yeast cells in a solitary nodule need to be differentiated from endospores of *Coccidioides immitis*, from *Cryptococcus neoformans* and some forms of *Blastomyces dermatidis*.

Variations in the pathology of histoplasmosis do occur. In patients recovering from disseminated histoplasmosis there may be wide-spread calcific lesions which histologically resemble the solitary nodule. Tiny granulomatous lesions are sometimes seen in the liver and spleen as incidental findings. With special stains some of them do demonstrate the fungus.

Histoplasma duboisii causes a variety of histoplasmosis in which the clinical features are skin lesions, subcutaneous abscesses and osteolytic lesions of cranial bones. This fungus is limited to tropical Africa.

Epidemiology

Histoplasmosis in man results from the exposure of a susceptible individual to an environment peculiarly suitable to the growth of the infecting fungus. Anything which disturbs this environment, such as excavations, tearing down abandoned buildings or cleaning chicken coops, increases the number of spores dispersed into the air. The number of people infected and the severity of infection appear to be related to the nearness of individuals to the environmental source, the quantity of spores inhaled, and the state of health of the people exposed.

The limits of human infection are geographically determined by the unique ecological arrangements which permit the growth of *H. capsulatum*. In general, the major river valleys of the United States, the Mississippi, Missouri, and Ohio have been recognized as the major regions of histoplasmosis infection. Throughout the world, this geographical association of human infection by *H. capsulatum* with large river valleys persists. The Amazon, Orinoco, and La Plata River valleys of South America and the Congo and Niger river valleys of Africa maintain similar suitable environments for the growth of this fungus.

Most infections in man have been limited to latitudes between 45° north and 30° south of the equator. Climatological maps superimposed on population areas with high skin reactivity to histoplasmin indicate strong correlations to the number of days with temperatures between 66–90°F and relative humidity in excess of 50 percent.

Maps of population which depict the high percentage of skin reactions in certain locations fail to show, however, the truly splotchy environmental characteristics of human infection. Adjacent counties, even adjacent farms, will vary among their inhabitants from nearly uniform skin reactivity to histoplasmin to virtually none. This means that the environmental foci responsible for fungus growth and subsequent human infection are small and sharply demarcated. Not surprisingly, epidemics often occur in areas of low skin reactivity to histoplasmin following exposure of susceptible individuals to a suitable environment harboring the fungus. As already mentioned, the spores of *H. capsulatum* are not airborne for any distance. There is either a mechanical disruption of the growing fungus or else man must come in very close contact with the fungus in order to inhale the spores.

Residents of South Carolina have less than a three percent incidence of skin reactivity to histoplasmin. Sellers and coworkers, however, reported in 1964 an epidemic of acute histoplasmosis among residents of Greenwood, South Carolina, following land excavation for a golf course. Erythema nodosum and multiforme were prominent manifestations of infection in nearly 40 patients. Local school children were skin tested with histoplasmin and the percentage of positive reactors varied from 0 to 98. The differences in positive skin reactions correlated with the distance the children lived from the golf course and the relation of their houses to the prevailing winds at the time of construction. This illustrates how a major epidemic of histoplasmosis occurs in an area of low endemicity.

In Florida there are virtually no individuals among life-time residents of the state who demonstrate positive skin reactions to histoplasmin. Recently, however, Johnson *et al.*, reported a college student at the University of Florida who contracted acute pulmonary histoplasmosis while exploring a cave in Northern Florida known to contain many bats. Some of the bats and bat guano in the caves in this region were cultured and found to have *H. capsulatum*. Members of the University Cave Explorers Club were found to have 71 percent incidence of skin sensitivity to histoplasmin. There was essentially no skin reactivity to histoplasmin found among the rural residents in the vicinity of the cave. These studies confirm the relationship between specific environmental foci and infection in man only after close exposure to these locations.

In 1949 Emmons made the first isolation of *H. capsulatum* from soil adjacent to a rodent burrow in Loudon County, Virginia. Since then there have been numerous isolations of the fungus from the soil. Some of these isolations have occurred in locations which correlated closely with either family or community epidemics of histoplasmosis. There is a definite relationship between the frequency of positive soil samples for *H. capsulatum* and the incidence of positive skin reactions to histoplasmin by nearby residents. This skin reactivity includes not only man but domestic animals such as dogs, cats, cattle, horses, and sheep. The percent of skin reactivity to histoplasmin among these animals closely parallels that of man when compared to the similar years of exposure to a common environment.

Soil isolations of *H. capsulatum* have been associated with the habits of birds, particularly starlings and chickens. The fungus is commonly recovered from soil that has been contaminated with excreta from these birds. Histoplasmosis has not been demonstrated in any avians, perhaps because their basic temperature, 40 to 42°C, does not permit the growth of the fungus. The fungus has never been isolated from fresh bird excreta. This has led to the postulation that the excreta enriches the soil to favor an environment capable of sustaining the growth of the fungus.

There have been numerous family epidemics related to cleaning an old chicken coop or silo or moving into a long-standing empty house. No longer, however, is histoplasmosis considered an infection of only rural inhabitants. Emmons has cultured the fungus in downtown Washington, D.C., usually from soil beneath trees which serve as starling roosts. During the fall of 1962 an epidemic of histoplasmosis occurred in Mason City, Iowa. The source of the infection was a large starling roost near the central business district. The epidemic was precipitated by cutting down trees which served as starling roosts and clearing the area with bulldozers. Two years later another epidemic of histoplasmosis occurred when a second attempt was made to clear the land.

Several years ago the source of infection of an infant with disseminated histoplasmosis was traced to the presence of the fungus in a feather pillow. Investigators were subsequently able to show that the fungus is recoverable from the tips of feathers of chickens injected intravenously with *H. capsulatum*. The temperature of the feathers of chickens is significantly less than body temperature and may account for the growth of the fungus. The epidemiological significance of this is speculative, however, as the fungus has never been cultured from feathers of birds in normal situations.

Pigeon habitats have been incorrectly identified with histoplasmosis. There have been no isolations of *H. capsulatum* from either pigeons or pigeon droppings encrusted on buildings. *Cryptococcus neoformans* is, however, commonly recovered from these locations.

Within the last ten years, studies have suggested that the bat may play an important relationship to histoplasmosis infection of man. The bat, a mammal, does become infected with the fungus which can be isolated from its liver, lung and spleen. Freshly excreted bat guano frequently contains *H. capsulatum*. The migratory habits of some species of bats appear to be superimposable upon the geographical regions with populations with high percentages of skin reactivity to histoplasmin. Bats live in caves and the major caves of the United States also coincide with the large river valleys. Speleologists demonstrate high incidence of positive histoplasmin skin reactions. "Cave fever," in retrospect, could very well have been a descriptive term for acute pulmonary infection in man caused by *H. capsulatum*. House bats have also been found to be infected with this fungus. This would represent another source of infection in both rural and urban areas.

The exact ecologic arrangements among bat, *H. capsulatum* and environment remain unclear. There is uncertainty whether the bat is infected, much like man, from exposure to the fungus, or whether the infection of the bat, and excretion of the fungus by the bat contributes significantly to the establishment of the fungus in nature and subsequent infection of man.

Some of the epidemiological characteristics described for histoplasmosis are similar for other fungi. Most fungal infections in man are the result of certain environmental contacts. The geographical limitation to the southwest of infection by *Coccidioides inimites* is comparable to the relationship between a special environment and infection by *H. capsulatum*. *Candida albicans* is an opportunistic pathogen normally found on human mucus membranes. Candidiasis occurs only in the gravely ill patients with obviously impaired host defense mechanisms. The environmental source of the fungus in blastomycoses remains obscure. Cryptococcosis in man probably results from exposure to the fungus which is commonly associated with pigeon excreta.

Clinical Patterns of Histoplasmosis

The manifestations of illness resulting from the infection of man by *H. capsulatum* result from the interaction of the infecting organism and the host defense mechanisms of man. The variation of clinical illness, therefore, depends partly on the quantity of infecting fungus and the state of health of the individual infected.

Any organ or group of organs may be infected. The literature is replete with case reports describing such clinical entities as mediastinitis, endocarditis, choroiditis and meningitis caused by *H. capsulatum,* clearly indicating the ability of this organism to invade any tissue. Nevertheless, there are common patterns of histoplasmosis infection in man that do permit, albeit arbitrary, clinical classifications of this disease.

Inapparent Infection

Estimates vary, but there are probably greater than 30 million people in the United States who demonstrate a positive skin reaction to histoplasmin. It is unusual, however, for a physician practicing in even a highly endemic area, to recognize more than an occasional person with histoplasmosis. The obvious conclusion is that virtually all infections go undiagnosed. When recent individuals who have converted from a negative to positive histoplasmin skin test are followed by serial chest x-rays, approximately one-third will develop calcified pulmonary lesions. In epidemics of histoplasmosis with a known point source of infection, many individuals experience only a brief "flu-like" illness. Others are totally asymptomatic and their infection is inapparent except for the development of skin test reactivity to histoplasmin.

Acute Pulmonary Histoplasmosis

This represents the most commonly diagnosed type of histoplasmosis. Approximately two weeks after exposure to a source of fungus, patients will manifest any collection of symptoms and signs heralding pulmonary infection. There may be cough, hemoptysis, pleuritic chest pain and dyspnea. Non-specific symptomatology includes weakness, fever, myalgia and weight loss. X-ray findings are equally variable. There may be diffuse infiltrates, scattered nodules, consolidation, but rarely pulmonary effusion. The x-ray findings often mimic either atypical pneumonia or miliary tuberculosis. Thrombophlebitis is a common complication and pulmonary infarction is not rare.

In epidemics of acute pulmonary histoplasmosis erythema nodosum may in some patients follow the pulmonary symptoms or by itself be associated with subsequent positive histoplasmin skin test and complement fixation titers. Erythema nodosum is markedly more common in women although histoplasmosis is more common in men.

Although the major symptomatology reflects the predominant pulmonary involvement of acute histoplasmosis, subsequent splenic calcifications indicate hematogenous dissemination occurs during the infection. The pulmonary lesions either resolve completely or calcify. The latter leads to either diffuse miliary califications or occasional solitary lesions, histoplasmomas, which will be discussed separately. Clinically patients may appear desperately ill, but invariably they recover completely after an illness lasting several weeks.

Chronic Pulmonary Histoplasmosis

Chronic lung infection from H. *capsulatum* is common. It mimics chronic pulmonary tuberculosis in every way. It favors the apices of the lung, may develop thick or thin walled cavities, causes the production of mucopurulent sputum and results in chronic cough, chest pain, weight loss, malaise and fatigue. Bronchiectasis is common in the involved lung areas. Pleural effusion also occurs. Hemoptysis, unlike tuberculosis, is rare in chronic pulmonary histoplasmosis.

This type of histoplasmosis develops insidiously and does not appear to be a progression from the acute pulmonic infection. The disease is frequently mistaken for tuberculosis despite negative acid-fast cultures and tuberculin tests. Sputum cultures for the fungus are usually positive. Approximately 50 percent of patients with proven diagnosis of chronic pulmonary histoplasmosis are dead within five years. The majority of infections are slowly progressive and often fatal if untreated. Pulmonary disorders such as emphysema and pulmonary hypertension do develop if the disease remains progressive and involves large portions of pulmonary tissue.

In the early 1960's it was estimated that between one and two percent of patients admitted to tuberculosis sanatoriums in Missouri and Tennessee actually had pulmonary histoplasmosis. An awareness of this confusion has hopefully led to the use of appropriate diagnostic tests to distinguish between these illnesses. Some patients do have both infections simultaneously.

Histoplasmoma

Patients recovering from acute pulmonary histoplasmosis frequently develop pulmonary calcifications. Residual infiltrates on chest x-ray may be either small diffuse miliary lesions or an individual "coin-like" lesion. These "coin-like" lesions caused by *H. capsulatum* are called histoplasmomas. The importance of pulmonary histoplasmomas are that they are sometimes indistinguishable from lung tumors. In areas where histoplasmosis is endemic, lung resection because of a possible malignant lesion often yields tissue which on appropriate staining gives evidence of histoplasmosis. Relying on calcification as a sole measure of benignity is not possible because the host response to some bronchogenic tumors occasionally produces calcium. Previous x-rays and positive histoplasmin skin tests may give helpful evidence as to whether surgery is indicated. Nevertheless, prudent judgment will still result in surgical resection of many of these benign lesions.

Acute Disseminated Histoplasmosis

Human infection with *H. capsulatum,* particularly among the very young or those patients with decreased host resistance, is occasionally a rapidly, overwhelming disseminated infection. The blood stream distribution of the fungus results in at one time or another involvement of virtually every organ system. Characteristic of acute disseminated histoplasmosis are miminal pulmonary manifestations. Spiking daily temperatures of 104 or more are common. Hepatomegaly and splenomegaly are usually present. Symptomatology reflects the varying organ involvement and may present as Addison's disease, meningitis, endocarditis, mediastinitis and so on. Acute disseminated histoplasmosis causes no specific hematological response. Leukopenia with relative lymphocytosis is most common but rarely a gamut of apparent blood dyscrasis may coexist. A hematological picture compatible with pancytopenia, acute leukemia or infectious mononucleosis has also been reported in disseminated histoplasmosis. Clinical presentations are virtually limitless. At one time this form of histoplasmosis was considered invariably fatal with the outcome determined in six weeks. Treatment is now successful in preventing fatality. Also, patients are being recognized who have recovered spontaneously from this illness.

Skin tests are usually negative. This is not surprising if one considers it may take up to six weeks for the patient to demonstrate skin reactivity. Serological tests are positive. Cultures of blood, bone marrow or biopsy material are frequently positive.

Chronic Disseminated Histoplasmosis

The breakdown of disseminated histoplasmosis into acute and chronic illness is obviously arbitrary, similar to the old descriptions of acute and subacute bacterial endocarditis. Although this form of histoplasmosis may occur at any age, it is more common over the age of 40. Symptomatology is similar to any chronic infection. Fever, weakness, fatigue, anorexia and weight loss are common. Other symptoms represent the specific organ involved. This form of histoplasmosis occurs commonly as an opportunistic infection, complicating such clinical problems as bronchogenic carcinoma, diabetes mellitus, lymphomas, and prolonged therapy with corticosteroids and immunosuppressive agents. If this infection is recognized and treated with appropriate dosage of amphotericin, and death from a complication of underlying illness does not ensue, most patients will recover from their infection. Without treatment, prognosis is poor and death occurs within weeks or months.

With pulmonary involvement, sputum cultures are usually positive. Between two-thirds or three-fourths of the patients will demonstrate significant complement fixation titers. Skin tests are variable, more becoming positive as the illness is prolonged. Frequently the diagnosis is made through biopsy of superficial ulcers, bone marrow or lymph nodes. All biopsy material should be cultured for fungi. The scalene nodes often yield positive results with pulmonary involvement. Although liver involvement is considered a common finding, a recent report of 25 patients with progressive disseminated histoplasmosis showed hepatic disease in only two of nine patients autopsied.

Miscellaneous

There remains a varied collection of patients infected with histoplasmosis who defy any rigid or simple classification. Occasionally patients are reported with ulcers of the lips, larynx, glottis or skin caused by *H. capsulatum*. Although these lesions may rarely represent a primary cutaneous form of histoplasmosis, more commonly they are associated with a disseminated form of disease. Histoplasmosis may involve the adrenal glands and, in fact, is probably the leading cause of Addison's disease in endemic areas. Mediastinal fibrosis with subsequent obstruction of the superior vena cava is another histoplasmosis curiosity. This particular clinical picture may or may not be associated with discernible pulmonary lesions.

Ocular lesions in the uveal tract have been suggested as another clinical manifestation of histoplasmosis. The evidence remains circumstantial as the fungus has never been cultured from the uvea and uveitis is not more frequent in patients with proven histoplasmosis.

Histoplasmin Skin Test

Histoplasmin is prepared from a broth filtrate of a culture of *H. capsulatum* and standardized against reference products obtained from the National Institutes of Health. 0.1 ml. of standardized material is injected intradermally into the forearm. The test is interpreted similarly to the tuberculin test. A positive reaction is induration of 5 mm. or greater 48 or 72 hours after testing.

There is cross reactivity between histoplasmin antigens and antigens included in the skin test materials for blastomycosis and coccidioidomycosis. Usually skin reactivity appears four or more weeks after infection. Once a person has acquired skin sensitivity to histoplasmin, it persists for a lifetime. Rarely it may be suppressed by severe or terminal illness.

In endemic areas skin reactivity to histoplasmin is uncommon among infants. It begins to appear around age three and in some locations the annual conversion rate of the population is 10 percent. It is not unusual for more than 80 percent of the adult population to demonstrate a positive histoplasmin reaction. There is evidence that there may be a slight decrease in skin reactivity among the aged.

Histoplasmin skin testing has been of greatest use in epidemiological studies. Persons demonstrating positive skin reactions to histoplasmin usually reside in humid, temperate or equatorial climates. There are few reactors to histoplasmin in Europe, eastern Mediterranean countries or in Asia. Animals demonstrate skin reactivity to histoplasmin in geographical settings similar to man.

Between 1945 and 1951 the Public Health Service reported on 68,452 young adult men and women who had positive skin reactions to histoplasmin and were lifetime residents of single counties in the United States. The greatest number of individuals with histoplasmin skin sensitivity reside in the east central United States. In some localities more then 80 percent of the residents react to histoplasmin. Histoplasmin sensitivity is uncommon among lifetime residents of New England, the northwest and south atlantic states.

Skin sensitivity to histoplasmin among residents of the Southwest, usually represents cross reactions resulting from coccidioidomycosis rather than infection from *H. capsulatum*.

Recently a histoplasmin tine test has been developed. The major advantage of the tine test is the ease of administration. Studies comparing it to the standard intradermal Mantoux test are inconclusive. Some demonstrate good correlation between the two tests. Others indicate that the intradermal histoplasmin test may yield more positive reactors than the tine histoplasmin test when both are given to the same group.

Serological Reactions

Patients infected with *H. capsulatum* demonstrate changes in their serum which are detectable by classical serological techniques. Tests vary according to the antigen used and the type of antibody reaction performed.

Antigens are derived from both the yeast and mycelial growth forms of the fungus. The antigen obtained from the mycelial phase is similar to the histoplasmin used for skin testing. Yeast cells are used as antigens either intact or disrupted.

Complement Fixations Tests

Complement fixation tests are commonly used to aid in the diagnosis of histoplasmosis. Either the intact yeast cell or histoplasmin is used as antigen. In patients with acute pulmonary histoplasmosis, complement fixation titers appear within three weeks, peak at six weeks and decline rapidly by four months. In patients with chronic disseminated or chronic pulmonary infection, high titers persist for long periods of time. In severe, overwhelming infections low or negative titers are frequently present. The exact level of a significant titer depends on the test performed. A four-fold increase in titer during an acute infection with *H. capsulatum* is strong evidence of infection. A positive histoplasmin skin test in a healthy individual can result in a positive titer or a rise on a low titer, particularly when histoplasmin is used as the testing antigen for complement fixation.

Precipitin Test

In the majority of patients with acute histoplasmosis, serum precipitating antibodies are present to antigens of *H. capsulatum*. Highest and most prolonged titers are to histoplasmin. This antigen, therefore, is commonly used in this test. Significant titers appear in two weeks and reach their peak around three weeks. In patients known to have histoplasmosis, titers of 1:8 appear significant although a changing titer is more conclusive. Titers persist for six or more months.

Agglutination Tests

These tests are accomplished by coating colloidion or latex particles with histoplasmin. Positive sera cause these particles to clump visibly. Titers in acute histoplasmosis parallel those of the complement fixation according to time of appearance. There is little reaction to these antigens with sera from patients with chronic histoplasmosis.

Unfortunately these serological tests used to identify histoplasmosis are not specific. There is significant crossover to blastomycosis and less to coccidioidomycosis. Antigens from these two fungi do react with sera from patients with histoplasmosis and *H. capsulatum* antigens react with sera from patients with either *Blastomyces dematitidis* or *Coccidioides immitis* infections. In fact, there may be comparable titers in sera from patients with histoplasmosis to either *H. capsulatum* or *B. dermatitidis* antigens.

Generally 80 percent of patients with acute histoplasmosis will have a measurable antibody by any one of the tests. This approaches 90 percent if more than one test is used. Most important is the demonstration of a changing titer over a period of time which may often be the strongest or only evidence of recent infection with *H. capsulatum*.

Many infectious diseases elicite a predictable immunoglobulin response. Characteristically there is an initial rise in IgM antibody levels, a subsequent increase in IgA, and later a rise in IgG. Human immunoglobulin reactions to mycotic infections differ.

Immunoglobulin response in patients with acute histoplasmosis reveals an early rise of IgM followed by an increase in IgA and IgG. Patients with chronic histoplasmosis have very high IgA levels and normal IgM and IgG. Latex agglutinating antibody is in the IgM fraction; precipitating antibody in the IgG; complement fixation antibody predominantly in the IgG with a little in the IgM.

Diagnosis

The greatest asset to the diagnosis of histoplasmosis is suspicion on the part of the attending physician. If the physician understands the epidemiology of the disease, the relationships of the peculiar environmental foci which permit the fungus to produce human infection, the diagnosis will be facilitated.

The majority of human infections with *H. capsulatum* go unrecognized. A practicing physician in a highly endemic area sees only a few patients with histoplasmosis. Most of these represent acute and chronic pulmonary disease. Half a million people in this country convert yearly from negative to positive histoplasmin skin reactions. Virtually all of them manifest no significant clinical illness. A survey of elementary school children in Frederick County, Maryland, revealed that 26 percent of the second graders and 42 percent of the sixth graders had positive histoplasmin skin reactions. There were 1,924 students tested in this study. Any illness which apparently involved 16 percent of this defined population group during a four year period is nearly of epidemic proportions. Yet there were no clinical correlations of any kind despite this immunological evidence of human infection.

Any acute pneumonitis whose etiology remains unknown and which fails to respond to antibiotics suggests histoplasmosis. Sputum cultures are of little help in diagnosing acute pulmonary histoplasmosis, but occasionally the urine culture will yield the fungus, illustrating the fungemia which invariably occurs with this infection. At times it is difficult to differentiate the pneumonitis from pulmonary infarction or primary atypical pneumonia. The history of possible exposure (exploring a cave, recent nearby excavation) in a young adult male is helpful. Serological titers are often the only recourse to establish a presumptive diagnosis of histoplasmosis. There are no characteristics of the pulmonary infiltrate on x-ray which give a clue to the cause of this infection.

Chronic pulmonary histoplasmosis mimics chronic tuberculosis. Symptomatology is similar in both. Skin tests which are positive for one or the other infection are helpful. Sputum cultures do give positive results particularly in cavitary disease. Gastric and bronchial washings are also sometimes helpful in yielding positive cultures for *H. capsulatum.*

Disseminated histoplasmosis is a rare disease. With lymphadenopathy and hepatosplenomegaly, it is often mistaken for a lymphomatous process. Frequently it represents an opportunistic infection in individuals with a lymphoma or other debilitating disease. Biopsy material from bone marrow, liver or lymph node is frequently diagnostic. Fungal cultures of the biopsied material should also be done along with cultures of the blood and urine. Scrapings from superficial ulcers often yield *H. capsulatum* on smear and culture.

Not only must the clinician suspect the diagnosis of histoplasmosis, but it is equally important for the microbiologist working in the clinical laboratory to be skillful in handling cultures of fungi. *H. capsulatum* is a fastidious microorganism, slow to grow and difficult to culture.

Treatment

There was no therapeutic agent of any significant value in the treatment of histoplasmosis until 1955 when amphotericin B was isolated from a strain of streptomyces. Before the use of this drug in histoplasmosis infection, disseminated disease was uniformly fatal. A follow-up study of 100 untreated patients with chronic pulmonary disease revealed a 50 percent 5-year mortality and progression of disease in another 18 percent of patients.

Improvement in prognosis of patients with these forms of histoplasmosis will vary from series to series depending on the selection of patient treated with amphotericin B. In one report 238 patients with chronic pulmonary disease were treated with amphotericin alone. Five-year mortality of these patients was reduced to 28 percent. Patients treated with amphotericin and surgery or surgery alone did not fare any better than those treated only with amphotericin. Another recent study documented the effectiveness of amphotericin in 25 patients with desseminated histoplasmosis. Of 14 treated with adequate amphotericin, only one died from the infection. With incomplete courses of amphotericin or no drug, there were seven deaths among the other nine patients.

Adequate amphotericin dosage requires approximately 35 mgm. per kilogram of body weight. The drug is given intravenously starting with 5 to 10 mgm. of drug in 500 cc. of 5 percent glucose in water given slowly over a five-hour period. The drug is increased by 5 or 10 mgm. a day until 50 mgm. a day is given. Then the drug is administered 3 times a week for 16 to 20 weeks until the required amount of drug has been given.

Amphotericin is toxic to the patient and inconvenient to administer because it requires a prolonged course of intravenous therapy. Benign and transient side effects, often disappearing as the patient develops tolerance, include chills, fever, headache, nausea, vomiting and diarrhea. Aspirin given a few hours before therapy frequently lessens the pyrexic reaction. The other side effects may require symptomatic therapy. Phlebitis is a troublesome complication as it makes intravenous therapy increasingly difficult. Skin eruptions and hypokalemia also occur.

Nearly three-fourths of all patients treated with amphotericin will demonstrate nephrotoxicity with increased blood urea nitrogen or decreased creatinine clearance. Fortunately in most all patients the clinical evidence of renal disease induced by amphotericin disappears within six months after the drug is stopped. Autopsies and kidney biopsy material from patients treated with amphotericin, however, do reveal varying degrees of permanent parenchymal kidney damage. A few patients will also demonstrate some bromsulfalein retention.

Sulfonamide drugs have shown some *in vitro* inhibition of *H. capsulatum.* A controlled study comparing the effectiveness of amphotericin alone and amphotericin and sulfonamides, however, gave no evidence of additional benefits.

In Mason City, Iowa, there were two epidemics of histoplasmosis following efforts to clear land in a downtown area which was the site of starling roosts. Finally the land was sterilized using a three percent formalin solution. Before the application of formalin 65 percent of soil samples yielded *H. capsulatum* on culture. After formalin treatment of the soil there was only one of 572 surface soil samples and 9 of 78 below surface soil samples positive for the culture. This technique may be useful as a method of preventing epidemics of histoplasmosis when environments known to contain *H. capsulatum* are to be disturbed.

If a person is going to work in a place where the fungus may be present, certain precautions, such as wetting down the area and wearing a mask, may be helpful in decreasing the inhalation of the spores. If acute pulmonary histoplasmosis does occur, the disease is self limiting. Complete recovery usually occurs without specific therapy.

SELECTED REFERENCES

Christie, A. and Peterson, J. C.: Pulmonary calcification in negative reactors to tuberculin. Amer. J. Pub. Health, *35*:1131, 1945.

Darling, S. T. A.: A protozoan general infection producing pseudotubercles in the lungs and focal necroses in the liver, spleen and lymph nodes. J.A.M.A., *46*:1283, 1906.

Parker, J. D., Sansi, G. A., Doto, I. L., Bailey, R. E. and Tosh, F. E.: Treatment of chronic pulmonary histoplasmosis. A national communicable disease center cooperative mycoses study. N. Eng. J. of Med., *283*:225, 1970.

Reddy, P., Gorclick, D. F., Brasher, C. A. and Larsh, H.: Progressive disseminated histoplasmosis as seen in adults. Am. J. of Med., *48*:629, 1970.

Sellers, T. F., Price, Jr., W. N. and Newberry, Jr. W. M.: An epidemic of erythema multiforme and erythema nodosum caused by histoplasmosis. Ann. of Int. Med., *62*:1244, 1965.

Sweaney, H. C., ed.: *Histoplasmosis.* Springfield, Charles C Thomas, 1960.

Chapter
18

WOUND INFECTIONS

It is likely that virtually all wounds—whether resulting from the accidental trauma of everyday life, the misfortunes of the battlefield, or the painstaking incision of the surgeon—become contaminated to some degree with microorganisms. Whether such microbial contamination leads to significant disease (or "clinical infection") depends upon the interaction of a number of variables, including the particular species and quantity of organisms involved, the state of local tissue susceptibility, and the general systemic resistance of the patient.

Surgical wounds generally are induced in the "aseptic" environment of the operating room, through an area of skin relatively (but probably never *completely*) devoid of bacteria, and in a patient who has resided for a period of time in the specialized environment of the hospital where he may have been confronted with particular types of bacteria and treated with antibiotics which tend to alter the ecology of his indigenous microbial flora. In contrast, the battlefield wound of the previously healthy, well-immunized young man is likely to be contaminated with a multitude of soil bacteria, will probably have considerably more devitalized, necrotic tissue and will undergo variable delays in receiving medical attention. "Clean" *surgical wounds, traumatic injuries* (whether inflicted in war or peace) and a third category, major *burns* (involving more than about 20 percent of the body surface) all possess unique attributes and accordingly warrant separate consideration.

Surgical Wounds

Post-operative surgical infections differ statistically from hospital-acquired infections of medical patients with respect to the age, general condition and systemic resistance of the patient, and the frequency of

This paper was also published in Postgraduate Medicine, Nov. 1971, McGraw-Hill, Inc.

particular routes and types of infection. In both groups, however, important roles must be ascribed to inoculum size and type of the infecting microorganism, to local and systemic host resistance factors and to the epidemiological features of the spread of bacteria within hospitals.

Characteristics of the infecting bacteria.

Relatively few bacterial species make up the flora of normal human skin and of these, the only true pathogen which persists with any frequency is *Staphylococcus aureus,* which together with the more prevalent *Staphylococcus epidermidis* (the coagulase negative *S. albus*) may be found in virtually all regions of the skin. On occasion, *S. epidermidis* may also be pathogenic. Along with the Corynebacteria, these gram-positive organisms constitute the dominant bacterial inhabitants of the skin. The pathogenic gram-positive streptococci are by contrast among the rarest of organisms found on normal skin. Gram-negative bacteria, increasingly significant causes of certain types of wound infections, are also relatively rare on normal skin despite their great numbers in the intestinal tract.

There are striking quantitative regional differences in the concentrations of bacteria on the skin. Nasal and perineal carriage of staphylococci have been particularly implicated in the epidemiology of hospital infections, but it appears that almost all areas of the body, certainly the hands, may occasionally be important carriage sites. A shift in the normal predominance of gram-positive over gram-negative bacteria is the result usually of antibiotic treatment or of prolonged alterations in the moisture of the skin surface. The normal resident flora exert a "territorial imperative" which enables them to resist colonization by competing species. Eradication of the resident flora by antibiotics, however, will produce an ecological vacuum and facilitate the establishment of new (often antibiotic-resistant) species.

This phenomenon of bacterial "interference" may play an important role in protection against colonization by pathogens in diseased skin as well. Thus, in experimental skin burns, bacterial strains applied initially to the burn establish a priority which tends to prevent subsequent colonization by other species.

Efforts to utilize the principle of bacterial interference in blocking colonization of new-born infants by pathogenic staphylococci in the nursery have been successful. Widespread application of this technique, however, depends upon finding truly non-pathogenic interfering strains. Instead of interference, however, bacterial species may interact to produce effects of greater virulence than seen with either species alone (synergism). The best known example, perhaps, is the fortunately rare condition of "progressive synergistic bacterial gangrene" of the abdominal wall in post-operative patients described and studied by Meleney. In this instance a microaerophillic streptococcus combines with *Staphylococcus aureus* to produce a particularly destructive lesion. In general, however, very little is understood about the possible significance of the finding of "mixed bacterial flora" in skin wounds.

The number of microorganisms deposited in a wound is of considerable significance in determining the outcome since most species must be able to survive and multiply to a critical quantity before exerting their pathogenic effects. A small number of organisms can usually be dealt with adequately by host defense mechanisms. Very large numbers of staphylococci in fact must be injected into normal skin to produce a pustular lesion. The precise minimal inoculum size required to establish a clinical wound infection varies, however, not only with particular species but especially with such factors as the presence of foreign bodies or devitalized tissue in the wound.

Host Factors—Local

A surgical incision (or other trauma) obviously produces an interruption in the protective epidermal barrier. Previously diseased skin, as in patients with exfoliative dermatitis or burns, also shows alteration in local resistance. Staphylococci and other indigenous bacteria, in fact, very rarely infect skin without some form of preceding injury. The presence of a foreign body in the lesion markedly alters local resistance as shown dramatically by the reduction in the minimal dose of organisms required to produce a pustular lesion from several million to several hundred when introduced along with a silk stitch.

Acutely inflamed skin, whether caused by abrasions, burns or reactions to antigens, chemicals or microorganisms, is more susceptible than normal skin to infection during the first three days. Thereafter the inflamed skin often is more resistant than normal skin to infection. Vascular flow, serous exudation and phagocytes undoubtedly contribute to the changes in resistance in inflamed tissue, but the precise mechanisms are not known. Clinically, however, these phenomena are important, as wounds, uninfected during the first three days, are probably more resistant to infection after this time.

Necrotic tissue such as third-degree burns are extremely likely to be infected by indigenous microorganisms. The avascularity of necrotic tissue diminishes phagocytic exudation. Antibacterial immunity, however, probably is important in controlling these infections, particularly those caused by staphylococci and pseudomonas. Experimentally, antitoxin to staphylococcal leucocidins actually facilitates phagocytic activity in infected third degree burns.

Another consideration related to local resistance is the finding of significant differences in regional susceptibility to infection. Thus in humans, the thigh and especially the leg show significantly less resistance to experimental staphylococcal and streptococcal infection than do the trunk and arms.

Host Factors—Systemic

The immune status of the host may be an important determinant in development of wound infections, as mentioned. Specific opsonins which "coat" microorganisms and facilitate phagocytosis are of considerable significance in protection against many infections, including streptococcal and staphylococcal disease. The importance of antibody immunity in these infections is particularly dramatic in the diseases in which antibody production is deficient or absent: hypogammaglobulinemia and multiple myeloma.

In addition to antibody-mediated immunity it is possible that cell-mediated immunity, which depends upon the interaction of specifically sensitized lymphocytes and macrophages, may also play a role in resistance to staphylococcal infection. The development of delayed hypersensitivity (of the tuberculin type), however, may have an adverse effect on the evolution of skin infections in some circumstances. For example, patients with repeated staphylococcal skin infections show progressively intense inflammatory reactions with successive infections. The significance of hypersensitivity in human staphylococcal infection is not clear, but humans regularly show positive skin reactions to staphylococcal products, including toxoid antigens and it is likely that hypersensitivity influences the inflammatory reaction to skin infection.

The importance of circulating granulocytes in defense against staphylococcal skin infection is seen in patients with agranulocytosis who are at risk of acquiring serious skin infections. Furthermore, in granulomatous disease of childhood intracellular digestion of staphylococci within granulocytes is defective and serious staphylococcal infections are a constant problem.

It follows that conditions which adversely affect phagocyte function lead to increased susceptibility to staphylococcal infection. Processes which interfere with the mobilization of granulocytes via vascular channels (such as hypotensive shock, epinephine injection or small blood vessel disease in diabetes) as well as situations which impair phagocytic function (including keto-acidosis, insulin deficiency, and hyperosmolarity), all tend to increase susceptibility to staphylococcal and other bacterial skin infections. It is of interest that a cyclic defect in granulocyte phagocytic function has been detected in burned patients and appears to correlate with times of increased risk of septicemia.

In addition, a variety of other physiologic and pharmacologic factors can be incriminated as potentially altering host resistance to cutaneous infections. These include electrolyte disturbances, glucocorticoids, and alcohol.

Studies of surgical patients have identified several features which are associated with predisposition to the development of wound infection. These include the type of surgical procedure, the duration of operation, the age of the patient and the presence of cardiac disease or hypotension. A seasonal variation in staphylococcal wound infections has also been noted. It is highly likely that these factors operate principally through alterations of local and systemic resistance as described above. An additional feature, however, relates to the spread of organisms within hospitals.

Epidemiological Factors in Postoperative Wound Infection

In most hospitals, staphylococci are still the most common single cause of post-operative wound infections (45 percent in a large British series and 31 percent in a combined American series), but it is apparent that *E. coli*, Proteus, Pseudomonas and other gram-negative bacilli are becoming increasingly frequent causes. The source of infecting organisms in non-epidemic situations is frequently the patient himself, whose own indigenous bacteria (possibly acquired through colonization in the hospital) produce the wound infection. One study of 50 patients revealed that 92 percent had a coagulase-positive staphylococci culturable from the wound at the end of the operative procedure. In 68 percent of instances the staphylococcus was also in the air of the operating room, and in 50 percent represented the patients' own carrier strain. In contrast the hands and noses of the operative team very rarely yielded the strain found in the wound. The chief source of wound contamination *occurring at the time of operation* appeared, therefore, to be the patient himself and possibly the "non-scrubbed" personnel entering the room.

In specific instances, usually taking the form of a "common source" epidemic, a surgeon or assistant with a draining lesion may be the source of operative infection. Improperly sterilized equipment is also clearly a potential but rare cause of infections.

In addition to "self-infection" the other major route of wound infection represents "cross-infection" acquired from personnel or other patients on the ward. Environmental factors—bedding, blankets, water pitchers, etc. —have been studied intensively as possible sources of infection but it appears that such reservoirs principally reflect the organisms of the *people* in the environment and are themselves relatively unimportant sources of infection. It seems likely that the air serves as a vehicle for transmission of infecting organisms only through relatively short distances since there is evidence that staphylococci in the dust of the patient's room, though culturable show little virulence. Nevertheless, the air may be an important route of cross-colonization leading to the acquisition of carrier strains by patients newly admitted to the hospital. The hands of personnel must continue to be considered as important potential reservoirs of infection as emphasized by studies in a newborn nursery. This route was found to be important both in the dissemination of staphylococci from personnel who were nasal carriers and also in the spread of organisms between babies.

Finally with respect to possible routes of infection, it is of interest that experimental induction of bacteremia can be shown to lead to contamination of clean surgical wounds by the bacteremic organism. The indwelling intravenous polyethylene catheters frequently used in surgical patients have in fact been shown to be a common cause of staphylococcal bacteremia.

Prevention and Control

The determinants of surgical wound infection are multiple and differ with respect to relative importance from time to time and place to place. Until the relative significance of these multiple factors is better understood, it will probably continue to be necessary to carry out a lengthy set of precautions, some of which may ultimately prove to be of little value.

Good aseptic technique in the operating room is now widely practiced and hopefully needs little emphasis here. It is worth remembering, however, that it is virtually impossible to achieve *complete* sterility of the skin by scrubbing techniques. Even if it were, wound infections would continue to occur as a result of contamination from other sources in the operating room or after the patient returns to the ward. The use of proper exhaust ventilation in the operating suite, the exclusion of surgeons or assistants with infected lesions, and restriction of all nonessential "traffic" through the operating room are measures to be highly recommended. Ultraviolet light sterilization is more controversial and less clearly indicated.

On the wards, isolation of patients with active infections (and possibly carriers also) as well as protective isolation of highly susceptible patients, and emphasis on hand-washing by personnel are recommended.

The use of prophylactic antibiotics as a general measure to prevent surgical wound infection has in most studies been ineffective and in fact may have adverse effects including facilitating the colonization of the patient by antibiotic resistant strains. While the incidence of infection usually is unchanged, prophylaxis assures that infections which develop are due to antibiotic-resistant organisms. Such practice has the further disadvantage of increasing the risk of sensitizing the patients and of promoting the evolution of antibiotic resistant strains. Limited indications for the judicious routine use of antibiotics are probably valid in special circumstances (e.g., certain operative problems associated with a high incidence of infection). Even here prophylaxis appears to be most effective when directed against a specific organism (e.g., anti-staphylococcal drugs in cardiac surgery) rather than efforts to erect a broad antibiotic "umbrella."

Treatment of wound infections once they have occurred requires appropriate drainage and debridement, and selection of a proper antibiotic (utilizing culture and antibiotic sensitivity testing).

Burn Infection

Studies of severe third-degree burns in humans have revealed that virtually all burn wounds become colonized with bacteria in a fairly consistent sequence. The burn is initially sterile. Over the first two to three days, however, rapid surface colonization by staphylococci occurs with some invasion through the superficial parts of the lesion. By the fourth or fifth day gram-negative bacilli appear in increasing numbers (especially under the influence of antibiotic therapy) and by the end of the first week thorough involvement of the eschar by organisms such as Pseudomonas, Klebsiella and Proteus has usually occurred. Invasion of the surrounding viable tissue produces "burn wound sepsis." In one half the cases of fatal burn sepsis there is no evidence of distant metastatic spread of the infection, pointing to the importance of local resistance factors. Utilizing the appearance of verdoglobinuria as an indication of Pseudomonas "exotoxemia," a study of 1921 major burns revealed that 291 had Pseudomonas infection of which 187 showed verdoglobinuria and 51 developed Pseudomonas bacteremia. The appearance of verdoglobinuria proved to be a reliable sign indicating probable progression to fatal septicemia. Pseudomonas "toxemia" was in fact associated with 100 percent mortality until the institution of gentamicin therapy in this series.

Once the scourge of burn wounds, streptococcal infections have largely been controlled by the use of penicillin. More recently, severe staphylococcal infections have also been more easily manageable with the availability of penicillinase-resistant anti-staphylococcal drugs. The result has been the emergence of gram-negative infections, especially with Pseudomonas, as the most difficult therapeutic problem. Virus infection is also a potential threat.

Despite improvement in the management of burn patients through better use of fluids, electrolytes and colloids, mortality of burn wound sepsis has remained significant. Recently, however, improved therapeutic results have been achieved through the utilization of two major approaches: the use of topical antibacterial treatment, and enhancement of the patients' immunity against Pseudomonas by both active immunization and passive administration of antibody.

The most effective topical measures have been the application of silver nitrate (0.5%), mafenide (Sulfamylon, Winthrop) and gentamicin. Each of these measures has certain disadvantages, and search for additional agents continues.

Enhancement of the burn patient's antibacterial immunity has been attempted through the use of pooled human gamma globulin. Antibody to staphylococcal anti-hemolysin is protective in experimental burn infections in rabbits. A problem with immunity to Pseudomonas is the relative lack of cross protection between antibodies to heterologous Pseudomonas strains. A new heptavalent Pseudomonas vaccine appears promising. Good results have also been obtained using hyperimmune human plasma plus active immunization.

An additional potential therapeutic approach for the future is the utilization of bacterial interference to block colonization of the burn wound by pathogenic strains.

Traumatic Wounds

Accidental wounds and especially battlefield wounds are much more likely to undergo significant initial bacterial contamination than operative wounds. Nevertheless, in a study of minor industrial wounds, the source of staphylococcal infection appeared to be the patient's own carrier strain in 50–60 percent of cases.

War wounds along with major accidental crush injuries are likely to contain a significant quantity of devitalized or necrotic tissue as well as foreign bodies. In this type of lesion, anaerobic infection becomes a major threat. The fact that tetanus is no longer a military problem is attributable to the high level of effective immunization with tetanus toxoid achieved in the armed forces. Clostridial gas gangrene can be prevented by the use of early debridement and delayed closure of such wounds, techniques carried out most effectively in the Vietnam conflict. Accordingly organisms most frequently implicated in military wounds in Vietnam have been staphylococci, Pseudomonas and *E. coli*.

The effectiveness of early debridement, followed by delayed secondary closure, in the treatment of military wounds is indicated by the remarkably low wound infection rate of 2.58 percent reported from Vietnam. This can be contrasted to infection rates of 3–11 per cent in 5 University Hospital series of "clean" surgical cases—although in different types of patients. Experimental studies indicate the optimum time for delayed closure to be on or after the 4th day. A possible role for topical antiseptic treatment of war wounds has been suggested, particularly when early debridement cannot be carried out. A similar situation might apply to mass civilian casualties. Irrigation of contaminated experimental wounds with a variety of antiseptic agents including 70 percent ethanol, benzalkalonium and iodine preparations produced significant protection while silver nitrate *enhanced* the infection rate. Carbolic acid in effective concentrations led to fatal phenol poisoning.

The use of topical antibiotic sprays in experimental crush wounds led to significant reduction in mortality, as did the use of methenamine salts. In these experiments, however, maximum effectiveness required the use of the agent within five minutes after contamination and little effect was noted if delayed for four hours or more. Systemic antibiotics also reduced mortality in the experimental model. Potential hazards of topical antibiotic therapy include sensitization of the patient and the absorption of toxic quantities of certain agents. For example, deafness has resulted from topical irrigation of wounds with drugs such as neomycin.

The desirability of utilizing topical antibiotic treatment of human traumatic wounds requires further study.

Summary

The development of infection in *surgical, traumatic* or *burn* wounds is a resultant of the interaction of the dose and characteristics of the contaminating microorganisms and of local and systemic host resistance factors. Especially in surgical operative wounds these factors are influenced by epidemiological aspects of the spread of bacteria within hospitals. Indiscriminate use of antibiotics may lead to the facilitation of the colonization of patients with antibiotic resistant strains and to the development of infection with such strains. The type and duration of operation, and the patient's age and underlying diseases play a role through effects on local and sytemic resistance. Knowledge of the determinants of infection permits the rational application of prophylactic measures.

Infections in burns and in traumatic wounds present special problems. Recent advances in therapeutic techniques have led to improvements in the prevention and management of these infections.

SELECTED REFERENCES

Anthony, B. F., Wannamaker, L. W.: Bacterial interference in experimental burns. J. Exp. Med., *125:*319, 1967.

Burke, J. F.: Identification of the sources of staphylococci contaminating the surgical wound during operation. Ann. Surg., *158:*898, 1963.

Cluff, L. E.: The inflammatory response of skin to bacterial infection. In Maiback, J. J., and Hildick-Smith, eds.: *Skin Bacteria and Their Role in Infection.* 1965, New York, McGraw-Hill, p. 95.

Cohen, L. W., Fekety, F. R. and Cluff, L. E.: Studies on the epidemiology of staphylococcal infection. VI. Infection in surgical patients. Ann. Surg., *159:*321, 1964.

Duncan, W. C., McBride, M. E. and Knox, J. B.: Experimental production of infection in humans. J. Invest. Derm., *54:*319, 1970.

Edlich, R. F., Rogers, W., Kasper, G., Kaufman, D., Tsung, M. S. and Wangensteen, O. H.: Studies in management of contaminated wounds. I. Optimal time for closure of contaminated open wounds. II. Comparison of resistance to infection of open and closed wounds during healing. Am. J. Surg., *117:*323, 1969.

Goshi, K., Cluff, L. E., and Johnson, J. E., III: Studies on the pathogenesis of staphylococcal infection. III. The effect of tissue necrosis and antitoxic immunity. J. Exp. Med., *113:*259, 1961.

Johnson, J. E., III: Immunity in staphylococcal infection: Effect of gamma globulin on burn infection. Proc. Soc. Exp. Biol. & Med., *122*:584, 1966.

Johnson, J. E., III, Cluff, L. E. and Goshi, K.: Studies on the pathogenesis of Staphylococcal infection. I. The effect of repeated skin infections. J. Exp. Med., *113*:235, 1961.

Marples, M. J.: *The Ecology of the Human Skin.* Charles C Thomas, Publisher, 1965.

Matsumoto, T. and Dobeck, A. S.: Systemic antibiotics in contaminated crust wound without debridement. Arch. Surg., *99*:103, 1969.

Meleney, F. L.: *Treatise on Surgical Infections.* New York: Oxford University Press, 1945.

Miles, A. A., Miles, E. M., and Burke, J. F.: The value and duration of defense reactions of the skin to the primary lodgement of bacteria. Brit. J. Exp. Path., *38*:79, 1957.

Moncrief, J. A.: Topical treatment of the burn wound: present status. Clin. Pharm. Therapeut., *10*:439, 1969.

Stone, H. H.: Diagnosis and treatment of *Pseudomonas* sepsis in major burns. J. Inf. Dis., *119*:504, 1969.

Wangensteen, O. H.: Military surgeon and surgery, old and new: An instructive chapter in the management of contaminated wounds. Surg., *62*:1102, 1967.

Welch, W. H.: Conditions underlying the infection of wounds, Congress of Amer. Phys. Surg., Transactions, *2*:1, 1891.

Williams, R. E. O., Blowers, R., Garrod, L. P. and Shooter, R. A.: *Hospital Infection: Causes and Prevention.* London, Lloyd-Luke, 1966.

Williams, R. E. O. and Miles, A. A.: Infection and sepsis in industrial wounds of the hand. Spec. Rep. Med. Res. Coun. (London) No. 266, 1949.

Williams, R. E. O., Noble, W. C., Jerons, M. P., Lidwell, O. M., Shooter, R. A., White, R. G., Thom, B. J. and Taylor, G. N.: Isolation for the control of staphylococcal infection in surgical wards. Bul. Med. J., *2*:275, 1962.

Chapter 19

STAPHYLOCOCCAL DISEASE

Resistance to antimicrobial drugs, infection in persons with serious associated diseases or subjected to extensive surgery, and epidemics in hospital nurseries have increased concern about staphylococcal infections over the past 15 years. Decreasing concern recently is attributable to control of nursery outbreaks and development of drugs effective against staphylococci which were resistant to previously available antibiotics. Problems with staphylococcal disease, however, have not, and probably will not, disappear as long as individuals experience circumstances reducing their resistance to infection by indigenous and ubiquitous microorganisms, among which the staphylococcus is prominent.

The epidemiology and pathogenesis of staphylococcal infection now are better understood. This understanding has facilitated a more rational approach to prevention and control of epidemic infection, but has had little impact upon sporadic, non-epidemic disease. More effective antimicrobial drugs have reduced mortality from staphylococcal disease but have had little influence upon the frequency of infection. Whether or not sporadic infections are completely preventable is questionable. In fact, prevention of infection by any indigenous microorganism is difficult.

Epidemiological Features

Staphylococcus aureus (coagulase and mannitol positive) is a more important cause of infection than *Staphylococcus albus* (coagulase and mannitol negative). The latter also may cause serious disease but clinically resembles infection caused by *S. aureus*. *S. aureus* is a constant or intermittent colonizer of human skin and mucous membranes. Thirty percent of adults harbor staphylococci in their anterior nares. Some of these persons are chronic or persistent carriers; others are intermittent or transient carriers. Chronic upper respiratory disease may be a factor determining the persistence of carrying staphylococci, but in most instances, the responsible factors are not known.

Chronic nasal carriers of staphylococci probably are more likely to acquire staphylococcal infection, such as boils and furuncles. Very often, however, the staphylococci isolated from furuncles and boils differ by bacteriophage typing from staphylococci found in the anterior nares. The importance of the asymptomatic nasal carrier as a source of infection in others is controversial, but probably limited.

Staphylococci also are found on skin; more frequently in some sites, such as the perineum, than in others. These bacteria also can be isolated frequently from feces of normal persons.

The staphylococci harbored by individuals are often characteristic of the setting in which these persons live or work. Hospital personnel and patients usually carry antibiotic resistant staphylococci, often belonging to particular bacteriophage types. Individuals having no contact with hospitals often carry antibiotic sensitive staphylococci usually of other bacteriophage types. Those patients in hospitals receiving antibiotics—particularly tetracycline—acquire drug resistant staphylococci more rapidly than others, but the overall frequency of colonization of patients with staphylococci usually is not appreciably higher in those receiving antibiotics.

Certain types of staphylococci, particularly bacteriophage type 80/81, have been incriminated in outbreaks of infection among newborn infants and among other hospitalized patients. These types also are most prevalent in the hospital environment and most commonly found as the carrier strain in hospital personnel. For these reasons the "hospital" staphylococci, specifically type 80/81, have been said to have "epidemiologic virulence." Investigation of the virulence of different strains of staphylococci by experimental infection of animals and man, however, reveals little variation between strains in their ability to initiate an infection. In fact, experimental staphylococcal infection of normal man or animals requires enormous numbers of organisms, indicating rather low virulence under these conditions. Relatively small numbers of staphylococci, however, may cause infection when inoculated into animals with deranged systemic or local resistance.

During the past 10 years, the relative importance of air, fomites, and direct contact in transmission of staphylococci has been clarified. Direct contact—particularly via the hands—is the single most important route of transmission of these bacteria. Transmission of staphylococci in a nursery from a colonized infant or from a nurse who is a carrier can be avoided by nurses and others washing their hands before handling newborn infants. Control of air or clothing possibly harboring staphylococci is less important.

Common source outbreaks of staphylococcal infection in surgical patients and newborn infants have most often been related to an infected surgeon or nurse having contact with the affected patients. Exclusion of those with overt staphylococcal disease is important in prevention of such outbreaks of infection; but control of asymptomatic carriers has usually proven unnecessary.

Everyone develops staphylococcal infections at one time or another, usually characterized by boils or furuncles. Serum antibodies directed towards staphylococcal antigens can be detected in almost all children and adults. Serious staphylococcal disease, however, is relatively uncommon, and infection, when it occurs, usually is in previously infected individuals.

Accidental and surgically induced skin trauma are the most important precipitating causes of staphylococcal infection. Pneumonia, upper respiratory infection, endometritis, omphalitis and urinary tract infection are much less common sites of invasion, and collectively account for less than one-half of the patients.

The frequency of infection of different surgical wounds varies depending upon the type of surgical procedure. Patients undergoing herniorrhaphy or appendectomy, for example, have a wound infection rate of less than one percent, while abdominal-perineral resections, colon resections and esophageal operations are followed by staphylococcal wound infection in 10 to 40 percent of cases. Abdominal surgical procedures account for the largest proportion of postoperative wound infections. The reasons for this association are not known, but indigenous skin and fecal staphylococci may be an important source of the bacteria causing infection. Prolonged surgery predisposes to these infections but of equal significance are the occurrence of hypotension or cardiovascular failure. Controlled diabetes mellitus is not associated with an increased rate of postoperative staphylococcal infection. Administration of antibiotics to prevent surgical infection has a limited effect upon staphylococcal surgical wound infection rates, but does increase the likelihood of the infection being attributable to antibiotic resistant bacteria.

Insertion of foreign bodies into tissues predisposes to infection. Foreign materials, such as intravascular prostheses and intravenous plastic catheters, provide a nidus for vascular infection, bacteremia, and its many complications. Surgical sutures also may serve as a nidus for infection, but are less often sources of serious consequences. Removal of foreign bodies is necessary to control these infections, as antimicrobial therapy alone may reduce the severity of, but will not terminate the infection.

Recurrent furuncles and boils occurring only in specific locations may be attributed to recurring trauma. For example, recurrent infection in the axillae may be caused by shaving; recurring perineal infection may be caused by the abrasive effects of sanitary napkins used during menstruation. Avoiding the trauma may result in termination of the recurrent infections.

Staphylococcal bacteremia in children 10 years old or younger is more common than in any other decade, and one-half of infections in the first decade are in infants under one year of age, usually in the first weeks of life. Umbilical infection is a common source of bacteremia in newborns and bacteremia often leads to metastatic pulmonary infection and osteomyelitis. Ventriculo-atrial shunts, meningomyelocele and severe skin disease also are important predisposing causes of serious infection in infants. Although bacteremia in the first decade of life is more common, the mortality rate in these patients is lower than in other decades. The children, however, are less likely to have other serious associated diseases impairing resistance to infection.

Staphylococcal bacteremia occurs most frequently in persons with cardiovascular disease, diabetes mellitus, granulocytic disorders, and immunological deficiency. It is uncommon to observe staphylococcal bacteremia in individuals without an associated disease predisposing them to infection.

Acidosis and vascular disease are associated with the increased occurrence of bacteremia in diabetics, and are responsible for an inadequate granulocyte inflammatory reaction. Patients having controlled diabetes mellitus without vascular disease probably have no increased susceptibility to staphylococcal disease.

Leukemia and lymphomatous diseases predispose to staphylococcal infection if there is granulocytopenia—attributed to lymphoblastic or lymphocytic neoplasia or chemotherapy.

Immune deficiency as observed in hypogammaglobulinemia and multiple myeloma is associated with increased susceptibility to staphylococcal bacteremia. In contrast, patients with osteomyelitis and the highest antistaphylococcal antibody titers have the lowest mortality of any group of patients with bacteremia. These findings suggest that circulatory immunoglobulins play a role in host resistance to staphylococcal disease.

Patients with ulcerative or granulomatous colitis are susceptible to staphylococcal bacteremia and may develop gangrenous skin lesions (pyoderma gangrenosum). The reasons for this relationship are unknown.

The serious associated diseases predisposing patients to staphylococcal infection also increase susceptibility to infection by other commensal indigenous organisms such as enterobacteriaceae, bacteroides, listeria, cytomyegalovirus, and pneumocystis. Therefore, as might be expected, mixed infection and bacteremia with more than one microorganism at the same time are often observed.

Antibiotic usage alters the commensal bacterial flora, and the magnitude of this effect is related to the dosages of antibiotics administered. Patients with chronic respiratory disease given large doses of antibiotics may be infected by dominating indigenous microbes with development of suppurative bronchopulmonary disease. Similarly, administration of oral antibiotics, particularly tetracyclines, to patients with gastrointestinal diseases, particularly those undergoing surgery, may precipitate staphylococcal enterocolitis by allowing replacement of the normal indigenous bacteria by antibiotic resistant enterotoxigenic staphylococci. Otherwise, antibiotic usage probably does not increase the frequency of staphylococcal disease, but determines whether or not the infection is caused by antibiotic resistant or susceptible bacteria.

Increased use of an antibiotic in the hospital can result in appearance of staphylococci resistant to that antibiotic but may not alter the rate of infection in hospitalized patients. Controlled use of an antibiotic may preserve it as an effective drug for treatment of staphylococcal infection by limiting its influence upon the antibiotic resistance of prevalent strains. The widespread use of antibiotics in hospitals, however, has resulted in emergence of resistant organisms. In addition, the widespread use of antibiotics outside hospitals, and frequent contact of individuals with hospitalized persons or employees, has led to an increased prevalence of antibiotic resistant staphylococci outside hospitals.

Seasonal variations of staphylococcal pneumonia and surgical wound infections have been observed. In Boston, Baltimore, and Miami, pneumonia with bacteremia has been observed most frequently in May-June and November-December. The explanation for this seasonal variation is unknown, although the increased frequency in November-December may be related to viral respiratory diseases, particularly influenza.

Almost one third of surgical wound infections were observed in January-February in Baltimore, and could be related only to the very low humidity in hospitals at that time of year, and was not related to frequency of respiratory infection. Possibly, the effect of humidity upon skin dryness and exfoliation are important factors.

Contamination by food handlers infected with enterotoxin-producing *S. aureus* can result in bacterial growth in improperly refrigerated products. Cream-filled pastries, custards, cottage cheese, milk products or meats are the common offenders. The ingested toxin elaborated by the staphylococci produces an acute diarrhea (food poisoning) often with vomiting and abdominal discomfort, but no fever unless associated with profound dehydration. Infection of the gastrointestinal tract ordinarily is not found and the illness is an intoxication. Symptoms begin within a few hours after ingestion of the food and is of brief duration. Correction of hydration is the therapeutic measure required. Most persons ingesting the infected food become ill and commonly large numbers of persons are affected simultaneously, indicating a common food source. The staphylococci may be isolated from the food but rarely from the feces.

Pathogenetic Considerations

S. aureus is ubiquitous on body surfaces, benign staphylococcal skin infections, common, but serious staphylococcal disease, infrequent, illustrating the usual effectiveness of local resistance of skin and mucous membranes to invasion by these bacteria. The integity of these surfaces must be interrupted before infection can develop. Third degree burns, exfoliative dermatitis, decubitus or trophic ulcers, traumatic or intentionally induced incisions are a few of the many such events predisposing patients to staphylococcal infection. Conceivably, the normal mucous membrane and skin provide only mechanical protection against invasion by staphylococci. What keeps these surface bacteria from replicating uncontrollably, however, is not known. In the respiratory, gastrointestinal, and genitourinary tracts, the secretory immunoglobulins, macrophages, and nonspecific antibacterial substances such as lysozyme may play a role in control of commensal indigenous microorganisms. In addition, an increasing body of evidence indicates that these microorganisms maintain a balance between themselves (bacterial interference). Disturbance of this balance by administration of antibiotics which eliminate one bacterium but not another provides a mechanism for superinfection.

Once staphylococci have penetrated the skin or mucous membranes, the resulting inflammatory reaction facilitates phagocytosis of the bacteria by granulocytes. This is a most important mechanism for controlling extension and further development of infection. Circumstances interfering with granulocytic exudation, phagocytosis or intraphagocytic killing of staphylococci result in enhancement of infection. Necrotic tissue, as in third degree burns; foreign bodies such as splinters, sutures or prostheses; pharmacologic or biologic agents such as bacterial endotoxin, adrenalin, and corticosteroids; acidosis, as in diabetes mellitus or uremia; heritable abnormalities of granulocytes, as in granulomatous disease of childhood; and granulocytopenia, as in lymphoid leukemia and drug induced bone marrow suppression, all are responsible for increased susceptibility to staphylococcal disease because of deficient granulocyte exudation or defective intraphagocytic killing of the bacteria.

The reticuloendothelial cells, particularly of liver, remove staphylococci from blood, but they are less important than granulocytes in resistance to staphylococcal infection. Fixed and wandering macrophages may influence infection in the immune host but their precise role in staphylococcal disease is unclear.

The frequency of immune deficiency diseases in patients with serious staphylococcal infection, and the low mortality rate from bacteremia in patients with osteomyelitis and high antibody titers, indicate the probable importance of acquired immunity in these infections. Induced immunity does not greatly affect susceptibility to experimentally induced staphylococcal infection of normal skin, but can prevent infection of experimental necrotic burns, and control bacterial replication in the kidney during experimental bacteremia. The antileucocidins are probably responsible for immunity to experimental staphylococcal disease by preventing granulocytolysis caused by leucocidal staphylococcal toxins and thereby allowing phagocytosis of the bacteria to occur.

Some strains of staphylococci have a particular polysaccharide surface antigen which resists phagocytosis except in presence of specific opsonins. Most adults possess this antipolysaccharide antibody but it probably plays no role in resistance to infection by the many bacterial strains not having the surface antigen.

The necrotizing, leucocidal, lethal, hemolytic and enterotoxic effects of some staphylococcal infections are attributable to toxins elaborated by the bacteria. Antibodies to these toxins probably are important, as indicated before, in experimental disease, but their importance in human infection still is unclear.

Recurrent staphylococcal disease of the skin often is accompanied by exaggeration of the inflammatory reaction during recurring infection. This is associated with development of delayed hypersensitivity to antigens of the organisms. This inflammatory reaction may nonspecifically increase susceptibility to infection. Other acute inflammatory reactions of skin can lead to transient increases in local susceptibility to infection. Chronic inflammatory lesions, however, are more resistant to infection, possibly associated with enhanced macrophage reaction and phagocytosis.

Staphylococcal bacteremia may lead to selective localization of infection in kidney, bone, and lungs. The preference of this infection to localize in these organs is not understood, but may be related to organ vascularity. The granulocytic inflammation following injury to the renal medulla is not brisk and this may be a factor facilitating localization of infection to this organ.

Clinical Features

S. aureus causes pyogenic lesions almost invariably, and is probably responsible for more pyogenic diseases than other bacteria. The most frequent staphylococcal infections involve the skin, but infection of the sinuses, ears, lung, and gastrointestinal tract also occurs. Systemic or local spread of these infections can result in renal or perinephric abscess, osteomyelitis, acute endocarditis, and multiple lung abscesses.

Skin Infections

Furuncles and boils occur commonly in the axillae (hydradenitis suppurativum) and perineum of women, the posterior cervical hair line (carbuncle) or beard area (sycosis barbae) of men, the umbilicus of newborns, in occluded sebaceous glands, at sites of trauma or injury, about toe or finger nails (paronychia), and following insertion of splinters or other foreign bodies. The characteristic feature of each of these infections is a local abscess, surrounded by varying degrees of cellulitis and lymphadenitis, and occasionally associated with fever and leucocytosis when the lesion is extensive.

Respiratory Infections

Acute sinusitis is commonly caused by staphylococci. Acute pharyngitis or tonsillitis caused by staphylococci, however, is seen largely in patients with granulocytopenia or agranulocytosis.

Staphylococcal pneumonia most often is associated with antecedent severe respiratory viral infection such as influenza. The radiological lesion in the lungs is characterized by confluent areas of consolidation, rapidly leading to abscess or cavitation, and usually associated with recurrent chills and bacteremia. In children, the radiological lesions often appear as multiple cysts with little apparent surrounding inflammatory reaction. Lung abcesses, often multiple, may also complicate staphylococcal bacteremia. Such metastatic involvement of the lung may be associated with septic embolism when occurring as a complication of acute endocarditis or septic thrombophlebitis.

Osteomyelitis and Pyoarthritis

Although once quite common, staphylococcal osteomyelitis is now uncommon except as it may complicate orthopedic surgical procedures. These infections most often involve long bones, usually at their diaphyseal ends, but also may affect flat bones, vertebrae and joints. Vertebral staphylococcal disease with perivertebral involvement is now a more important cause of psoas abscess and Pott's disease than is tuberculosis. A patient with localized vertebral or back pain with fever and leucocytosis must be investigated carefully for vertebral or perivertebral infection.

Staphylococcal pyoarthritis is almost invariably a complication of periarticular osteomyelitis and may be a complication of bacteremia or follow joint injections, particularly in patients with rheumatoid arthritis given cortico-steroids intraarticularly. Acute monarticular involvement in patients with rheumatoid arthritis should always be suspected as due to staphylococcal pyoarthritis.

Staphylococcal joint infection is destructive of articular cartilage and may result in permanent joint deformity. Aspiration of the joint, particularly to relieve increased joint pressure, is essential to avoid this consequence.

Renal Abscesses

Staphylococcal bacteremia may lead to perinephric or renal abscesses. Renal cortico-medullary abscesses will usually be accompanied by pyuria or hematuria and staphylococci can be isolated from the urine. Perinephric abscess, however, may cause no urinary abnormalities, and be manifested only by flank pain and tenderness, fever, chills, and leucocytosis. Even pyelography may not reveal perinephric abscess.

Miscellaneous

Staphylococcal meningitis, empyema, pericarditis, hepatic abscess, dural abscess, testicular and prostatic abscesses are usually complications of surgery, bacteremia, or spread from contiguous sites. Multiple abscesses or widespread metastatic infection is not uncommon in patients with bacteremia. The significance of this relates prominently to the importance of long-term antimicrobial treatment, the requirement of prophylactic administration of antimicrobial drugs before, during, and following incision and drainage of staphylococcal abscesses, and the need for diligent search for metastatic infection in patients who have staphylococcal bacteremia.

Staphylococcal food poisoning has been discussed as an epidemiological problem.

Management

All staphylococcal infections do not require administration of antimicrobial drugs. Furthermore, attention towards clinical factors responsible for precipitating or influencing the course of infection may be more important than administration of an antibiotic in managing the patient's disease.

Clinical Factors

Foreign bodies present at the site of infection must be removed if successful resolution of the lesion is to be assurred. This includes removal of splinters, ingrown hairs or nails, dirt, suture material, grafts, prostheses, bone sequestra and others.

Obstruction to drainage of an abscess, small or large, in a solid tissue, duct or tube, must be removed. Antimicrobial drugs may control spread of infection from an abscess but will not reliably influence bacteria in the abscess and certainly will not facilitate resolution of the contents of the abscess. The failure of antibiotics in acting upon bacteria in an abscess are not clearly understood but in most instances cannot be attributed to lack of drug penetration. Only sulfonamides are appreciably inactivated by pus. The bacteria in pus, however, are usually in high concentration, in a static growth phase, and in this form are less susceptible to antibiotic action.

The associated illnesses usually present in patients acquiring serious staphylococcal disease, including agranulocytosis, leukemia, peripheral vascular disease, acidosis, and immunological deficiency, must be appropriately dealt with, and this may contribute more to management of the infection than any other measure.

Local treatment, including incision and drainage of an abscess, including empyema, application of warm soaks or heat, debridement, frequent cleansing, rest of the affected part, and avoidance of local trauma may be the major requirement in treatment of a skin infection unassociated with cellulitis or systemic symptoms.

Selection of antibiotic

Several important considerations are necessary in initial selection of an antibiotic and in determining duration of treatment for staphylococcal infection. Antibiotic sensitivity testing will be required for precise antibiotic selection and in evaluating the course of the infection.

Skin infections not likely to require therapy for longer than one week may be treated with antimicrobial drugs to which staphylococci may acquire resistance after that period of treatment. Erythromycin and novobiocin, for example, are effective against most staphylococci causing infection outside the hospital and in other settings where erythomycin and novobiocin are not used frequently. Resistance to these antibiotics, however, is acquired by the infecting staphylococci in most instances after 7 to 10 days of treatment. If treatment is continued beyond this time, therefore, another antibiotic should be selected. Ordinarily a dose of 1.0 to 2.0 grams of erythromycin or novobiocin is necessary for treatment of simple staphylococcal infections.

Treatment planned for longer than seven days, or given to a patient with serious staphylococcal infection, should begin with a penicillinase resistant antibiotic, such as methicillin, oxacillin, cloxacillin, dicloxacillin, nafcillin, cephalothin or cephalexin. Lincomycin has also been used, particularly in treatment of osteomyelitis, but should not be preferentially used except possibly in that instance.

Only about 30 percent of staphylococcal infections acquired outside hospitals, and 80 percent or more infections acquired in the hospital, are attributable to penicillin resistant or penicillinase producing bacteria. Therefore, penicillin should not be the initially selected antibiotic for treatment of serious staphylococcal infections. Penicillin resistance is not usually acquired by penicillin sensitive or penicillinase negative staphylococci during the course of treatment, however, and if infecting strains prove to be sensitive to penicillin this drug then becomes the drug of choice for continued therapy. If *in vitro* sensitivity tests are not done, however, the penicillinase resistant drug should be continued instead of changing to penicillin.

Most serious staphylococcal infections, particularly those associated with bacteremia, should be treated for at least four to six weeks. Otherwise, there probably is greater threat of emergence later of a metastatic staphylococcal abscess. Similarly, parenteral therapy should be given at first, but oral therapy may be given after the first week or two if the infection seems under control and the patient is recovering. Blood levels by measuring serum antibacterial activity, are particularly important if oral treatment is used.

The dose of the penicillinase resistant drugs and of penicillin in treating serious staphylococcal disease should be reasonably large, for example, 6 to 12 grams methicillin or oxacillin, and 6 to 20 million units penicillin in adults. At the moment, cloxacillin or oxacillin probably are the preferred drugs resistant to penicillinase but any of those mentioned are satisfactory.

Only one antibiotic is required or desired in treatment. The oral absorption of oxacillin is limited if administered with sulfonamides. Methicillin is unstable in solution and at acid pH; therefore, it must not be administered continuously as an intravenous drip and cannot be given orally.

Resistance to the penicillinase resistant drugs, particularly methicillin, has been described. Its rarity at the moment, however, presents no great threat to their effectiveness in treatment of staphylococcal diseases.

Prevention of infection

Handwashing and disposal of materials contaminated by pus from staphylococcal infections are essential to prevent spread of staphylococci in the hospital or the home. Air control is important largely with patients having respiratory staphylococcal disease, and then primarily to avoid contamination of others with sputum or droplets.

Skin cleanliness and hygienic care are essential in prevention or control of recurrent staphylococcal infection of the skin. Use of hexachlorophene containing soaps, frequent washing, avoidance of cutaneous trauma or irritation are equally important in these patients.

Isolation, separation or segregation of asymptomatic carriers of staphylococci is generally unnecessary. Antibacterial creams or ointments applied to the nasal mucosa or skin alone have little if any effect in controlling colonization with staphylococci. Skin preparation prior to surgery is important but even this does not reliably eliminate staphylococci from skin surfaces or from subaceous glands or ducts and hair follciles. Reduction of the bacterial mass, however, will probably reduce the possibility of infection.

There is limited evidence that patients undergoing certain types of surgery uniquely predisposing to frequent or serious post-operative infection should receive penicillinase resistant antimicrobial drugs just before, during and for a short time after surgery. This practice, however, is not generally accepted as effective in preventing surgical staphylococcal infection.

SELECTED REFERENCES

Cluff, L. E., Reynolds, R. C., Page, D. L. and Breckenridge, J. L.: Staphylococcal bacteremia and altered host resistance. Ann. Int. Med., *69*:859, 1968.

Cluff, L. E. and Reynolds, R. C.: Management of staphylococcal infections. Am. J. Med., *39*:812, 1965.

Cluff, L. E.: Cellular reactions in the pathogenesis of staphylococcal infection. Ann. N. Y. Acad. Sci., *128*:214, 1965.

Mudd, S.: A successful parasite: parasite-host interaction in infection by *Staphylococcus aureus,* in *Infectious Agents and Host Reactions,* ed. by Mudd, S., Phila., W. B. Saunders Co., 1970.

Cohen, L. S., Fekety, F. R., and Cluff, L. E.: The changing ecology of hospital staphylococci. N. Eng. J. Med., *266*:367, 1962.

Elek, S. D.: *Staphylococcus pyogenes,* Edinburgh and London, E. and S. Livingstone, Ltd., 1959.

Koenig, M. G.: Staphylococcal infections, treatment and control. Disease-a-Month, April, 1968.

Chapter 20

STREPTOCOCCAL INFECTIONS AND THEIR SEQUELAE

The wide spectrum of diseases caused by β-hemolytic streptococci is often overshadowed by the widely recognized association between "strep" and sore throat (Table 20.1). Although many of these diseases, such as erysipelas, were probably described by Hippocrates, the etiological role of the streptococcus was not demonstrated until less than a century ago. Of major importance was the recent recognition that rheumatic fever and acute glomerulonephritis were sequelae to anticedent infection by a specific group of β-hemolytic streptococci, the *group A* streptococcus. Another major contribution was the advent of penicillin, an antibiotic that shortly after its discovery was found to be effective against the group A streptococcus, and that at this writing, no *group A* streptococcal strain has been proven to be resistant to penicillin. The fact that this microorganism has resisted the vagaries of overuse and misuse of penicillin and remained sensitive to this antibiotic is a prime factor in the role that penicillin has played in control of streptococcal infections and their sequelae.

Bacteriology and Immunology

Streptococci are gram-positive organisms that grow in chains. They are sub-divided on the basis of the kind of hemolysis produced on sheep blood agar. Organisms that produce a green or incomplete hemolysis are called *α-streptococci,* while those that produce a completely clear, golden hemolysis are *β-hemolytic streptococci.* Some streptococci do not produce any hemolysis on culture and are called *γ-streptococci.*

The characteristic hemolysis produced on blood-agar plate helped identify the pathogenic streptococci, β-hemolytic. However, it soon became apparent that not all β-hemolytic streptococci were pathogenic to man. It was through the work of Lancefield in 1933 that a serological classification evolved which helped differentiate the β-hemolytic streptococci into distinct groups and demonstrate that a single group, the *group A streptococcus,* was associated with most of the acute streptococcal infections in *man* and the *only* group responsible for the late sequelae of acute rheumatic fever and acute glomerulonephritis. In addition to the group A streptococcus, 12 other groups have been identified (groups B, C, D, E, F, G, H, L, M, N, O). While many of these groups of β-hemolytic streptococci are responsible for diseases in lower animals (e.g., group B, bovine mastitis; group C and G, canine disease), some of these groups have been associated with acute infection in man and can be recovered from about five percent of nasopharyngeal cultures obtained from normal individuals. It is important to emphasize that *none* of these groups leads to rheumatic fever or glomerulonephritis.

The antigen responsible for the serological specificity of each group is a carbohydrate, the C-carbohydrate, which is usually part of the streptococcal cell wall. In the case of the group A streptococcus the polysaccharide is a polymer composed of rhamnose (50–60%) and N-acetylglucosamine (25–30%), in which the N-acetylglucosamine is the specific antigenic determinant. Mutant strains have been found which lack the N-acetylglucosamine and where the polysaccharide is composed almost completely of rhamnose. In these mutant strains, the A-variant strains, the antigenic determinant of the polysaccharide is rhamnose. Minor differences in the C-carbohydrate often account for differences in group specificity, such as in the case of the group C where the difference from group A is no more

TABLE 20.1

Diseases associated with β-hemolytic streptococci

Acute (purulent) infections	
Pharyngitis-tonsilitis	Vaginitis
Peritonsillar abscess	Pyoderma-impetigo
Otitis media	Erysipelas
Mastoiditis	Cellulitis-(perianal)
Sinusitis	Scarlet fever
Pneumonia-empyema	Septicemia (puerpural sepsis)
Pericarditis	Endocarditis
Arthritis-osteomyelitis	Meningitis
Non-purulent sequelae	
Acute rheumatic fever and sydenham's chorea	
Acute glomerulonephritis	

than the presence of N-acetylgalactosamine instead of N-acetylglucosamine in the C-carbohydrate.

Division of the group A streptococcus into several serological *types* is based on the presence of a protein antigen, the M-protein or *type specific antigen,* in the cell wall. More than 50 types with antigenically different M-proteins have been described. Of importance is the role of the M-protein in virulence and immunity.

The presence of M-protein on the surface of the streptococcal cell allows the organism to resist phagocytosis. Removal of the M-protein, which can be achieved while maintaining the viability of the organism, results in deletion of this resistance and enhancement of phagocytosis. Neutralization of the anti-phagocytic effect of the M-protein can also be achieved by adding antibody specific to the M-protein. In the presence of type specific antibody, phagocytosis occurs readily. Immunity in the host is predicated on the presence of type specific antibody. These specific antibodies are formed in response to infection by each type and may persist for upwards of 20 years, but their formation is readily suppressed by treatment with antibiotics very soon after onset of infection.

The carbohydrate and M-protein fractions of the group A streptococcal cell wall constitute the most prominent antigenic components. Other structures that have been identified are listed on Table 20.2. The hyaluronic acid capsule imparts the mucoid characteristic to the colonies of some strains. The T-protein, part of a mosaic of several proteins, is of importance because of the recent popularization of an alternate technique in the serological typing of group A streptococci, the T-typing. This technique is of value in epidemiological studies, especially of skin infections, in which the isolated strains are not easily identifiable by M-typing. A mucopeptide is the structural component that imparts rigidity to the cell wall. Underlying the cell-wall and surrounding the fluid protoplasm inside the cell is a lipoprotein membrane forming the envelope of these organisms, the streptococcal protoplast membrane. Of interest is the recent implication of some of these components in cross-reactive antigen-antibody systems with human cardiac tissues and the suggestion that these systems might play a role in the pathogenesis of rheumatic fever and glomerulonephritis.

As the living organisms grow and metabolize in culture medium or tissue, they release several extracellular products. Most of the identified *extracellular products* (Table 20.2) are enzymatic proteins.

The erythrogenic toxins are thought to be responsible for the rash of scarlet fever. The streptolysin S (stable) is responsible for the β-hemolysis produced by the organism on the surface of blood agar plates, while the streptolysin O (oxygen labile) is active under conditions of low oxygen tension and produces the hemolysis seen in the "stab" areas of the plate.

TABLE 20.2

Cellular components and extracellular products of group A streptococcus

Cellular components	Extracellular products
Capsule:	Erythrogenic toxins (A, B, C)
Hyaluronic acid	Hemolysins:
Cell Wall:	Streptolysins ("O" and "S")
Proteins (M, T, R)	Deoxyribonucleases (A, B, C, D)
C-Carbohydrate (Group A polysaccharide)	Nicotinamide adenine dinucleotidase
	Streptokinase
Mucopeptide	Hyaluronidase
Polyglycerophosphate	Ribonuclease
Protoplast:	Amylase
Membrane	Esterase
Protoplasm	

The other products are identified by their enzymatic activity and, as in the case of the deoxyribonucleases, several antigenically different products have been separated which possess the same enzymatic function (isozymes).

While the role of these extracellular products in the metabolic activities of the streptococcal cell have not been defined, their presence serves a practical role in demonstrating infection. With the known exception of streptolysin S, these products are antigenic to man and their release into the tissue during infection results in the formation of specific antibodies. This has served as a basis for antibody tests to determine the occurrence of infections by the group A streptococcus. The prototype of these antibody tests is the anti-streptolysin O (ASO). Because these products are not formed uniformly by all infecting group A streptococci, a significant antibody response to any one occurs in 80 to 85 percent of individuals infected by group A streptococci. Again, certain of the isozymes are produced at a higher frequency and in greater concentrations by group A streptococci. For example, deoxyribonuclease B isozyme is produced in greater amounts than the other isozymes by the majority of group A streptococci. This accounts for the finding of higher incidence of elevated antibody titers to this product following group A streptococcal infection and the low frequency of antibodies to the three other streptococcal deoxribonucleases. It should be emphasized that while some individuals may not show antibody response to one of the streptococcal products, there is a very good probability that they will show a good response to one of the other products.

In contrast to the function of antibody to the M-protein, antibodies to the various extracellular products do *not* play a role in immunity to streptococcal infections. Neither are these extracellular products or their antibodies involved in the pathogenesis of the non-purulent complications of group A streptococcal infections.

Acute (Purulent) Infections

The group A streptococcus is responsible for a variety of acute purulent infections (Table 20.1). The most common locus is the pharynx and its associated lymphoid tissue. While many of the acute purulent diseases listed are direct extensions or simultaneous infections of adjacent tissues, other infections are the outcome of bacteremia or primary infections at different sites and are unrelated to streptococcal pharyngitis. Thus, in the case of streptococcal pyoderma, evidence points to infection of the skin prior to or in the absence of colonization of the pharynx by the infecting organism.

Although it can occur at any age, group A streptococcal infection is rare in early infancy and less common in late than early adulthood. Upper-respiratory infections occur predominantly during the winter months while skin infections peak during summer. Transmission of group A streptococci is primarily via the infected individual or the human carrier, with contagiousness being higher in the case of the nasal carrier. Epidemics of streptococcal infections acquired from contaminated foods have been described. The mode of transmission and acquisition of skin infection has not been clarified, although studies show cultures obtained from normal skin of individuals with susceptibility to pyoderma are often positive for the infecting organism. The spread of respiratory infection is affected by crowding and stressful conditions, while acquisition of skin infection seems to be related to injury of the skin and poor hygienic conditions.

Acute Tonsilitis and Pharyngitis

The group A streptococcus usually invades and establishes an infection in the lymphoid tissue of the pharynx. The result is a set of characteristic symptoms, although not specifically diagnostic, of the disease. These manifestations vary with the age of the individual. In the young infant the findings may be somewhat similar to those of a common cold associated sometimes with an exfoliative dermatitis of the upper lip. In the older child fever and pain on swallowing with refusal to eat solid foods might be the main presenting symptoms. In the young adult and adult the symptoms are more severe. The onset of the disease is manifested by sore throat, fever, chilliness, headache and muscular aches. Swallowing aggravates the soreness of the throat. Nasal discharge is not a prominent feature. Hoarseness may be present, but loss of voice rarely occurs. A dry, hacking non-productive cough may be present.

There is usually a high fever and varying degrees of prostration. The tonsils are enlarged, severely congested or covered by a rather confluent yellowish or gray-white exudate. The exudate is easily removed upon swabbing the tonsils. Petechiae may be seen on the soft palate. Cervical adenitis is usually prominent, with enlargement and *tenderness* to palpation of the anterior cervical nodes.

Laboratory findings consist of a leukocytosis in the majority of patients during the early stages of the disease. Urinalysis may reveal a mild and transient proteinuria or hematuria.

The above symptoms and findings persist for only 2 to 3 days in 60 to 80 percent of the patients and subside within a week in most others. Cervical adenitis may persist for a longer period of time. Recovery occurs in most patients without antibiotic therapy and antibiotics tend to shorten the course of illness only to a minor extent.

The diagnosis of streptococcal pharyngitis can only be established with certainty by obtaining a *throat culture*. While the clinical findings can be highly suggestive, especially in association with epidemiological data, the infection produced by streptococci can be mimicked by other etiological agents. Several viral agents, especially adenovirus and infectious mononucleosis, can produce exudative pharyngitis. The differentiation of streptococcal pharyngitis from diphtheria can sometimes pose a problem. The exudate in diphtheria is cream-colored and not easily removable from the underlying tissue: when removed it usually leaves a raw, bleeding surface. Although streptococcal pharyngitis presents a characteristic clinical picture, chances of determining the underlying etiology on *clinical grounds alone* is no better than a 50 percent probability.

Scarlet fever can be defined as streptococcal pharyngitis associated with a rash. This disease was described about three centuries ago by Sydenham, and its relationship to streptococcus proven two centuries later. That the rash is due to a toxin produced by the streptococcus was suggested by the studies of Schultz and Charlton and confirmed by Dick and Dochez shortly thereafter.

Twenty-four hours after onset of pharyngitis an exanthem and an enanthem may appear. The exanthem is a diffuse, erythematous rash covering the whole body but characteristically absent around the mouth (*circumoral pallor*). In areas of skin creases, the rash appears accentuated (*Pastia's sign*). The rash blanches on pressure and the involved skin feels like "sandpaper." The enanthem involves the pharynx and tongue. Initially there is papillary hypertrophy giving rise to the description of "strawberry tongue," followed in two to three days by a deep reddish coloration described as the "raspberry tongue." The rash persists for three to five days and then begins to fade. The regression is associated with peeling of the skin in the involved areas, and in severe cases the skin of the palms and soles may be shed as casts.

The clinical picture and findings are classical for scarlet fever. Confirmation of the diagnosis can be made by throat culture positive for group A streptococcus. In confirming a scarlatinal rash, the Schultz-Charlton test is useful and consists of injecting 0.1 ml. antiserum against the erythrogenic toxin(s) into an area of affected skin and noting disappearance of the rash in that area. The Dick Test, performed to assess immunity against the erythrogenic toxins, is carried out by injecting the toxin(s) intradermally. The formation of erythema in that area indicates the absence of circulating antibody against the toxin. Most adults show a negative Dick test.

Treatment of acute streptococcal pharyngitis or scarlet fever, while effective in the prevention of the acute suppurative complications, should be directed primarily at the prevention of rheumatic fever. The most effective therapeutic regimen is a single injection of 600,000 to 1,200,000 units of benzathine penicillin. Oral therapy can be given in the form of penicillin G 250,000 units or penicillin V 250 mg. to 400 mg., 4 times daily for a minimum of 10 days. The main hazard of oral therapy is discontinuation of medication before 10 days. If the antibiotic level is not maintained for at least 10 days rheumatic fever may not be prevented.

Patients sensitive to penicillin should receive erythromycin in doses of 250 mg. 4 times daily. Because of failure to prevent rheumatic fever, sulfonamides should *not* be used in the treatment of acute streptococcal infections.

Skin Infection

The second common site of streptococcal infection in man is the skin. *Pyoderma* and *Impetigo Contagiosa* indicate superficial infections of the skin while *Erisypelas* is a more deep-seated infection involving subcutaneous tissue.

Erysipelas is now a rare disease. The onset is abrupt and associated with fever. There is an elevated, edematous, purplish discoloration of the skin with a sharp border surrounded by normal skin. When on the face, a common site, it may assume a butterfly distribution around the nose. Bacteremia occurs during the peak of infection. Cultures of the nasopharynx or from the margin of the skin lesion and the blood often yield group A streptococcus. Penicillin therapy is highly effective and the lesion regresses in two to three days.

Perianal cellulitis is similar to erysipelas. It occurs predominantly in boys five years or less of age. The affected child is fussy and complains of pain on defecation. There is marked erythema around the anus. A culture of this area is positive for group A streptococcus. These patients respond promptly to penicillin therapy.

Impetigo contagiosa is a form of pyoderma that results from infection of the skin, usually superimposed on an abraded area (scratch, bite). It is common in the southern part of the U. S. and in hot climates, with a high incidence in late summer and early fall. In certain areas of high prevalence it has acquired its local nomenclature, e.g., Florida sand sore. Children of preschool age are commonly involved. It is more frequent in low socio-economic populations. Initially, there is a vesicle, thin-roofed and underlying the horny layer of the skin. Within one to two days pus replaces the fluid in the vesicle which breaks and becomes covered by a light brownish crust. Constitutional and subjective symptoms are usually minimal. Regional lymphadenopathy may occur. Unlike erysipelas, bacteremia is rare. Cultures of the lesion, performed by swabbing the lesion area with alcohol, elevating the crust and applying the swab to the underlying area, yields either pure cultures of streptococci or a mixed culture of streptococci and staphylococci. The group A streptococci isolated from such lesions belong to a certain number of types that are poor M-producers and are better identified by their "T-agglutination pattern," T-typing.

Staphylococcal impetigo differs from streptococcal impetigo by the persistence of bullae and a transient whitish, rather than amber crust.

Intramuscular benzathine penicillin appears to be the most effective form of therapy in streptococcal impetigo. Oral therapy may be given for 10–14 days. Scrubbing of the lesions with hexachlorophene soap, removal of the crust and swabbing with alcohol may offer some additional help in healing. Proper and frequent baths are a requisite in the prevention of recurrences.

While it is not the intent to under-emphasize the importance of other purulent infections due to group A streptococci, these diseases occur rather infrequently. Their manifestations are peculiar to the type of tissue involved. The streptococcal etiology is determined by recovering the organism on culture of the infected site. Treatment for localized infection is similar to that prescribed for streptococcal pharyngitis, while more severe systemic infection requires more intensive therapy with high doses of penicillin. The major reason for emphasizing throat and skin infection is the well documented evidence that these common infections are responsible for one or both sequelae, rheumatic fever and acute glomerulonephritis, that occur if these acute infections are not recognized and treated adequately.

Non-Purulent Sequelae of Acute Streptococcal Infection

Acute Rheumatic Fever

Rheumatic fever is a disease of protean manifestations that follows untreated group A streptococcal infection of the pharynx in susceptible individuals. Although the relationship of this disease to streptococcal pharyngitis and scarlet fever was noted over a century ago, the specific relationship to antecedent group A streptococcal infection was established only about three decades ago. Rheumatic fever was previously thought to be limited to temperate zones until recent studies showed that it was highly prevalent in subtropical areas. The incidence of the disease is highest in winter and spring. While the prevalence of streptococcal pharyngitis in this country has been steady over the past 3 decades, the number of reported cases of rheumatic fever has constantly declined. There has been a shift in the affected population in certain areas of the U. S., with a decreased incidence in the white and a predominant incidence (60–80%) in the black population. The reason for these changes are not clear.

Rheumatic fever is always preceded by a group A streptococcal infection. The infection may be clinically apparent with acute pharyngitis or scarlet fever, or inapparent. Rheumatic fever "never, or certainly very rarely," follows streptococcal pyoderma. Rheumatic fever occurs in about three percent of individuals with documented group A streptococcal pharyngitis. However, the rate of *recurrence* of rheumatic fever after infection with streptococci in patients affected previously with rheumatic fever is about 50 percent. This high recurrence rate suggests an individual predisposition to this poststreptococcal sequela and supports the adage: "Once a rheumatic, always a rheumatic." The reason for this susceptibility is unclear and the mechanism by which the streptococcal infection precipitates rheumatic disease has not been determined.

There is a *latency* of about three weeks following streptococcal pharyngitis before rheumatic fever appears. The onset of acute rheumatic fever is characterized by one or several of the major clinical manifestations of the disease listed on Table 20.3.

Polyarthritis: The more common presenting manifestion is migratory polyarthritis involving several large joints, showing pain, heat, redness, and swelling. Sometimes the arthritis does not progress and may be limited to one joint. This is to be differentiated from "joint aches and pains" or arthralgia which is a minor manifestation of the disease.

Carditis: The acute carditis of rheumatic fever varies with the severity of the disease. Most commonly there is an apical murmur (grade 3/6 or more) transmitted to the anterior axillary line. It is blowing and high pitched and not altered by respiration or change of position. This murmur is indicative of mitral insufficiency and regurgitation, due to dilatation of the mitral annulus. Aortic regurgitation is indicated by a high-pitched, early diastolic murmur in the third or fourth intercostal space at the left sternal border. Murmurs of mitral or aortic stenosis are rarely encountered during an initial acute attack. The presence of murmurs, evidence of cardiomegaly, pericardial rub and congestive failure are elements of pancarditis.

Chorea: Sydenham's chorea or St. Vitus Dance is manifest by spas-

TABLE 20.3

Jones criteria (revised) for guidance in the diagnosis of rheumatic fever

Major manifestations	Minor manifestations
Carditis	Clinical:
Polyarthritis	Previous rheumatic fever
Chorea	Arthralgia
Erythema Marginatum	Fever
Subcutaneous Nodules	Laboratory:
	Acute phase reactions:
	ESR, CRP, leukocytosis
	Prolonged P-R interval

Requirements for diagnosis:
2 major manifestations *or* 1 major and 2 minor manifestations
plus
Supporting evidence of streptococcal infection

modic, purposeless movements often resembling "nervous tics," involving the skeletal muscles and including the tongue. These may be unilateral, hemichorea, but usually are bilateral. Choreiform movements can be controlled or exaggerated by concentrated effort. The tongue shows wavy contractions and phonation is impaired. Constant, "wormian" muscular contractions can be felt if the patient grasps the fingers of the examiner. Writing is wavy and irregular in upward and downward strokes. Severe cases may present with uncontrollable convulsions of the trunk.

Erythema marginatum: A flat, maculopappular, nonpruritic rash with irregular borders on trunk and extremities may occur in conjunction with other manifestations. It may be accentuated by warming the skin in a suspicious area.

Subcutaneous nodules: Firm nodules, about one cm. in size can be felt in the extensor surfaces of tendons, near bony prominences. They are usually associated with chronic valvular disease.

Of the above criteria, arthritis is the most frequent manifestation, while carditis occurs in about 50 percent, chorea in 10 percent, and erythema marginatum or subcutaneous nodules in about 5 percent of the patients.

DIAGNOSIS OF ACUTE RHEUMATIC FEVER. There is no single clinical or laboratory criterion that unequivocally establishes the diagnosis of acute rheumatic fever. Although an "Aschoff" body in myocardial tissue from a patient with the clinical diagnosis of rheumatic fever may help substantiate the diagnosis, this also may be found in patients with no history of rheumatic fever and conversely may be completely absent in patients with well documented disease.

The diagnosis of *acute* rheumatic fever is based, at present, on the revised Jones Criteria, shown in Table 20.3. It should be emphasized that these criteria do not apply to the diagnosis of chronic rheumatic fever. A patient presenting with two major manifestations or one major plus two minor manifestations is assumed to have acute rheumatic fever. Arthralgia should not be used as a minor criterion when polyarthritis is present as a major manifestation.

Although utilization of these criteria is the mainstay of the diagnosis of rheumatic fever, the diagnosis should be substantiated by evidence of antecedent group A streptococcal infection. This evidence can be clinical: sore throat with positive culture or scarlet fever, bacteriological (throat culture positive for group A streptococcus) or serological (elevation or rise in the streptococcal antibodies, i.e., ASO, anti-DNAse B, etc.).

TREATMENT. Management of the patient with acute rheumatic fever varies with the severity of the illness. All patients should receive a therapeutic course of penicillin. Salicylates should be avoided if the diagnosis is not firmly established, especially if mono-articular arthritis is the only manifestation. Once the diagnosis is substantiated, salicylates are the drug of choice for arthritis and mild or moderate carditis. The response of rheumatic arthritis to salicylates is usually prompt. In severe myocarditis or pancarditis, steroid administration may be lifesaving. Salicylates are given in a dose of 100 mg./Kg./day, maximum dose 10 gm./day. Bed rest is needed only as desired by the patient and by physical limitations. Supportive therapy with digitalis and diuretics should be given cautiously to patients in heart failure. Anti-inflammatory drugs are gradually withdrawn when relief of arthritis is achieved or the carditis stabilized, usually after four to six weeks. A sleeping pulse rate of 100/min. or less and a stable or regressing erythrocyte sedimentation rate are suggestive of stabilization of carditis.

All patients should be started on a regimen of streptococcal prophylaxis. This insures protection against streptococcal infection and prevention of rheumatic recurrences and added heart damage that such patients are highly susceptible to. Monthly injections of long acting benzathine penicillin offer the best prophylaxis. Oral penicillin or sulfonamides, given twice daily, are also effective but somewhat less so. Patients allergic to these drugs should be placed on oral erythromycin. Penicillin prophylaxis is available free in many states through state programs, and patients should be encouraged to register in these programs. At present it is recommended that rheumatic patients be advised to receive prophylaxis for their lifetime, especially if heart disease were present during the acute episode or is a residual lesion.

Acute Glomerulonephritis

In contrast to rheumatic fever, acute glomerulonephritis may follow streptococcal impetigo as well as pharyngitis. As expected, nephritis following impetigo occurs in the late summer and early fall while that complicating pharyngitis occurs in the late spring. Nephritis has been associated with epidemics of pharyngitis due to group A streptococci of M-types 1, 4, 12, 25, and impetigo due to M-type 49 (Red Lake) and T-agglutination patterns 3/13/B3264, 5/27/44 and 8/25/Imp. 19. These types are called *nephritogenic*. The attack rate is about 15 percent following infection with a nephritogenic strain. A notable difference is that the latency period before onset of nephritis is longer (three weeks) following impetigo than following pharyngitis (10 days). Otherwise, there are no differences in the clinical or pathological characteristics of the disease.

The pathogenetic mechanism underlying acute glomerulonephritis is believed to be due to the formation of soluble immune complexes. Experimental evidence as well as histological studies showing deposition of "immune-complexes" in the glomerular basement membrane lend support to this hypothesis. Although antibody to the group A streptococcal protoplast membrane has been shown to cross-react with glomerular basement membrane, this probably is not an important pathogenetic mechanism of the disease.

Acute post-streptococcal glomerulonephritis may be associated with several variable signs and symptoms. Gross or microscopic hematuria is the most constant finding. Periorbital or peripheral edema, oliguria and marked hypertension are found. Proteinuria and hematuria, often with granular casts in urine, are common. The blood urea nitrogen is elevated. The serum complement level, reflected by β_{1C}, is usually decreased during the early acute phase of the disease.

As in rheumatic fever, the diagnosis of post-streptococcal acute glomerulonephritis has to be substantiated by evidence of antecedent group A streptococcal infection. Throat cultures are positive in about 60 percent while cultures of impetigo lesions are positive in about 95 percent of patients who have not received antibiotics. If isolation of an organism from the patient is not successful, cultures taken from members of the immediate family usually are positive. In the performance of streptococcal antibody tests, special attention should be given to the type of infection with which the nephritis is associated. In pharyngitis-associated nephritis the ASO, anti-DNAse B or anti-NADase tests are almost equally effective. However, in nephritis associated with impetigo, the anti-DNAse B most reliably yields evidence of antecedent streptococcal infection, while the ASO and anti-NADase tests are less reliable.

During the acute stage, hypertensive encephalopathy requires prompt antihypertensive treatment. The prognosis, especially in children, is excellent with a recovery rate of 95 percent or better. Available evidence indicates that post-streptococcal nephritis in children heals completely, while the same disease in adults may lead to chronic nephritis.

Infections by Non-Group A Hemolytic Streptococci

Neonatal sepsis may be caused by group B streptococcus, although this organism is usually innocuous. Group C and G streptococcus have been found responsible for outbreaks of pharyngitis similar to those described with the group A streptococcus. Group D streptococcus, Streptococcus faecalis or enterococcus and Streptococcus viridans are frequent causes of subacute bacterial endocarditis. The group D streptococci are not uniformly sensitive to penicillin, but usually are sensitive to ampicillin or a combination of penicillin and streptomycin.

Diagnostic Laboratory Tests

Familiarization with the technique of culturing and identifying group A streptococci is important to the management of streptococcal disease. Swabbing the throat should be carried out under clear vision and in a deliberate fashion. Plating or inoculation of the culture swab should not be delayed more than one hour, as this results in a poor yield of the streptococcus. Sheep blood agar plates, and no other blood substitute, should be used. The swab is spread over 1/6 of the blood agar plate and streaked over the rest of the plate with a flame-sterilized loop. The agar in the area of the original spread and in other streaked areas should be stabbed with the inoculating loop. The stab allows streptolysin O to effect hemolysis under anaerobic conditions and produce the characteristic β-hemolysis which otherwise might be missed.

Further identification of a β-hemolytic organism can be performed by subculturing the β-hemolytic colonies on another blood agar plate and placing a standard bacitracin disk (Taxos) on the area of the subculture. β-hemolytic streptococci that are sensitive to bacitracin, i.e., show a zone of growth inhibition around the disk, are in all likelihood group A streptococci, while those that are resistant usually are not group A streptococci. This technique is quite satisfactory and is widely used in office laboratories. Another method for group identification is by the fluorescent antibody technique, commonly used in state-wide programs. Definitive identification utilizes the serological technique of Lancefield where hot acid extracts of the cells are tested for reaction with specific antisera. This technique is used also for M-typing of the organism.

Streptococcal antibody tests are particularly useful in providing evidence for antecedent streptococcal infections in patients with acute rheumatic fever and acute glomerulonephritis. As described before, antibodies for the various products of the group A streptococcus are formed during infection by this organism and released into the tissue of the host. Antibodies to certain streptococcal cell components are also formed. The antibody tests available against the streptococcal products are the ASO (anti-streptolysin O), the anti-DNAse B (anti-deoxyribonuclease B), anti-NADase (anti-nicontinamide adenine dinucleotidase, also called anti-DPNase), ASK (anti-streptokinase) and ASH (anti-streptococcal hyaluronidase). Of these tests, the ASO is the most widely used. The other tests have proven to be good adjuncts to the ASO in those cases where the ASO is not elevated in the face of a clinical picture diagnostic of the disease, or in conditions where an ASO response does not occur at a high frequency, as in streptococcal pyoderma or impetigo-associated nephritis.

As with other antibody responses, a certain lapse of time from the onset of infection is required before the antibody level reaches a maximum. For most of the above antibodies this period is three to four weeks. That is why these tests when performed during the acute infection will in all probability be normal, but will become elevated during convalescence or at the time of the onset of the non-purulent sequelae. As mentioned before, an antibody response to any one of these antigens occurs only in 80 to 85 percent of individuals following well documented group A streptococcal infection. Thus, in 15 to 20 percent of cases, a "false" normal value may be encountered. This accounts for the unreliability of using a normal value obtained with *one* antibody test and points to the necessity of performing more than one test before ruling out antecedent streptococcal infection.

The *type-specific* antibody test is of value in determining previous infection with, or immunity to, a specific streptococcal type. Because this antibody cannot be detected before two to three months after an infection and may persist for several years thereafter, its presence does not carry the same significance as the above antibody tests.

Another recently introduced antibody to a cell component is the antibody to the streptococcal group A carbohydrate, the A-antibody. Recent studies have shown this test to be useful in patients with chronic rheumatic valvular heart disease.

Other tests that are commonly used in patients with acute rheumatic fever are the erythrocyte sedimentate rate (ESR) and the C-reactive protein (CRP). These tests, like the leukocyte count, are acute phase reactants and reflect an ongoing inflammatory or tissue destructive process. They are *not* specific for any disease and should not be used as evidence for antecedent streptococcal infection.

It should be re-emphasized that a diagnosis of streptococcal pharyngitis based on clinical criteria alone is often no better than a toss of a coin. The availability of a simple and inexpensive aid for the accurate identification of such infections should compel any physician to have access to the ready performance of throat cultures. The primary prevention of rheumatic fever and rheumatic heart disease, a preventable disease, is predicated on the recognition and proper treatment of acute streptococcal infections.

Again, the diagnosis of acute rheumatic fever should be based on meeting satisfactorily the required Jones Criteria, which were initially proposed to avoid the overdiagnosis of this disease. A hasty diagnosis, particularly one based on the presence of fever and an atypical arthritis, may carry eventually a far more detrimental effect on the patient, socially and psychologically, than the disease itself.

SELECTED REFERENCES

Ayoub, E. M.: Cross-reacting antibodies in the pathogenesis of myocardial and valvular disease. In *Streptococci and Their Diseases.* Symposium held at the University of Minn., May 12–14, 1971. Academic press, to be published.

Brink, W. R., Rammelkamp, C. H., Jr., Denny, F. W. and Wannamaker, L. W.: Effect of penicillin and aureomycin on the natural course of streptococcal tonsillitis and pharyngitis. Am. J. Med., *10*:300, 1951.

Commission on Acute Respiratory Diseases: The role of Lancefield groups of β-hemolytic streptococci in respiratory infections. N. Eng. J. Med., *236*:157, 1947.

Dixon, F. J.: The pathogenesis of glomerulonephritis. Am. J. Med., *44*:493, 1968.

Dudding, B. A. and Ayoub, E. M.: Persistence of streptoccal group A antibody in patients with rheumatic valvular disease. J. Exp. Med., *128*:1081, 1968.

Feingold, D. S., Stagg, N. L. and Kunz, L. J.: Extrarespiratory streptococcal infections. Importance of the various serologic groups. N. Eng. J. Med., *275*:356, 1966.

McCarty, M.: The hemolytic streptococci. In *Bacterial and Mycotic Infections of Man.* R. J. Dubos and J. G. Hirsch (Eds.), 4th Ed., Philadelphia, J. B. Lippincott Company, p. 356, 1965.

Markowitz, M. and Kuttner, A. G.: *Rheumatic Fever*—Diagnosis, Management and Prevention. Philadelphia, W. B. Saunders Company, 1965.

Rammelkamp, C. H., Jr.: Epidemiology of streptococcal infections. The Harvey Lectures, Series 51, p. 113, 1955–56.

Rammelkamp, C. H., Jr.: Etiology of glomerulonephritis. In Black, D.A.K.(Ed.), *Renal Disease.* Philadelphia, Davis, p. 173, 1962.

Stillerman, M. and Bernstein, S. H.: Streptococcal pharyngitis. Evaluation of clinical syndromes in diagnosis. Am. J. Dis. Child., *101*:476, 1961.

Taranta, A.: Rheumatic fever: pathology, etiology, epidemiology and pathogenesis. In Hollander, J. L. (Ed.), *Arthritis and Allied Conditions,* Philadelphia, Lea and Febiger, 1966.

Wannamaker, L. W. and Ayoub, E. M.: Antibody titers in acute rheumatic fever. Circulation, *21*:598, 1960.

Wannamaker, L. W.: Differences between streptococcal infections of the throat and of the skin. N. Eng. J. Med., *282*:23, 78, 1970.

Chapter 21

MENINGITIS

Bacterial meningitis is an acute medical emergency. In patients with signs and symptoms suggestive of meningitis, the physician must first confirm the diagnosis; secondly, identify those patients with bacterial disease; and thirdly, institute appropriate antimicrobial and supportive therapy. Delay in any of these three phases of activity subjects the patient to an increasing risk of significant morbidity or mortality.

Recognition of Meningitis

Recognition of meningitis is seldom difficult if most of the classical signs and symptoms are elicited. Clinical findings that should alert one to the possible presence of the disease are outlined in Table 21.1. Delays in diagnosis occur most frequently with neonates and the elderly or debilitated, in the presence of other infections or neurologic disorders, and in early meningitis. Typical signs and symptoms of infection and meningeal irritation may be minimal or absent in infants; full or bulging fontanelles, lethargy, vomiting and failure to feed are the only usual clinical findings. Sudden or unexpected alterations in mental state and neurologic findings may be the only clues to the presence of the disease in elderly or debilitated patients. Early meningitis may mimic influenza, with only slight nuchal pain and stiffness, headache and low-grade fever. Head trauma, mental aberrations, neurological abnormalities, otitis, sinusitis, mastoiditis, pneumonia, and bacteremia may produce signs and symptoms of sufficient severity to obscure the diagnosis or divert the physician's attention. Each of these should, in fact, alert one to the possible presence of infection of the meninges. If a thorough personal and epidemiologic history and physical examination do not exclude the presence of meningitis, a lumbar puncture should be performed.

Confirmation of the Diagnosis of Meningitis

The clinical diagnosis of meningitis may be substantiated only by careful examination of the cerebrospinal fluid (CSF). This fluid should be

TABLE 21.1

Clinical findings that signal the possible presence of meningitis

---

Classical description:

Evidence of infection: fever (100–106° F), tachycardia (may be slow relative to degree of temperature elevation), chills, lethargy, malaise and skin rash.

Signs of meningeal irritation: headache, stiff neck, stiff back, Brudzinski's sign—resistance to passive neck flexion (may be demonstrable only with patient seated in bed, bending forward at the hips; or with flexion of both knees and hips) and Kernig's sign—difficulty due to pain in extending the leg on the thigh when the latter is flexed to a 90° angle with the trunk.

Disturbances of mental function: lethargy, confusion, delirium, stupor, or coma.

Other neurologic abnormalities: seizures, cranial nerve palsies, hemiparesis, hemiplegia, alterations in superficial or deep tendon reflexes, or other focal neurologic signs.

Early meningitis:

May be flu-like with only a sore and minimally stiff neck, headache, low grade fever and lethargy.

Neonatal meningitis:

Signs of infection and meningeal irritation may be minimal or absent.

Temperature varies—may be low-grade only, normal or subnormal.

Full or bulging fontanelles, lethargy, vomiting, failure to feed or grimacing may be the only suspicious signs.

Meningitis in the elderly or debilitated:

Many, if not all, of the classical signs of infection and meningeal irritation may be absent. Sudden or unexpected alterations in mental status and changes in the neurologic examination may provide the only clues.

---

obtained by lumbar puncture. In the presence of signs of increased intracranial pressure, only the minimum necessary amount of fluid should be removed through a narrow gauge needle. Cysternal or ventricular taps may be required in unusual circumstances, such as a failure to obtain fluid in the lumbar area due to obstruction above.

Recommended studies for confirmation of the diagnosis of meningitis are enumerated in Table 21.2 The cell count and gram stain on the cerebrospinal fluid are of paramount importance. Both of these should always be performed, since inflammatory cells may be absent in early bacterial meningitis, or in fulminant pneumococcal and meningococcal disease in the very young or the elderly. The gram stain, if positive, will provide the basis for initial selection of antimicrobial therapy. It is, therefore, imperative that each slide contain a control sample of mixed flora, such as scrapings from one's teeth, to ensure adequacy of the technique.

TABLE 21.2

Diagnostic studies in patients with meningitis in approximate order of their importance to prompt institution of antimicrobial therapy

Studies imperative for the diagnosis of meningitis:

Cell count on cerebrospinal fluid (CSF).

Gram stain on spun sediment, even in the absence of imflammatory cells. Appropriate control material (e.g., teeth scrapings) should be included on the same slide.

Studies imperative for the recognition of immediately life-threatening, bacterial meningitis:

Cell count on CSF or *gram stain*, or both, should indicate the presence of meningitis, as above. Total cell counts above 1000/cu.mm. are highly suggestive. If initial gram stain is negative, repeat after 6–8 hrs. incubation at 37°F in 3–10% CO_2.

Differential cell count. Granulocytic cells predominate, except in partially treated bacterial meningitis or established infection due to mycobacteria, *Listeria*, or in leptospirosis or syphilis.

Simultaneous blood and CSF glucose. CSF sugar is usually less than 40 mg/100 ml or less than one-half that in blood.

Studies imperative for identification of the etiologic agent in septic meningitis of all causes:

Bacterial culture of CSF. Include warm chocolate agar plate, incubated immediately for meningococci and hemophilus.

Blood cultures. Preferably two.

Acid-fast stain and India ink preparation. Always perform if initial gram stain is negative, or if mononuclear cells predominate and CSF sugar is low.

Culture of CSF for mycobacteria. Always perform if gram stain is negative, even if granulocytic cells predominate.

Culture of CSF for fungi.

Other studies of value in determining the etiology of aseptic meningitis:

CSF serologic test for syphilis.

Acute and convalescent serum for leptospirosis serology.

Culture of CSF for virus isolation.

Acute and convalescent serum for viral antibody determinations.

Stool specimen for virus isolation.

CSF tumor cytology, if indicated.

Recognition of Immediately Life-Threatening Bacterial Meningitis

Having confirmed the presence of meningitis, attention should be directed immediately to recognition of possible life-threatening pyogenic infection. Recommended studies are listed in Table 21.2. If the gram stain reveals the presence of bacteria, one must assure that appropriate cultures are planted and therapy should be instituted at once. If the initial gram stain is negative, pyogenic meningitis is by no means excluded. A total cell count above 1000 per cu. mm., predominance of granulocytic cells and decreased glucose content of the CSF constitute sufficient evidence to begin antimicrobial therapy. Initial selection of therapeutic agent in this setting is based upon the distinctive clinical features of the illness and the most probable etiologic agents for the patient's age and prior state of health (see below). Failure to observe predominance of granulocytic cells, by itself, does not exclude the diagnosis of bacterial meningitis. Partially treated pyogenic meningitis and infections due to mycobacteria, listeria, leptospira, and treponemes may result in a mononuclear inflammatory response in the CSF. If doubt remains regarding the presence or absence of bacterial meningitis at this point, both antimicrobial therapy and further diagnostic studies should be begun promptly.

Identification of the Etiologic Agent in Meningitis

Having attempted to recognize the presence of life-threatening pyogenic infection, attention should then be directed to precise identification of the etiologic agent. The more serious, potentially remedial causes of meningitis are afforded priority. The appropriate laboratory studies are listed in Table 21.2. Cultures of CSF for pyogenic bacteria should be performed in all patients with meningitis. Blood cultures should be obtained, since they are frequently diagnostic in patients with bacterial meningitis. Occasionally, cultures of blood will yield the infecting microorganism, while those of CSF remain negative. If the initial gram stain has been unrevealing, stains and cultures for acid-fast microorganisms and fungi are next in order of importance. Granulocytic cells may be present early in the course of tuberculous meningitis. Therefore, this diagnosis should be strongly considered in any patient with negative studies for other bacteria and low CSF glucose. Diagnosis of viral, leptospiral, or syphillitic meningitis may be confirmed by appropriate cultures or serologic study.

Distinctive Clinical and Epidemiological Features of the Various Meningitides

Heretofore, rapid identification of the more serious, potentially remedial causes of meningitis has been emphasized. This is clearly the most useful approach in the emergent situation. The various meningitides have been traditionally categorized as *septic* or *aseptic*. (The meningitides have also been classified as *granulocytic* or *lymphocytic,* and *suppurative* or *serous*. These are synonymous with septic or aseptic, respectively.) *Septic meningitis* is associated with a granulocytic response or a low glucose in the CSF. *Aseptic meningitis* is characterized by predominance of mononuclear cells and normal glucose. It must be understood that these terms are not synonymous with *treatable* or *non-treatable* with regard to specific antimicrobial therapy. As noted above, certain patients may present with meningeal infection due to common pathogens, that may mimic aseptic meningitis. Thus, in the absence of microorganisms in stained specimens, no single test, or combination of laboratory studies, is infallible in immediately distinguishing remedial from non-remedial causes of meningitis. In order to make this distinction, the physician must rely upon his clinical judgment which is based upon a composite of distinctive clinical and epidemiological features of the patient's illness, plus the results of appropriate laboratory studies. The unique clinical and epidemiologic characteristics of the various meningitides are outlined in Table 21.3, and the more commonly encountered clinical entities are described below.

Meningococcal Meningitis

Meningococcal meningitis may be a rapidly lethal disease. Death occurs occasionally within a few hours of onset of symptoms. Prompt recognition and aggressive therapy are imperative to ensure a favorable outcome.

Meningococci are gram-negative diplococci belonging to the genus Neisseria. They are frequently observed intracellularly in clinical specimens. They grow poorly in routine culture media and may not survive prolonged exposure to air or ambient temperature. For these reasons, clinical specimens should be inoculated promptly onto warm enriched medium, such as sheep's blood or chocolate agar plates. Incubation at 37°C in 3 to 10 percent CO_2 in air will ensure optimal recovery of the microorganisms from clinical specimens.

Meningococci may be classified into at least 10 distinct groups on the basis of agglutination in specific antisera. Strains of serogroups A, B, and C account for the majority of cases of meningitis. Meningitis may occur as an epidemic disease or sporadically. Major epidemics due to group A strains tend to occur in 14 to 21 year cycles. Smaller, more protracted epidemics due to groups B and C meningococci occur in intervening years. Disease due to all serogroups is most frequent in winter and early spring. Children and young adults are most commonly afflicted. Epidemic disease is more likely to occur among individuals living in crowded conditions. Military recruits are especially vulnerable during their first 90 days of training.

Meningococci are spread from person to person by aerosol, or occasionally by direct contact. Initial infections occur in the nasopharynx. The vast majority of these are asymptomatic, and are followed by an antibody response that appears to be protective within several weeks. Infected individuals may carry and shed the organisms for weeks or months despite the appearance of group-specific antibodies in their serum. There are no known reservoirs of the organisms in nature other than man.

TABLE 21.3

Distinctive clinical and epidemiological features of the various meningitides and their therapy

Type	Distinctive features	Optimal therapy in adults
	A. Potentially remedial meningitides	
Pneumococcal	Primary site of infection frequently found in lungs, ears, sinuses. Frequent in elderly, alcoholics, and patients with head trauma or myeloma.	Penicillin G, 15–20 million units/da.
Meningococcal	Primary site of infection in nasopharynx. Petechial skin rash common and may yield the microorganism on stain or culture. Purpuric skin lesions. Waterhouse Freiderichsen syndrome. More common in winter. Epidemic disease seen among crowded individuals.	Penicillin G, 15–20 million units/da.
Hemophilis influenzae, Type B	Originates in respiratory tract and contiguous structures in children, age 3 mo. to 6 yrs., and alcoholics. Antecedent infection, such as croup or epiglottitis, often apparent. Transient, unilateral VI cranial nerve palsy occurs early in 20% of patients. Secondary cases in family contacts occur rarely.	Ampicillin, at least 150 mg./kg./da.
Staphylococcus aureus	May originate in skin or respiratory tract and contiguous structures. Almost always associated with bacteremia and abscesses in central nervous system. Wound infection may be present. Not common.	Methicillin or other penicillinase-resistant penicillin, 12 gm./da.; or penicillin G, 20 million units/day, depending on susceptibility.
Staphylococcus albus	Frequent skin contaminant in CSF cultures. One of more common causes of meningitis originating on artificial valves or shunts used in control of hydrocephalus.	Depends on susceptibility. Replacement of valve or shunt may be necessary.
Listeria monocytogenes	Occurs most commonly in the debilitated, alcoholics, or diabetics. May be associated with lymphocytosis in CSF or peripheral blood. May be confused with contaminant diphtheroids in CSF.	Penicillin G, 15–20 million units/da.
Leptospirosis	Illness may be diphasic. Suffusion conjunctivae, hepatitis, myositis common. Diffuse erythematous skin rash, vasculitis may occur. Peak incidence in summer. Follows exposure to rodents, dogs, farm animals or water contaminated by their excreta. Granulocytic pleocytosis in CSF early, becomes mononuclear. CSF sugar may be normal. CSF bilirubin approximates that in blood.	Penicillin G, 15–20 million units/da.
Acute syphilitic	Genital or other lesions may be noted. Varies from asymptomatic to severe meningitis. Blood and CSF serologic test for syphilis positive. Lymphocytic pleocytosis and normal sugar in CSF.	Penicillin G, 15–20 million units/da.
Partially treated bacterial meningitis	Mononuclear cells predominate and sugar in CSF may be nearly normal. Untreated patients often relapse to septic meningitis with granulocytic pleocytosis and low sugar in CSF.	Appropriate to infecting organism. Usually penicillin G.
Tuberculous	Usually originates in lung, although lesions may not be apparent on X-Ray. Tuberculomas in choroid. Focal neurological signs common—may predominate. Lymphocytic pleocytosis follows initial granulocytic response in CSF. Glucose in CSF usually low. Acid-fast bacilli may be demonstrable in sputum, pellicle in CSF sample, exudates, bone marrow aspirate or liver biopsy.	Isoniazid, 300 mg./da., streptomycin, 1 gm./da., and PAS, 12 gm./da., or ethambutol, 15 mg./kg./da. Adrenal steroids may be a useful adjunct.

TABLE 21.3—*Continued*

Type	Distinctive features	Optimal therapy in adults
Cryptococcal	Originates in lung, although lesions may not be apparent. Onset insidious. Focal neurologic signs may predominate. Lymphocytic pleocytosis and low sugar in CSF. Organisms demonstrable on India ink preparation of CSF and may be recovered from blood, urine or other tissues.	Amphotericin B or 5-fluorocytosine
	B. Reactions to parameningeal inflammation-potentially remedial	
Brain abscess	Often originates in lungs. Follows bacteremia. Patients with cyanotic heart disease are especially prone. Focal neurologic symptoms may predominate. Mononuclear cells in CSF rarey exceed several hundred—numbers in excess of 500 indicate impending or actual rupture of abscess. CSF sugar normal.	Antimicrobial depends on infecting microorganism. Surgical drainage or excision required.
Epidural abscess	Originates in structures abutting dura—skull, spine, mastoid, sinuses, ears. Local tenderness may be evoked. Focal neurological signs common. Mononuclear pleocytosis (<200 cells/cu. mm.) and normal sugar in CSF.	Surgical drainage, plus antimicrobial depending on susceptibility.
Thrombophlebitis of venous sinuses	Originates from infection in adjacent structures. Symptoms are focal. Patients are usually profoundly ill. CSF contains few mononuclear cells, normal sugar and occasionally red cells.	Antibiotics depending on susceptibility. Treat infection at site of origin.
	C. Other meningitides—seldom remedial by specific therapy	
Enteroviral	Originate primarily in alimentary tract. Mononuclear pleocytosis follows initial granulocytic response with normal sugar in CSF. Epidemics occur in summer and fall. Poliovirus infection may be followed by paralysis. Coxsackie group may cause herpangina, upper respiratory infections, orchitis, pleurodynia, pericarditis and rarely paralysis. ECHO viruses cause a variety of exanthems and occasionally encephalitis.	Symptomatic
Mumps	May precede or follow parotitis or orchitis. Asymptomatic meningeal reaction is common. Mononuclear cells and normal sugar found in CSF. Occurs primarily in winter and spring.	Symptomatic
Lymphocytic choriomeningitis	Flu-like illness may precede or occur simultaneously. Mononuclear cells predominate with normal CSF sugar. Occurs in autumn and winter. Follows exposure to mice.	Symptomatic
Other viruses	Occur infrequently. Symptoms depend on specific virus. Mononuclear cells and normal CSF sugar.	Symptomatic
Arboviruses	Encephalitis usually predominates. Serologic titres (HI test) are usually elevated at onset on symptoms. In an endemic area insect bite usually precedes disease.	Symptomatic
Tumor	Focal neurologic signs are commonly present. Cells in CSF are those of tumor, or mononuclear. Occasionally CSF sugar may be depressed.	Occasionally responds to antitumor therapy, especially if origin in hematopoietic or reticuloendothelial tissues.

A minority of infected individuals develop meningococcal disease. In patients who acquire meningitis, only a mild sore throat, slight fever and headache may be noted at the outset. Within hours, symptoms abruptly worsen; headache becomes more profound, fever increases and signs of meningitis evolve rapidly. Nausea and vomiting may occur. Occasional patients complain of agonizing joint pain. Shortly thereafter the characteristic skin rash appears. At first, it may be morbilliform or infrequently urticarial. Within approximately an hour the rash becomes petechial, and then purpuric. Cutaneous manifestations may be absent in some patients while petechiae are confined to the conjunctivae in others. Meningococci may be found within material obtained by puncture or scraping of petechial lesions.

Early neurological manifestations are variable. Extreme mania and hyperactivity occur more frequently in meningococcal meningitis, than in other meningitides. Cranial nerve palsies are common; bilateral involvement of the sixth, seventh or eighth nerves is most frequent. Damage to the eighth nerve is usually irreversible. The function of other cranial nerves more commonly returns to normal following recovery.

The Waterhouse-Friederichsen syndrome—massive purpura, hypotension, and overwhelming sepsis—may supervene. Few patients with this syndrome survive. Although it occurs most frequently in meningococcal disease, patients with meningitis or bacteremia due to other microorganisms may experience a similar syndrome. Adrenal hemorrhage is often noted. Consumptive coagulopathy occurs concomitantly, and may be etiologically related to many of the manifestations of this syndrome.

Infection may localize in the humors of the eye, joints or pericardium during the course of meningitis and bacteremia. Effusions of the joints and pericardium that occur early in the disease are often septic. Sterile effusions may be noted 10 to 14 days following the onset of meningitis and usually after the patient has recovered from the acute infection. These are almost always self-limited. Occasionally, pericardial effusions are of sufficient size to necessitate pericardiocentesis.

Pneumococcal Meningitis

The pneumococcus is the most common cause of bacterial meningitis in adults and of recurrent meningitis in patients of all ages. Most patients who acquire the disease experience antecedent symptomatic infection in the respiratory tract or contiguous structures. Sinusitis, otitis, mastoiditis, and pneumonia are the most frequent antecedents. Head trauma, alcoholism, sickle cell disease, debility, multiple myeloma and dysglobulinemias predispose to pneumococcal infection and meningitis. Recurrent meningeal infection occurs primarily in patients with multiple myeloma or skull fractures with cerebrospinal fluid rhinorrhea. There are few other distinctive clinical features of pneumococcal meningitis.

Occasional patients with pneumococcal meningitis and bacteremia develop petechial or purpuric skin lesions. The lancet-shaped, gram-positive diplococci may be identified in material obtained from petechial lesions. Consumptive coagulopathy and a clinical picture resembling the Waterhouse-Friederichsen syndrome of meningococcal disease may occur. Secondary cases among contacts of patients with pneumococcal meningitis seldom occur.

Meningitis due to Hemophilus Influenzae

Pathogenic strains of *Hemophilus influenzae* are pleomorphic, encapsulated gram-negative rods. Because of the high degree of pleomorphism, stains of clinical specimens are frequently misinterpreted. Coccoid forms may resemble meningococci in adequately stained preparations; while pneumococci may be suspected in slides that have been insufficiently decolorized. The proper identification of these three genera in stained specimens has important therapeutic and epidemiologic implications.

Strains of *Hemophilus influenzae* are common inhabitants of the respiratory tract of man. Few children escape contact with these microorganisms in their early years. Most infections in children are confined to the respiratory tract and contiguous structures. Pharyngitis, otitis, sinusitis, mastoiditis, epiglottitis and pneumonia are most frequently seen. The initial encounter with hemophilus is followed by a brisk rise in serum antibodies directed against the capsular polysaccharide of the infecting strain. Thus group-specific immunity is conferred. Most school-age children possess antibodies against the Group B organisms, which cause the majority of serious hemophilus infections. Meningitis due to hemophilus is therefore seen almost exclusively in children of ages less than six to eight years. Newborns are seldom infected because of the presence of maternal antibody in their serum.

Infections of the respiratory tract, sinuses, ears or mastoid air cells are frequently noted immediately before or coincident with the onset of hemophilus meningitis. These infections may be of sufficient severity to obscure the presence of meningeal symptoms. Skin rashes are less frequently encountered in hemophilus meningitis than in the meningitides due to meningococci or pneumococci. Unilateral palsy of the sixth cranial nerve may be seen in approximately 20 percent of patients with hemophilus meningitis. There are few other distinctive clinical features of the illness. Secondary cases of meningitis among household contacts are encountered rarely.

The Aseptic Meningitis Syndrome

The syndrome of aseptic meningitis (lymphocytic pleocytosis and normal or low cerebrospinal fluid sugar) may be caused by a variety of agents. That due to listeria, leptospira, spirochetes, mycobacteria, fungi, abscess in contiguous structures, or partially treated bacterial infection may be responsive to appropriate specific therapy. No specific treatment has been described for the remainder of the etiologic agents. Distinctive features of the remedial and non-remedial causes of this syndrome are outlined in Table 21.3.

Most cases of the aseptic meningitis syndrome result from viral infection. The mumps and enteric viruses are implicated in the majority of instances. Among the latter, most ECHO and coxsackie A and all poliomyelitis and coxsackie B viruses have been shown to cause meningitis. The arthropod-borne (Arbo), lymphocytic choriomeningitis (LCM), and herpes simplex viruses have been encountered less frequently. Typically, illnesses are self-limited, seldom exceeding 3 to 10 days in duration. Prolonged illness (weeks to months in duration) may result occasionally from infection with the LCM virus. CSF cell counts per cu. mm. in viral meningitis usually range from 10 to 500, although counts as high as 5000 may occur. Although a mononuclear pleocytosis is most common, a polymorphonuclear response may occur early in any of the viral meningitides. CSF glucose concentration is most often within the normal range; however, slightly low values have been observed in many viral meningitides, especially those due to mumps, LCM and herpes viruses.

Certain epidemiological characteristics may be useful in presumptive identification of the etiologic agent in the aseptic meningitis syndrome. Disease occurring in summer or fall in temperate climates suggest enteroviral, arbovirus or leptospiral infection. Peak incidence of LCM occurs in late fall or winter, while mumps meningitis is noted most frequently in winter and spring. Seasonal variations in the incidence of viral meningitides may be less pronounced in tropical or subtropical climates. Disease due to LCM virus follows exposure to infected mice, while leptospirosis follows contact with rodents, dogs, farm animals or water contaminated by their excreta. Patients with tuberculous meningitis may give a history of contact with infected patients, while patients with cryptococcal disease may report contact with pigeons or their excreta. Occurrence of viral meningitis in otherwise well patients over 40 years of age suggests infection with the arthropod-borne viruses.

Knowledge of the diseases extant coincidentally in the community may provide useful clues to the etiologic agent in the aseptic meningitis syndrome. Epidemic parotitis or orchitis indicate the presence of mumps or coxsackie viruses. Epidemic pleurodynia results from spread of certain coxsackie viruses, and appearance of cases of encephalitis may implicate the arboviruses.

Certain clinical and laboratory characteristics of the patient's illness may be sufficiently distinctive to provide useful diagnostic clues. A diphasic illness with conjunctival suffusion, jaundice and diffuse erythematous skin rash suggests leptospiral meningitis. A concentration of bilirubin in the CSF that approximates that found in the blood also may be indicative of infection with leptospira. Cerebrospinal fluid sugar content is seldom low in leptospiral meningitis.

Skin rash may occur with infections due to the enteroviruses, especially the ECHO group. The rash characteristically appears with the onset of fever and lasts four to five days. It is discrete, erythematous, maculopapular and non-pruritic. It may involve all body surfaces or remain confined to the face, neck and shoulders. Petechial or vesicular skin rashes may occur occasionally, especially with infections due to the coxsackie A9 and A17 viruses. Occurrence of paralysis suggests infection with the polioviruses or rarely the coxsackie group. Herpangina, pleurodynia, and pericarditis may be associated with coxsackie meningitis. Parotitis and orchitis occur commonly with mumps and occasionally with coxsackie meningitis.

A progressive illness with positive tuberculin skin test, characteristic chest x-ray and CSF cell count below 500 per cu. mm. is highly suggestive of tuberculous meningitis. However, occasional patients with tuberculous meningitis may not have abnormal chest roentgenograms. Diagnosis then depends upon demonstration of the tubercle bacilli in CSF, liver or bone marrow aspirates.

Chronic meningitis with insidious onset, fluctuations in severity of illness and focal neurologic signs is characteristic of infection with cryptococci. An increased susceptibility to cryptococcal meningitis has been noted in patients with poorly controlled diabetes, lymphomas and other diseases involving the reticuloendothelial system.

Therapy

The prompt administration of appropriate antimicrobial therapy is the single most important factor in determining the outcome of bacterial meningitis. It is thus not possible to await results of cultures and susceptibility tests before initiating treatment. If the etiologic agent has been presumptively identified by microscopic examination of the cerebrospinal fluid, the appropriate antimicrobial agent should be given immediately. The optimal therapy for the specific causes of bacterial meningitis is listed in Table 21.3.

Occasionally no etiologic agent is demonstrable on initial CSF stains, despite findings that suggest the presence of bacterial meningitis. In this situation, consideration must be given to the distinctive clinical and epidemiologic features of the patient's illness as well as his age. The more common etiologic agents in bacterial meningitis, listed according to age of the patient, are shown in Table 21.4. The antimicrobial therapy chosen should be of known efficacy against the most probable causative agents of

TABLE 21.4

Common etiologic agents in septic meningitis: occurrence by age and initial antimicrobial therapy

Age	Etiologic agents in approximate order of occurrence	Initial therapy, pending definitive diagnosis
Prematures to 3 mo.	*E. coli*, other enterobacteriaceae, streptococci, *H. influenzae*, listeria, pneumococci	Penicillin G or ampicillin, plus kanamycin or gentamicin
3 mo. to 6 yrs.	*H. influenzae* (type B), meningococci, pneumococci	Ampicillin
6 to 21 yrs.	Meningococci, pneumococci	Penicillin G
Greater than 21 yrs.	Pneumococci, meningococci	Penicillin G

the patient's illness. The drugs most likely to be effective for meningitis occurring in various age groups are listed in Table 21.4.

In meningitis of all causes, the ultimate outcome may depend in large part upon the prompt administration and careful maintenance of supportive care. The patient's vital signs and clinical status should be monitored frequently until significant improvement is noted. Fluid volume should be maintained. An indwelling central venous catheter should be employed to follow the patient's circulatory status if shock is present. Shock should be managed according to the principles outlined in Chapter 9. An adequate airway should be maintained. Occasionally ventilatory assistance may be required. The delirious or convulsing patient may require restraint or cautious sedation.

Antimicrobial therapy of acute bacterial meningitis should be continued until the patient has been free of signs and symptoms of meningitis for three to five days. In addition, the spinal fluid cell count should be less than 20 to 40 cells/cu. mm. and glucose content should be normal. Persistence of symptoms or abnormal findings in the CSF suggest the presence of phlebitis, abscess, subdural effusion, parameningeal infection or drug fever. Chemotherapy of tuberculous meningitis should be continued for six weeks with streptomycin and for one to two years with isoniazid and its companion drug.

Prevention

The occurrence of bacterial meningitis, particularly meningococcal, has frequently been considered an indication for chemoprophylaxis of all the patient's recent contacts. Chemoprophylaxis is useful in only specific circumstances. Secondary attack rates among contacts of patients with meningitis due to bacteria other than meningococci are insufficient to warrant the expense and risks of drug therapy. Among contacts of patients with meningococci, only the following are at sufficiently increased risk to warrant chemoprophylaxis: 1) military recruits among whose ranks meningococcal disease has developed; 2) ship or submarine crews who have been exposed and are likely to be at sea for prolonged periods; 3) case-contacts sleeping in crowded, unpartitioned quarters, such as dormitories, barracks or nursing homes; 4) contacts of cases in households in which three or more individuals share the same bedroom; and 5) medical personnel who have highly intimate contact, such as administration of mouth-to-mouth resuscitation. Other case-contacts appear to be at little or no increased risk, and should not receive prophylaxis. They are 1) casual contacts not sharing the same living quarters; 2) most adults residing in the same household; and 3) other medical personnel.

At present, only sulfadiazine (or other sulfonamides) and rifampin are likely to be efficacious in prevention of meningococcal disease due to susceptible strains. Many meningococci are now highly resistant to the sulfonamides and a few are resistant to rifampin. Other antimicrobial agents that inhibit meningococcal growth *in vitro* have been shown to be of little or no value in elimination of meningococci from asymptomatic subjects. They are 1) penicillin G—despite its proven value in treatment of meningococcal disease; 2) benzathine penicillin; 3) ampicillin; 4) erythromycin; 5) tetracycline; 6) chloramphenicol; and 7) cephalexin.

Currently, a recently marketed drug, minocycline, appears to be promising in elimination of meningococci from known carriers. Group specific polysaccharides of sero-group A and C meningococci have been extracted and purified. Injection of these into human volunteers has been followed by a brisk bactericidal antibody response. Early studies indicate significant protection against acquisition of infection with Group A and C microorganisms. The prospects for eventual immunologic or chemotherapeutic control of epidemic meningococcal disease appear promising.

Prevention of specific viral meningitides depends upon maintenance of immunizations with the appropriate available vaccines. Nosocomial meningitides may be prevented by prompt recognition and therapy of bacteremias and by proper use of devices, such as indwelling catheters, that may serve as potential sources of bacteremia.

Until more satisfactory techniques for prevention become available, control of meningitis depends primarily upon prompt recognition and aggressive therapy.

SELECTED REFERENCES

Fekety, F. R., Jr., and Johns, R. J.: Infections of the nervous system, in *The Principles and Practice of Medicine,* 17th Ed., A. M. Harvey, L. E. Cluff, R. J. Johns, A. H. Owens, Jr., D. Rabinowitz, and R. S. Ross, Ed., Appleton-Century-Crofts, N. Y., 1968, p. 762.

Lepow, M. L., Carver, D. H., Wright, H. T., Woods, W. A. and Robbins, F. C.: A clinical, epidemiological and laboratory investigation of aseptic meningitis during the four-year period, 1955–1958. I. Observations concerning etiology and epidemiology. N. Eng. J. Med., *266*:1181, 1962.

Lepow, M. L., Coyne, N., Thompson, L. B., Carver, D. H., and Robbins, F. C.: A clinical, epidemiological and laboratory investigation of aseptic meningitis during the four-year period, 1955–1958. II. The clinical disease and its sequellae. N. Eng. J. Med., *266*:1188, 1962.

Sanders, E. and Deal, W. B.: Prevention of meningococcal infections. J. Infect. Dis., *121*:449, 1970.

Chapter 22

ENCEPHALITIS

The traditional concept of a viral disease affecting the nervous system is that of an infectious illness which is initially manifested by signs and symptoms of a systemic malady and is followed, within days, by evidence of neural malfunction. Such a concept, however, needs to be modified in view of recent interpretation of possible infectious mechanisms causing certain, heretofore designated, degenerative central nervous system diseases. These latter conditions, subacute encephalitis, Jakob-Creutzfeldt disease and kuru are thought to represent a chronic viral infectious state implying that viruses or at least "filterable agents" persist in the CNS and cause a slowly evolving type of brain disease in contrast to the "hit and run" variety which is more readily recognized as acute encephalitis.

Acute Viral Encephalitis

Those viruses known to affect the central nervous system have been categorized according to their ecological characteristics (e.g., arthropod borne viruses), and their antigenic responses as well as their usual site of replication within the human body (e.g., enteroviruses). Moreover, identification has been made on the basis of viral predilection for the nervous system; those being neurotropic (e.g., polio) in contrast with others which only occasionally penetrate the CNS. Possibly a better definition is to be obtained by referring to the morphological, physical and chemical qualities of the virus, although the clinical observations do not lead the physician immediately to the conclusion that an RNA or DNA type of virus is involved with the disease being considered.

Clinical manifestations

A preceding upper respiratory or gastrointestinal infection is described by approximately one-half the patients who are seen with the signs and symptoms characteristic of acute encephalitis. Severe unlocalized headache, fever and vague mental changes ranging from lethargy to irritation and confusion characterize the complaints of the mildly affected patient. Symptoms of a more profound nature including delirium, convulsions and coma may occur within hours after the initial complaint of headache. The neurological examination may reveal evidence of meningeal irritation, photophobia as well as mild generalized weakness.

Focal neurological signs such as hemiplegia or aphasia are uncommon but, when present, imply a more serious illness. Furthermore, such focal involvement is more typical of an arthropod-borne or Herpes hominis viral disease. Increased intracranial pressure is another unusual finding, again apparent in the patient with severe encephalitis who presents with signs of a rapidly progressive illness.

Certain viruses are more likely to be suspect on the basis of selective findings on history or examination (Table 22.1).

Diagnostic Studies

Laboratory studies designed to confirm a diagnosis of viral encephalitis include a hemogram which may be normal or reveal a mild leucocytosis. Skull and chest roentgenograms are of help in excluding a chronic infectious locus in the sinuses or lungs as a source for cerebral mycotic emboli and abscess formation. The cerebrospinal fluid (CSF) pressure may be elevated; the fluid, however, is usually clear and colorless (rarely cloudy or xanthochromic), the protein content may be normal or mildly elevated, the sugar content is normal (rarely depressed), and the cell count is commonly elevated. Approximately 15 percent of patients with acute viral encephalitis have normal CSF findings in the initial diagnostic lumbar puncture fluid; subsequent CSF studies, however, usually reveal the more typical cellular response with 20 to 500 leukocytes/mm^3, primarily lymphocytes. Recent fluorescent antibody techniques have allowed a diagnosis of *Herpes simplex* infection to be made from the cells obtained at the time of lumbar puncture.

The differential diagnosis based on the spinal fluid findings include other infectious illnesses. Bacterial meningitis may be suspected, particularly if there is a predominance of polymorphonuclear leucocytes. The offending agent involved in the case of a partially treated bacterial meningitis may never be cultured and the physician must decide whether the clinical picture represents a viral or bacterial process. Elevated spinal fluid enzymes signifying a destructive process would point in favor of a severe encephalitis; however, in the mildly affected patient this test is of little help. It rests with the clinician to elect to use high doses of antibiotics or not.

Associated pulmonary findings, skin tests, and family history of disease would urge consideration for treatment with anti-tuberculous therapy

TABLE 22.1

Characteristics in acute viral encephalitis

Virus	History	Often seen general findings	Neurological features
1. DNA			
A. Pox virus: variola-vaccinia	Recent contact or immunization	Skin lesions	Severe, generalized encephalitis
B. Herpes virus a) *H. hominis* (simplex)	"Cold sores"	Skin lesions	Severe, often focal temporal lobe dysfunction may present as mass
b) *H. Varicella* (chicken pox)	Recent contact	Skin lesions	Cerebellar symptoms; combined encephalomyelitis
c) Cytomegalo virus	Immunosuppressive therapy; kidney transplant in adult	Petechiae and hepatosplenomegaly in newborn	Diffuse encephalitis with residual symptoms such as hydrocephalus in child
C. Adenovirus	Previous URI	Rash	Usually mild encephalitis or aseptic meningitis
2. RNA			
A. Myxovirus			
Mumps	Recent contact	Parotitis, orchitis, abd. pain	Mild encephalitis; hearing impairment
Measles	Recent contact	Exanthem	Severe generalized encephalitis
B. Reovirus	Upper respiratory tract infection	Occasional rash	Usually mild encephalitis or aseptic meningitis
C. Arthropod-borne (equine encephalitis, etc.)	Epidemic situation		Severe encephalitis in infants and elderly may present focal signs
D. Small RNA virus: enterovirus, coxsackie virus, polio	Gastrointestinal disease, respiratory disease	Occasional rash	Usually mild encephalitis except in infancy; cerebellar and myelitis signs
Rabies	Rabid animal bite	Pain and numbness at site of rash	Convulsions induced by swallowing

particularly if the duration of illness is somewhat prolonged. A positive serological and spinal fluid test for syphilis would likewise change the initial impression of a viral infection; and the presence of large numbers of cells would urge one to consider the possibility of a fungal infection which might be identified by the use of an India ink stain as well as by means of special culture media. Concomitant hepatitis or a history of rat bite indicates leptospirosis; splenomegaly and adenopathy would suggest infectious mononucleosis, or toxoplasmosis; and evidence of a collagen-vascular systemic illness would indicate an encephalitic vasculitis in the suspect patient with CSF pleocytosis. During the acute phase of the illness, irregular diffuse slow wave activity (Fig. 22.1) corresponds to the generalized cerebral dysfunction clinically apparent. Bitemporal lobe abnormalities imply infection with *Herpes hominis*. In association with the clinical improvement, the EEG will become more normal (Fig. 22.2), however, a normalization of the record will be seen when the acute phase of the illness recedes and the patient's condition has stabilized, thereby indicating that further clinical improvement may not be forthcoming to a significant degree.

Focal neurological deficits may indicate the need to pursue further diagnostic studies to exclude the possibility of an intracerebral or extradural abscess. Certainly if the history is vague and the patient is in coma, additional tests are vital if the interpretation of the deficit is inapparent. The echoencephalogram will confirm a shift of midline structures; however, the arteriogram is the definitive test. Localized encephalitic disease may cause intracranial vessel displacement often with the appearance of a vascular "blush" implying new vessel formation. This finding is indistin-

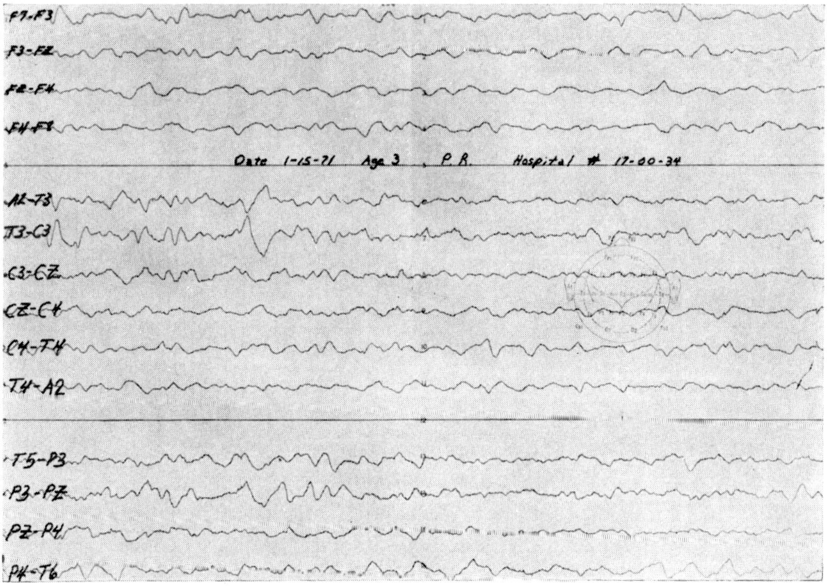

FIG. 22.1. EEG revealing diffuse slow wave forms in 3-year-old child with acute viral encephalitis.

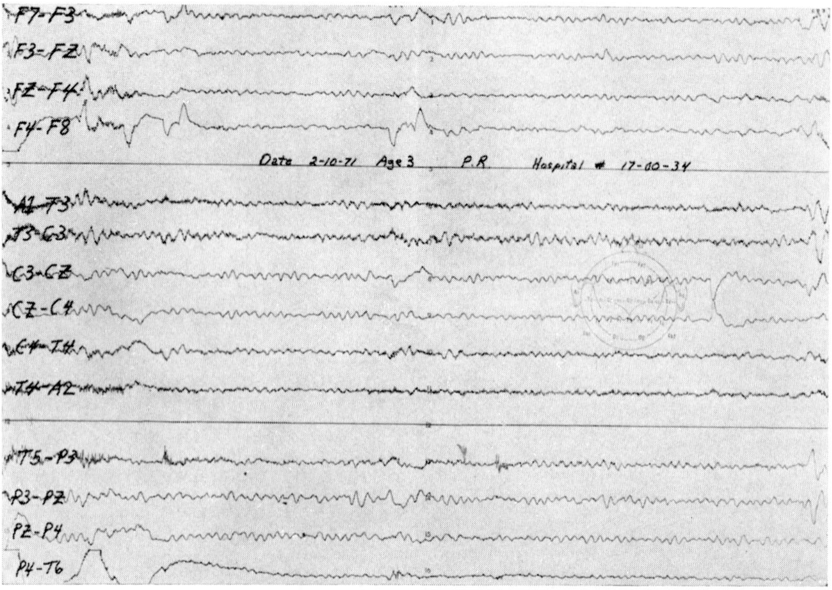

FIG. 22.2. EEG performed 25 days later in same patient as Fig. 22.1 revealing normal pattern.

guishable from a bacterial cerebritis or a malignant neoplasm. On the other hand, a normal arteriogram denies the existence of a mass as well as hydrocephalus, since lateral ventricular size can be estimated by this study.

Craniotomy has been undertaken in those circumstances where the mass effect is sufficient to cause significant intracranial hypertension since a mistaken diagnosis could lead to herniation of the temporal lobe through the tentorial notch and death. Biopsy of an encephalitic area in a so-called silent part of the brain does not insult the brain nor does it lead to a clinical deficit upon recovery. The presence of perivascular inflammatory round cells, glial clusters and inclusion bodies confirm the diagnosis of a viral encephalitis (Fig. 22.3); furthermore, immediate specific fluorescent antibody staining techniques can provide a rapid means of diagnosing *Herpes hominis* infection as a prelude to considering antiviral therapy. In addition, the tissue may be sent for virus isolation.

In general, regional state viral laboratories isolate a virus from the following tissues and body fluids in decreasing order of success: feces, brain, urine, cerebrospinal fluid. Serodiagnostic tests revealing a rise in antibody titers noted in specimens taken two or more weeks apart are more reliable since the mere presence of the virus in body tissue does not imply its disease-producing activity. Depending on the sophistication and facilities of the diagnostic laboratory the offending virus may be detected in up to 60 percent of those patients suspected of suffering from viral infections of the nervous system.

Treatment

General supportive measures include care of respiratory, bladder and bowel function, protection of the eyes from exposure keratitis, avoidance of pressure sores on the skin, gentle passive movement of the limbs to prevent contractures and the administration of appropriate fluid therapy with frequent monitoring of serum electrolytes. Maintenance of normal body temperature is appropriate and may be achieved by the rectal administration of aspirin if oral feeding is contra-indicated because of the fear of aspiration. Cool sheets on the skin or even isotonic saline enema may be required in the hyperthermic patient. Hypothermia therapy (ice blanket) to maintain subnormal temperature is not warranted.

Periodic urine cultures in the catheterized patient, chest roentgenograms in the obtunded patient, blood counts and cultures when indicated followed by the administration of appropriate antibiotic will prevent the development of serious superimposed bacterial infection. Anticonvulsant

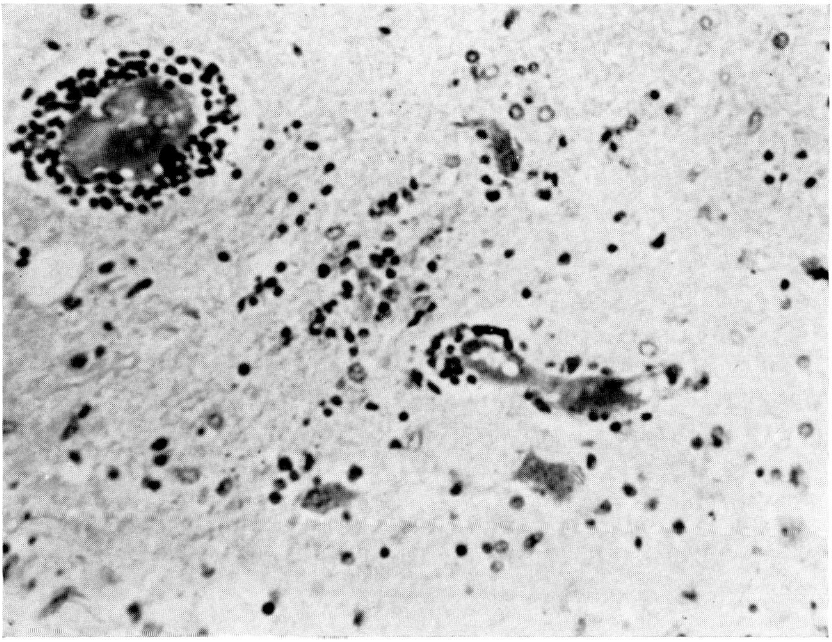

FIG. 22.3. Perivascular round cell and round cell clusters in brain of patient who died from acute viral encephalitis.

therapy is to be administered if seizures occur. Sodium phenobarbital given intravenously at the time of the seizure (1 to 4 mg./kg.) and then maintained (2 mg./kg./da.) until recovery is felt to be complete is the drug of choice. Status epilepticus may be treated also with diazepam, 5 to 10 mg. IV. Diphenylhydantoin sodium (200 to 400 mg./da.) may be substituted for or added to phenobarbital if the latter drug is felt to add to the obtunded state of the patient and prevent adequate assessment of his mental state.

Corticosteroid therapy has not proven to be of value. Moreover, the risk of worsening the virus infection is great. Gastric ulcers and hypertension are two other worries which may be eliminated if corticosteroid therapy is not given.

Specific antiviral therapy is available only in the instance where a rabid animal is known to have bitten the patient. According to an appropriate schedule depending on the severity of the bite, avianized rabies vaccine prepared from virus grown in duck embryo is administered. Hyperimmune rabies antiserum also may be given.

Other antiviral agents including those capable of inhibiting virus absorption and penetration (1-adamantanamine), inhibiting virus-directed biosynthesis (benzimidazole derivatives, isatin β-thiosemicarbazone, 5-iodo-2′-deoxyuridine), and inhibiting viral replication (penicillium mold constituents, interferon and interferon inducers) have not been proven to be successful in the treatment of human viral encephalitis. A possible exception to this is the report concerning the use of 5-iodo-2′-deoxyuridine (IUDR) in which the drug was given intravenously (430 mg./kg. over 5 da.) to patients with proven *Herpes hominis* encephalitis. In comparison with only one out of seven patients who survived and did well in the control group, four out of six treated patients were cured. In view of the generally accepted figure of about 50 percent mortality or serious morbidity in this disease, this treatment program should be considered if the diagnosis can be established early in the course of the illness (fluorescent staining of spinal fluid leucocytes, temporal lobe changes by EEG, biopsy) and appropriate precautions are used to guard against the drug-induced leucopenia and stomatitis.

Course and Prognosis

By and large an acute viral encephalitis will have run its course in 10 days to 2 weeks. Sequelae are directly proportional to the severity of the cerebral insult; however, it is wise to defer giving a prognosis until one year has elapsed. Treatment with anticonvulsants need not be continued if the neurological picture and the EEG are normal, even though seizures may have existed during the acute illness.

Mental changes are commonly described by the convalescing patient which are difficult to quantify; vague headaches, impaired concentrating ability, recent memory deficits, irritability and disturbance of sleep patterns. The family, likewise, will comment on the patient's short temper, his lack of oral responsiveness and his "dull" appearance. Many of these signs and symptoms eventually disappear.

Chronic Viral Encephalitis

The ability of a virus to persist in the nervous system and cause clinically evident disease at a time remote from the initial penetration is considered a mechanism responsible for post-infectious Parkinson's disease. Although a variety of viral agents have been implicated as responsible for the initial insult and the subsequent evolution of this clinical disease, the pathological findings do not in any way resemble that which is seen in acute encephalitis.

This lack of pathological correlation is evident in other diseases evolving as slowly progressive, central nervous system degenerative conditions. These diseases are to be distinguished from the low grade encephalitic response that persists for months after *Herpes hominis* encephalitis or congenital rubella, where, although the virus may be recovered from the brain, progressive neurological symptoms are not significant.

In subacute sclerosing panencephalitis (SSPE) a myxovirus antigenically identical with the measles virus is considered responsible for the childhood illness characterized by personality changes and myoclonic seizures and progressing to dementia, spastic quadriplegia and death within two years. Epidemiologic studies have demonstrated that a significant percentage of these children has acquired measles prior to their second year of life although SSPE becomes apparent several years later. The electroencephalogram is characteristic, demonstrating bursts of sharp wave forms corresponding to the myoclonic seizures followed by a brief suppression of electrical activity. A serological rise of measles antibody titer and an elevation in the cerebrospinal fluid gammaglobulin confirm the diagnosis. Supportive treatment is all that can be offered.

Jakob-Creutzfeldt disease and kuru are degenerative CNS illnesses in which a filterable agent (?virus) from the brains of such patients given via intracerebral inoculation is responsible for a similar clinical and pathological disease in chimpanzees. Progressive ataxia and dementia characterize kuru, an endemic disease in New Guinea. Jakob-Creutzfeldt is an uncommon grey matter disease diagnosed on the basis of a progressive encephalopathy with dementia, spasticity, rigidity, seizures and even evidence of anterior horn cell involvement. Again, no treatment is available.

Advances in laboratory techniques give promise to the discovery of other infectious agents which may solve the etiologic riddle in multiple sclerosis, amyotrophic lateral sclerosis and other malignant diseases of the nervous system.

SELECTED REFERENCES

Johnson, R. T., and Johnson, K. P.: Slow and chronic virus infection of the nervous system, in Plum, F. (ed.): *Recent Advance in Neurology*. F. A. Davis Co., Philadelphia, 1969, pp. 33.

Nolan, D. C., Carruthers, N. M., and Lerner, A. M.: *Herpes hominis* encephalitis in Michigan. N. Eng. J. of Med., *282*:10, 1970.

Webb, H. E.: Management of virus central nervous system disease. Brit. Med. J., *4*:603, 1969.

Chapter 23

VIRAL HEPATITIS

Viral hepatitis, as it is usually recognized clinically, is an acute disease of the liver characterized by inflammation and necrosis. Acute viral hepatitis is an extremely important disorder for an assortment of reasons including its high frequency, potential devastating effects, relationships to other varieties of hepatic diseases, and in its differential distinction from other diseases involving the liver.

Traditional Classificatons with Viral Hepatitis

Viral hepatitis has been associated with hepatic injury due to the effects of at least two viruses. The illness produced by these infective viruses have been traditionally referred to as *infectious hepatitis* (IH) and *serum hepatitis* (SH), resulting from hepatic injury damage to infection with the IH and SH viruses respectively. The virus responsible for infectious hepatitis has been also designated as virus A, and the virus responsible for serum hepatitis has been called virus B. Distinction between the IH and SH viruses have been made on the basis of epidemiological, clinical and behaviorial characteristics, some of which must be re-examined in light of newer knowledge concerning the etiologies of viral hepatitis (as will be discussed later).

Viral hepatitis due to infection with the IH virus has also been designated as short incubation hepatitis inasmuch as the period of incubation from exposure to initiation of clinical symptoms is usually within a period from two to six weeks. Conversely, viral hepatitis due to infection with the SH virus has also been referred to as long (or delayed) incubation hepatitis since the period of incubation from exposure to clinical symptoms is commonly within a period of from two to six months in duration.

The mode of transmission of viral hepatitis has also been utilized as a method of discriminating between serum hepatitis and infectious hepatitis. Infectious hepatitis is usually transmitted by the oral-fecal route, whereas serum hepatitis is usually transmitted by injection or by transfusion of blood or blood products. It should be emphasized, however, that recent evidence indicates that in some instances hepatitis associated with infection by SH viruses may follow oral viral transmission. Conversely, it has been clearly shown that hepatitis due to the IH virus may, and often does, result from transmission of the virus contained in injected materials, including blood and its products. In general, however, it appears, particularly in epidemic situations, that hepatitis due to the IH virus is usually transmitted by the oral-fecal route, and viral hepatitis following transfusion or injection is probably more commonly due to the virus which we have traditionally referred to as the SH virus.

Recognition of the fact that both the IH and SH viruses may be transmitted by injection and transfusion has led to the usage of the term post-transfusion (or post-injection) hepatitis in preference to the term serum hepatitis. Post-transfusion hepatitis has been associated with the transfusion with whole blood, single donor plasma and an assortment of blood derived products. High-risk products which have been particularly associated with post-transfusion hepatitis include preparations of fibrinogen, pooled plasma, and fractions prepared for the treatment of hemophilia. Viral hepatitis transmission is not associated with adequately prepared thrombin, serum albumin, and immune globulins.

It is not known at the present time what factors dictate the difference in mode of transmission of these two viruses: modifying mechanisms may include dose of the viral particles administered, varying of infectivity of individual strains of virus, host factors including perhaps immunological mechanisms. Major distinctions between viral hepatitis, resulting from that which has been traditionally designated as serum hepatitis, and infectious hepatitis may be made on the basis of the recognition that infection with one of the viruses (SH or IH) protects against subsequent infection by that, but not by the alternate, virus.

Clinical Manifestations of Acute Viral Hepatitis

Viral hepatitis is an acute infectious disease. Symptoms include almost invariable anorexia, nausea, and sometimes vomiting. Many patients experience revulsion at the sight or thought of food. When vomiting occurs, it is usually neither severe nor protracted. A distaste for cigarettes among smokers is common. The patient frequently experiences malaise, fatigue, and in approximately two-thirds of cases fever which seldom exceeds 39°C. When present, fever usually occurs in the first few days of illness.

Abdominal discomfort is frequent, although usually not severe, and is most commonly located in the right upper quadrant: it may be amplified by abrupt motions. Patients with acute viral hepatitis commonly note lightening of their stools and darkening of their urine which may precede visably recognizable jaundice. Darkening of the urine is a particularly frequent observation, being found in almost all patients with acute viral hepatitis who are visably icteric. Pruritus may occur especially in those instances in which cholestasis is a prominent feature of the disease.

Occasionally patients experience a minor illness, perhaps associated with initial viremia, with anorexia, nausea and sometimes vomiting which may precede clinical viral hepatitis from several days to several weeks. Occasionally abrupt hemolysis may contribute to rapidly deepening severe jaundice, frequently associated with erythrocyte glucose-6-phosphate dehydrogenase (G-6-PD) deficiency, with the hemolytic episode being triggered by the viral hepatitis. As with other episodes of hemolysis due to G-6-PD deficiency, erythrocyte abnormalities may not be detected during the acute episode due to the destruction of G-6-PD deficient red cells. Urticaria with or without arthralgia may occur in a small proportion of patients with viral hepatitis.

Physical examination usually reveals visible jaundice, which is variable in degree. Almost all patients with acute viral hepatitis have tenderness over the liver. The liver, although often normal in size, is commonly slightly to moderately enlarged. The liver is rarely massively enlarged: its margins are smooth and not irregular. The spleen is palpably enlarged in 5 to 15 percent of cases. Transient spider angiomata, palmar erythema or gynecomastia may appear, and should not be considered necessarily indicative of chronic liver disease.

Laboratory abnormalities usually include an elevation of the serum glutamic oxaloacetic transaminase (SGOT) and serum glutamic pyruvic transaminase (SGPT) which are almost always elevated above 200 (Karmen) units and most commonly above 500 units. Elevations of transaminase usually occur 7 to 10 days before onset of clinical symptoms and often reach their highest levels in the first week of illness. Bilirubinuria is common, particularly early in the course of the disease. Most patients with acute viral hepatitis, who are recognized clinically, become icteric with bilirubin levels which may vary widely from 3 mg./100 ml. to as high as 40 mg./100 ml., but are usually less than 10 mg./100 ml. The elevation in serum bilirubin is composed of both conjugated and unconjugated bilirubin species, although the proportion may vary substantially from patient to patient. The severity of the viral hepatitis may be reflected by the duration of the sustained substantial hyperbilirubinemia ($>$10 mg. percent) and to less degree to the height to which the bilirubin is increased. Prothrombin activity may also be reduced in acute viral hepatitis. The degree of reduction in prothrombin activity, particularly if of marked degree, may help to judge the severity of the viral hepatitis. Although modest reductions in serum albumin concentration may occur, when uncomplicated, acute viral hepatitis is not associated with substantial reductions in albumin levels. The serum alkaline phosphatase is usually modestly elevated. It may range, however, from normal levels to degrees of marked elevation, particularly in instances characterized by functional cholestasis.

Occasional patients with acute viral hepatitis may exhibit leukopenia and in smaller numbers marked leukocytosis. Usually, however, leukocyte counts are relatively normal.

In many instances it is impossible to differentiate the clinical and laboratory manifestations of infectious hepatitis from those of serum hepatitis. On the other hand, there are some clinical and laboratory characteristics which tend to distinguish the two major varieties of viral hepatitis. The onset of clinical symptoms in infectious hepatitis is frequently abrupt, and more commonly accompanied by fever. Fever is less common in patients with serum hepatitis and onset of symptoms is commonly insidious. Krugman has suggested that children with MS-1 viral hepatitis (probably IH) have sharp increases in serum IgM and thymol turbidity during their acute illness; and in contrast, in children with MS-2 viral hepatitis (probably SH), serum IgM is either normal or slightly elevated and thymol turbidity is less strongly positive.

Histological Features of Acute Viral Hepatitis

The histological features of acute viral hepatitis, as usually recognized clinically, are those of inflammatory change and necrosis within the liver. Areas of necrosis are usually small and may be limited to necrosis involving single hepatic parenchymal cells. These small areas of hepatocellular necrosis are scattered throughout the hepatic lobules, and do not distort the normal hepatic architecture. Areas of necrosis are not limited or confined to specific hepatic lobular regions. Hepatic parenchymal cells undergoing necrosis may undergo various morphologic changes during disintegration: these include balloon degeneration, hydropic degeneration, pycnosis, and forms of eosinophilic degeneration, sometimes with the formation of the characteristic eosinophilic "Councilman-like bodies." These morphological changes, although frequently occurring in acute viral hepatitis, are not limited to this disease and occur as well in other varieties of hepatic necrosis.

The nature of the cellular infiltrate which characterizes acute viral hepatitis is for the most part mononuclear, composed principally of lymphocytes, plasma cells, and macrophage-monocyte elements. Polymorphonuclear leukocytes and eosinophiles may also be seen, but in smaller numbers when compared with the mononuclear cell infiltration. The nature of the cellular infiltration is in contrast to that observed in alcoholic hepatitis, in which polymorphonuclear leukocytes predominate. Although in acute viral hepatitis limited numbers of eosinophiles may be seen as part of the inflammatory response within the liver, peripheral eosinophilia is not observed. Swelling and prominence of Kupffer cells of the liver may be seen in acute viral hepatitis. In addition, there may be inflammatory involvement of the central veins in the hepatic lobules. Variable degrees of cholestasis may also be recognized.

Occasional patients with acute viral hepatitis may present with a principally cholestatic picture, i.e., with deepening jaundice, dark urine, light stools, pruritus, marked elevation in serum alkaline phosphatase activity and little elevation in SGOT or SGPT levels. It is obvious that this syndrome must be distinguished from extrahepatic biliary tract obstruction. Occasionally cholestatic histologic changes are prominent in liver biopsy specimens from patients with this variant of acute viral hepatitis. Histologic examination of the liver in most such patients, however, is similar to that seen in more common varieties of acute viral hepatitis. This syndrome has been sometimes referred to as cholangeolitic hepatitis. A more accurate term is that of *hepatitis with cholestasis*.

Variants and Possible Sequelae of Acute Viral Hepatitis

Viral hepatitis should be viewed as a spectrum of clinical and morphologic expressions both in respect to severity and potential sequelae. The clinical features which lead to the recognition and identification of typical acute viral hepatitis have been described above. Acute viral hepatitis may range from *inapparent or nonicteric hepatitis* to usually fatal *massive hepatic necrosis*. Epidemiological studies and clinical experience indicate that a large proportion of patients experience inapparent or anicteric hepatitis with no clinical symptoms. In addition, patients with nonicteric hepatitis may, as the term indicates, be free of jaundice but develop nonspecific general symptoms which do not permit recognition of viral hepatitis as the etiology of their illness.

Often biochemical examinations, sometimes performed fortuitously, or performed during the investigation of hepatitis outbreaks, may indicate elevations of serum transaminase and perhaps subtle increases in serum bilirubin. Liver biopsy performed on such patients will commonly reveal mild but definite morphological abnormalities consistent with the diagnosis of acute viral hepatitis. Inapparent or nonicteric hepatitis is a frequent phenomenon and particularly among children may exceed the frequency of overt clinical viral hepatitis.

At the other end of the spectrum a small portion of patients with acute viral hepatitis will develop *acute hepatic necrosis* which is an ominous massively destructive variety of viral hepatitis with wide-sweeping necrosis of broad regions of the liver. In this disorder hepatocellular necrosis is diffusely extensive, with massive dropping out of hepatocytes and marked destructive distortion of hepatic lobular architecture. These morphologic abnormalities are accompanied by profound metabolic hepatic failure often with massively elevated levels of transaminase and markedly reduced prothrombin activity. This is usually accompanied by deep, persistent, progressive hyperbilirubinemia, with the frequent development of porto-systemic encephalopathy.

Massive hepatic necrosis represents the extreme in the severe expression of destructive hepatic disease in acute viral hepatitis. It is probable that that which by current terminology is designated as actue hepatic necrosis is similar to, if not identical to, that which by older and now discarded terminology was referred to as "acute fatty liver."

At least two varieties of chronic hepatitis may in certain instances follow viral hepatitis in a small proportion of patients. One form has been designated as *chronic persistent hepatitis* which appears to be a non-progressive benign disease in contrast to *chronic aggressive hepatitis* (equivalent to *chronic active hepatitis*). Chronic aggressive hepatitis is a chronic, destructive and inflammatory hepatocellular disease progressing inexorably, but at various rates, to the development of hepatic failure and post-hepatitic or post-necrotic cirrhosis. Extensive liver cell necrosis is found in chronic aggressive hepatitis. Piecemeal necrosis is often prominent: piecemeal necrosis is a morphological abnormality characterized by irregular distortion of the periphery of portal triads resulting from necrosis of adjacent hepatic parenchymal cells intermingled with the presence of mononuclear inflammatory cells. Large septae extend from abnormal portal triads with marked architectural distortion and reticulin collapse.

In contrast, in chronic persistent hepatitis, lobular architecture is preserved; there is some inflammatory infiltrate of the portal tracts with mononuclear cells but with little, if any, piecemeal necrosis. Reticulin collapse is not prominent. Chronic persistent hepatitis does not appear to progress to destructive cirrhotic liver disease. The role of the hepatitis virus, or viruses, in chronic aggressive hepatitis is not known. Possible autoimmune factors have been invoked for etiological consideration, particularly in view of the frequency of immunological markers in such patients: these include false positive serological tests for syphilis, hypergammaglobulinemia, a variety of antinuclear factors, LE cell phenomena, and antibodies to smooth muscle.

The true incidence of cirrhosis following viral hepatitis is not known. In a recent study Beebe and Simon examined the incidence of cirrhosis of the liver following the occurrence of recognized viral hepatitis in army enlisted men during World War II. This survey failed to demonstrate a subsequent increased incidence of cirrhosis of the liver in these patients. In that study the incidence of cirrhosis of the liver was no higher in those thought to have had serum hepatitis from those thought to have had infectious hepatitis. When large numbers of patients with prior viral hepatitis have been studied, it has been difficult to prove with certainty the suspected increased incidence of the development of post-necrotic cirrhosis. There is some other evidence suggesting that chronic destructive (cirrhotic) liver disease may be more frequent following that which has been thought to be serum hepatitis versus infectious hepatitis. The factors responsible for the development of chronic destructive liver disease with post-necrotic or post-hepatitic cirrhosis have to this point in time escaped complete clarification.

In general the deeper the jaundice in acute viral hepatitis the more probable that extensive hepatic necrosis has occurred and the more likely is the possibility of hepatic failure. Exceptions must be noted, however, inasmuch as in certain cholestatic varieties of viral hepatitis, hepatocellular necrosis may be relatively modest although jaundice may be profound. In additional instances of massive hepatic necrosis hepatic failure may be profound prior to the development of impressive jaundice.

In an additional severe form of acute viral hepatitis, indicated as *subacute hepatic necrosis*, large zones of hepatocellular necrosis bridge adjacent protal triads or central veins, or both, extending into contiguous hepatic lobules. Intralobular bridging of this variety may be accompanied by extensive destruction of whole lobules and may result in a fatal or progressively relentless destructive form of the disease. Reflecting the more extensive destruction of hepatic parenchyma, livers examined at autopsy in such patients are usually small. Boyer and Klatskin noted that 19 percent of patients with subacute hepatic necrosis died and 37 percent developed cirrhosis. This is in marked contrast to the relatively benign self-limited course of usual viral hepatitis. The development of subsequent cirrhosis appears to be highly correlated with the histological bridging features.

Thus, detection of the extensive bridging histological lesion, which characterizes subacute hepatic necrosis and distinguishes it from more common acute viral hepatitis, may be of great prognostic value. Later in surviving patients as the inflammatory response waned there was collapse and condensation of reticulin. Subacute hepatic necrosis appeared in their study to be somewhat more common following SH than with IH infection. In addition, a higher proportion of patients with this severe lesion were over the age of 40 when compared with other patients with typical viral hepatitis. An insidious onset is more common among patients with subacute hepatic necrosis. As one might anticipate by the extent of hepatic necrosis in these patients, liver function abnormalities are often greater than in patients with usual acute viral hepatitis. In particular, ascites, edema, and hepatic coma, which occur in approximately a quarter of patients with subacute hepatic necrosis, were clinical manifestations which, when present, might serve to distinguish between these patients and those with customary acute viral hepatitis.

Many of the features of subacute hepatic necrosis, particularly during stages of ongoing necrosis and subsequent development of cirrhosis, are remarkably similar to chronic aggressive hepatitis (chronic active hepatitis). It is possible that some patients who present the clinical syndrome of chronic aggressive hepatitis may represent sequelae from the relentless progression of subacute hepatic necrosis.

The Hepatitis Associated (Australia) Antigen

A most exciting and productive observation, which has led to enormous expansion of our knowledge of viral hepatitis, was recognition of the presence of the *Australia antigen* in the serum of some patients with and following viral hepatitis. Blumberg originally detected this antigen in serum from an Australian aborigine. Subsequently with his colleagues he described the presence of this antigen in sera from 27 percent of patients with viral hepatitis (in 22 percent of patients designated as having infectious hepatitis and in 41 percent of patients designated as having serum hepatitis by traditional criteria). This antigen, also referred to as the *hepatitis associated antigen,* has been found to be identical to that found by Prince in sera from patients with serum hepatitis, but not from those thought to have infectious hepatitis.

Hepatitis associated antigen has been found with frequencies from 50 to 95 percent in patients with well documented post-transfusion or post-injection viral hepatitis. It has been detected from 25 to 47 percent of patients with sporadic cases of viral hepatitis, in which no definite exposure to injection or transfusion could be obtained and were thereby considered to be infectious hepatitis. Hepatitis associated antigen is usually not found in so called "single source" outbreaks of short incubation viral hepatitis which are more clearly epidemiologically associated with that which has been traditionally referred to as the infectious hepatitis virus. A variety of studies have provided evidence that the hepatitis associated antigen reflects, or is associated with, infection by that which has been traditionally referred to as the serum hepatitis virus. The precise nature of the hepatitis associated antigen has not been defined. It has not been conclusively demonstrated to be an infectious agent. There is speculation that the particles which can be identified may represent an incomplete virus of some variety, perhaps a non-infectious empty virus coat.

Following ultracentrifugation, hepatitis associated antigen particles may be seen to aggregate and may be examined electronmicroscopically. The particles have a modal diameter of approximately 200Å. An occasional particle appears to have a central core and some conspicuously large spherical particles are observed. Tubular and filamentous forms of hepatitis associated antigen have also been observed. The spherical hepatitis associated antigen particles appear to be comprised of surface structure of 30Å diameter subunits without uniform arrangement. The concentration of hepatitis associated antigen particles, when present in serum, is exceedingly high, usually being greater than 10^{10}/ml.

The hepatitis associated antigen contains both protein and lipid. Small amounts of RNA, smaller amounts than are usually found in most RNA viruses, have been detected in preparations of hepatitis associated antigen.

In one study of patients with acute viral hepatitis, the incidence of hepatitis associated antigen was 45 percent whereas in control populations only 0.1 to 0.2 percent of hospital personnel and patients without liver disease had hepatitis associated antigen in their blood. Patients with liver disease clearly unrelated to viral hepatitis have no higher incidence of hepatitis associated antigen in their sera than do normal individuals.

Patients with acute viral hepatitis exhibit a variable frequency of positivity for hepatitis associated antigen in their sera dependant upon the variety of hepatitis being studied, the numbers of samples procured, the stage of the disease at which the serum samples are obtained, and also on the technique used to detect hepatitis associated antigen. Highest frequencies have been found when serum sampling is performed early in the course of the disease, rather than in convalescence or in the late active stages of viral hepatitis, and when more than one sample is procured per week. Initially testing for the presence of the hepatitis associated antigen was performed by use of immunodiffusion in agar gel. Higher frequency of positivity of hepatitis associated antigen is found when more sensitive immunological techniques, such as complement fixation or electrophoretic methods (e.g., electroendosmosis) are used, rather than simple immunodiffusion. Radioimmunoassay of Australian antigen is currently under development and may provide the most sensitive and specific means for identifying hepatitis associated antigen in serum samples.

Krugman and his associates have clearly identified infection by two distinct hepatitis agents: they have indicated these as a short incubation agent (MS-1) which produces hepatitis 35 to 47 days following injection or feeding of serum or stool filtrates; and a long incubation agent (MS-2) which, following feeding of infectious serum, produces hepatitis in 70 to 130 days, and following injection, in 41 to 108 days. It may be important to point out that the oral dose necessary to produce long incubation viral hepatitis was 50 times that required for induction of infection by parenteral injection. There is no cross-immunity between infections by MS-1 and MS-2 viruses. The studies of Krugman and Prince and their associates indicate that MS-2 infection is associated with the presence in the serum of the hepatitis associated antigen, whereas MS-1 infection appears not to be accompanied by serum positivity for the hepatitis associated antigen.

Hepatitis associated antigen, when positive in acute viral hepatitis, usually appears in the serum prior to clinical symptoms and other laboratory abnormalities including elevation of the serum transaminase. Hepatitis associated antigen may be present in the serum from two to four weeks prior to these abnormalities. The hepatitis associated antigen may be found in the serum of patients in the first week of clinical viral hepatitis and then may disappear in variable periods varying from a few days to many years. Some such individuals may be carriers of the hepatitis associated antigen. Hepatitis associated antigen may frequently persist in the serum of patients following mild or subclinical viral hepatitis; therefore a history of prior hepatitis may not be obtainable by historical examination.

Patients with chronic aggressive hepatitis (chronic active hepatitis) may have a 10 to 20 percent incidence of serum positivity for hepatitis associated antigen. This is less than the incidence with post-transfusion hepatitis but substantially exceeds the anticipated incidence in the general population. The hepatitis associated antigen may persist for long periods of time in the serum of patients with chronic active hepatitis as opposed to its rather transient presence in the serum of most patients with typical acute viral hepatitis. The precise role of the hepatitis associated antigen in chronic active hepatitis and the potential role of its persistence in the pathogenesis of the disease have not been defined. The incidence of hepatitis associated antigen appears to be substantially less among those patients with chronic active hepatitis who have prominent immunological features, including, among others, positive lupus erythematosus cell tests and substantial hypergammaglobulinemia. Patients with chronic active hepatitis who have hepatitis associated antigen in their blood are usually males as opposed to those with prominent immunological features who are more often females. Some patients with cryptogenic or postnecrotic cirrhosis have been noted to have hepatitis associated antigen in their sera, although the frequency is not as great as is found in acute viral hepatitis. The relationships between chronic destructive liver disease (cirrhosis) and persistence of the hepatitis associated antigen in the serum of some patients has not thus far been elucidated.

Treatment of Acute Viral Hepatitis

The therapeutic efficacy of bedrest and restricted activity has not been clarified in the treatment of acute viral hepatitis. Although traditionally bedrest and inactivity of various duration have been considered an integral part of the treatment of acute viral hepatitis, there is no conclusive evidence available at present that imposed inactivity benefits patients with acute viral hepatitis. Studies examining morbidity and mortality, both in respect to the acute infection and in regard to the subsequent development of chronic destructive liver disease, fail to provide support for the benefit of restricted activity. Most physicians, however, find that for many patients fatigue and intolerance to active pursuits are substantial during viral hepatitis and do restrict activity as required for the preservation of a sense of well-being in the patient. Prolonged restriction beyond such periods, however, may not really be necessary.

The question may then be posed—should all patients with acute viral hepatitis be admitted to the hospital? Clearly all patients with acute viral hepatitis are not presently admitted to the hospital and many, of course, escape diagnosis. It is probably not necessary to enforce hospitalization on all patients with acute viral hepatitis. It is important, however, for the physician to establish a diagnosis on the basis of clinical and biochemical data, to carefully follow the course of the patient and his illness, and to distinguish acute viral hepatitis from other similar diseases. It is also important to identify those patients who may develop complications of acute viral hepatitis which may require hospitalization and further treatment.

Decisions concerning discharge from the hospital during recovery from viral hepatitis must be individualized and are difficult to encompass with satisfactory broad statements. In general, discharge from hospital is considered when patients are free of fever, anorexia, nausea, vomiting, and when they are either distinctly improved or progressively improving. These areas of improvement in those patients who must be hospitalized generally occur from 10 to 20 days following initial hospitalization. Obviously the nature of the home setting into which the patient returns may favorably influence the possibility of early discharge from the hospital. Follow-up of patients with viral hepatitis, in addition to clinical assessment by history and physical examination, include measurements of serum bilirubin and SGOT levels. Progressive decreases in these values to <100 SGOT units and a bilirubin level of <2 mg./100 ml. several weeks following discharge would support continuing improvement. The physician must be alert to the possibility of recurrence, relapse, or perpetuation of progressive hepatocellular damage in unusual and complicated patients with viral hepatitis.

It is believed to be important that the patient with acute viral hepatitis be provided with an unrestricted nutritious diet. There is no persuasive evidence that diets unusually high in caloric or protein content are particularly preferable to a general unrestricted diet selected by the patient on the basis of taste and interest. Portosystemic encephalopathy may occur in certain patients, particularly those with severe and extensive hepatic necrosis, thereby requiring restriction or elimination of protein from the diet. Treatment of hepatic failure with impending or present portosystemic encephalopathy includes neomycin, four gms./day. Reduction in prothrombin activity may require the parenteral administration of vitamin K_1, 10 mg./day. The prothrombin time may respond in proportion to the cholestatic element of the disorder and in inverse proportion to the extent of hepatic parenchymal cell failure. Hypoglycemia which may accompany massive hepatic necrosis should be sought for and corrected when present. Inasmuch as ethanol is a hepatotoxic agent, it is probably desirable to eliminate or restrict ethanol intake in patients with acute viral hepatitis.

The role of corticosteroids in viral hepatitis is controversial. There is general agreement, however, that there is no benefit to the patient by the administration of corticosteroids in acute uncomplicated viral hepatitis. Some physicians elect to use corticosteroids in the treatment of certain patients with complications associated with acute viral hepatitis. These have included persistent and severe elevations of bilirubin, often associated with histologic development of submassive necrosis, and also in certain patients with acute hepatic necrosis, commonly with associated portosystemic encephalopathy. There is not a uniform opinion as to the efficacy of corticosteroids in these instances.

Massive hepatic necrosis is accompanied by fulminant hepatic failure with central nervous system deterioration, and clinical and laboratory evidence of massive interference with hepatic function. Such patients require glucose administration, protein restriction or elimination, control of gastrointestional bleeding, infection, etc. The use of sedatives, diuretic agents promoting hypokalemia and/or metabolic alkalosis, electrolyte abnormalities, and azotemia should be avoided. The mortality in patients with acute hepatic necrosis exceeds 75 percent. A variety of methods are being examined to treat patients with acute hepatic necrosis including hemodialysis, peritoneal dialysis, exchange transfusion, cross circulation with a donor subject, liver perfusion with liver from the same or different species, as well as liver transplantation. These modes of treatment are being investigated to assess their value in the treatment of patients with acute hepatic failure. It is anticipated that careful controlled studies will provide conclusions concerning the efficacy of these as yet experimental therapeutic procedures.

Prevention of Viral Hepatitis

In 1952 viral hepatitis was made a reportable disease in the United States. The Hepatitis Surveillance Unit of the U.S. Public Health Service was formed in 1960 and has collected and made available enormously valuable epidemiological data related to viral hepatitis. The incidence of viral hepatitis (particularly that which has been referred to as infectious hepatitis) appears cyclical. In various nations in which this has been examined incidence peaks occur (in temperate climates) at from 5 to 10 year intervals. In the United States incidence peaks have been observed at approximately seven year intervals. Modes of transmission of short incubation viral hepatitis are principally by person to person contact and by contaminated water and food. Recently there has been increased emphasis on the role of both raw and partially cooked clams and oysters from polluted bodies of sea water.

Prevention of viral hepatitis relies in great part on improved hygienic measures. These include instructions in hand washing, especially following defecation, and particularly in individuals concerned with food preparation. Cases of viral hepatitis should be reported to public health officials in order to identify sources of epidemic situations to permit diagnosis and applications of whatever measures are necessary to prevent further infection. The use of contaminated syringes and needles is strongly to be discouraged. The prevention of possible viral hepatitis transmission provides a persuasive argument for the use of disposable needles and syringes.

Immune globulin administration has been demonstrated to be effective in the prevention or attenuation of some varieties of viral hepatitis. There is no conclusive evidence indicating that immune serum globulin is beneficial in the prevention of post-transfusion hepatitis of the long incubation variety. The use of immune globulin is recommended in individuals exposed to that which appears to be IH hepatitis. It can be administered following exposure and is probably not indicated following five to six weeks after exposure. When indicated and possible immune serum globulin should be administered within two weeks of exposure.

There is no evidence that there is any benefit associated with administration of immune globulin to patients who have already developed clinical or laboratory evidence of acute viral hepatitis. A variety of dosage schedules have been proposed for those patients in whom immune globulin is indicated. Recommended dosages for immune globulin have ranged from 0.01 to 0.06 ml./lb. body weight. For practical purposes 0.5 ml. is given to children who weigh less than 50 lb., 1.0 ml. to children who weigh from 50 to 100 lb., and 2 ml. to all adults, and to children over 100 lb.

Individuals recommended to receive immune globulin are those who constitute household contacts of patients with viral hepatitis, contacts in prisons or institutions for the mentally retarded, and individuals exposed to an identified common source of infection such as water, food, etc. Immune globulin administration is not routinely recommended for school, office, factory, or hospital contacts except when associated with the accidental injection of blood or serum of patients with hepatitis. Immune globulin is also administered to individuals who are travelers to foreign countries in which their exposure constitutes a high risk for viral hepatitis. There appears to be no sufficient justification for routine administration of immune globulin preparations to patients receiving blood transfusions.

Post-transfusion or post-injection hepatitis, which of course may reflect transmission of either short incubation or long incubation viral species, is assuming increased importance. Transfusion of whole blood constitutes an important mode of transmission of this variety of hepatitis. Another important mode of transmission is by contaminated syringes and needles. Although disposable needles and syringes are increasingly being used by the medical profession, inadequately sterilized or non-sterilized needles and syringes constitute an important source of virus transmission among narcotics users, in which population viral hepatitis is rapidly increasing. The precise incidence of post-injection viral hepatitis among this population, for obvious reasons, is not known.

It is now recommended that all blood being considered for transfusion to patients be examined for the presence of the hepatitis associated antigen. It is anticipated that the elimination of transfusion of hepatitis associated antigen-containing blood will substantially reduce the incidence of post-transfusion hepatitis.

SELECTED REFERENCES

Becker, M. D., Scheuer, P. J., Baptista, A., and Sherlock, S.: Prognosis of chronic persistent hepatitis. Lancet, *1*:53, 1970.

Beebe, G. W., and Simon, A. H.: Cirrhosis of the liver following viral hepatitis, a twenty year mortality follow-up. Am. J. Epidem., *92*:279, 1970.

Berger, R. L., Liversage, R. M., Chalmers, T. C., Graham, J. H., McGoldrick, D. N., and Stohlman, F.: Exchange transfusion in the treatment of fulminating hepatitis. N. Eng. J. Med., *274*:497, 1966.

Blum, A. L., Stutz, R., Haemmerli, U. P., Schmid, P., and Grady, A.: A fortuitously controlled study of steroid therapy in acute viral hepatitis. Amer. J. Med., *47*:82, 93, 1969.

Blumberg, B. S., Alter, H. J., and Visnich, S.: A "new" antigen in leukemia serum. JAMA, *191*:541, 1965.

Blumberg, B. S., Sutnick, A. I., and London, W. T.: Australia antigen and hepatitis. JAMA, *207*:1895, 1969.

Boyer, J. L., and Klatskin, G.: Pattern of necrosis in acute viral hepatitis. Prognostic value of bridging (subacute hepatic necrosis). N. Eng. J. Med., *283*:1063, 1970.

Chalmers, T. C., Eckhardt, R. D., Reynolds, W. E., *et al.*: The treatment of acute infectious hepatitis. Comtrolled studies of the effects of diet, rest and physical reconditioning on the acute course of the disease and on the incidence of relapses and residual abnormalities. J. Clin. Invest., *34*:1163, 1955.

Chalmers, T. C., and Sebestyen, C. S.: Evidence against infectious hepatitis as a cause of cirrhosis. Trans. Amer. Clin. Climat. Ass., *74*:192, 1962.

Conn, H. O.: A rational approach for the management of hepatic coma. Gastroenterology, *57*:715, 1969.

Davis, M. A., Peters, R. L., Redeker, A. G., and Reynolds, T. V.: Appraisal of the mortality in acute fulminating viral hepatitis. N. Eng. J. Med., *278*:1248, 1968.

Dougherty, W. J., and Altman, R.: Viral hepatitis in New Jersey 1960-1961. Am. J. Med., *32*:704, 1962.

Fowinkle, E. W., and Guthrie, N.: Comparison of two doses of gamma globulin in prevention of infectious hepatitis. Pub. Health Rep., *79*:634, 1964.

Giles, J. P., McCollum, R. W., Berndtson, L. W., Jr., et al.: Viral hepatitis: relation of Australia/SH antigen to the Willowbrook MS-2 strain. N. Eng. J. Med., *281*:119, 1969.

Hirshchman, R. J., Shulman, N. R., Barker, L. F., and Smith, K. O.: Virus-like particles in sera of patients with infectious and serum hepatitis. JAMA, *208*:1667, 1969.

Klatskin, G.: Subacute hepatic necrosis and postnecrotic cirrhosis due to anicteric infections with the hepatitis virus. Amer. J. Med., *25*:333, 1958.

Krugman, S., Giles, J. P., and Hammond, J.: Infectious hepatitis: evidence for two distinctive clinical, epidemiological and immunological types of infection. JAMA, *200*:365, 1967.

Mallory, T. B.: The pathology of epidemic hepatitis. JAMA, *134*:655, 1947.

Mason, J. O., and McClean, W. R.: Infectious hepatitis traced to the consumption of raw oysters. Am. J. Hyg., *75*:90, 1962.

Matthews, J. D., and MacKay, I. R.: Australia antigen in chronic hepatitis in Australia. Brit. Med. J., *1*:259, 1970.

Mistilis, S. P., Skyring, A. P., and Blackburn, C. R. B.: Natural history of active chronic hepatitis. Austral. Ann. Med., *17*:214, 1968.

Nefszger, M. D., and Chalmers, T. C.: The treatment of acute infectious hepatitis: ten year follow-up of the effects of diet and rest. Amer. J. Med., *35*:299, 1963.

Prince, A. M.: An antigen detected in the blood during the incubation period of serum hepatitis. Proc. Nat. Acad. Sci. USA, *60*:814, 1968.

Prince, A. M., Hargrove, R. L., and Szmuness, W., et al.: Immunologic distinction between infectious and serum hepatitis. N. Eng. J. Med., *282*:987, 1970.

Rogers, A. I.: Therapeutic considerations in selected forms of acute and chronic liver disease. Med. Clin. North Amer., *55*:373, 1971.

Reisler, D. M., Strong, W. B., and Mosley, J. W.: Transaminase levels in the post convalescent phase of infectious hepatitis. JAMA, *202*:131, 1967.

Repsher, L. H., and Freebern, R. K.: Effects of early and vigorous exercise on recovery from infectious hepatitis. N. Eng. J. Med., *281*:1393, 1969.

Ritt, D. J., Whclan, G., Werner, D. J., Eigenbrodt, E. H., Schenker, S., and Combes, B.: Acute hepatic necrosis with stupor and coma. Medicine, *48*:151, 1969.

Scheuer, P. J.: *Liver Biopsy Interpretation.* Baltimore, Williams and Wilkins, 1968.

Shulman, N. R.: Hepatitis-associated antigen. Amer. J. Med., *49*:669, 1970.

Tisdale, W. A.: When to hospitalize the hepatitis patient. Hospital Practice, October 1967, p. 35.

Trey, C., Burns, D. G., and Saunders, S. J.: Treatment of hepatic coma by exchange blood transfusion. N. Eng. J. Med., *274*:473, 1966.

Wright, R., McCollum, R. W., and Klatskin, G.: Australia antigen in acute and chronic liver disease. Lancet, *2*:117, 1969.

Chapter 24

URINARY TRACT INFECTIONS

The widespread prevalence of urinary tract infections has been acknowledged only in recent years as clinical and epidemiological studies have uncovered the fact that bacteriuria is frequently "asymptomatic." In addition, experimental studies have added to understanding of the pathogenesis of urinary tract infections and the role of host-defense mechanisms. Some of these observations have furnished important clues to prevention and to long-term management.

The importance of urinary tract infections is indicated not only by their frequency, likelihood of recurrence and difficulty in management, but also by their potential to lead to serious renal disease with ultimate renal insufficiency, production of bacteremia, or by their possible role in pregnancy with associated fetal prematurity, and in the etiology of hypertension.

Definition

Urinary tract infection may be defined simply as the presence of significant numbers of pathogenic microorganisms anywhere within the urinary tract. Such infection is ordinarily detected by examination and culture of the urine. It is important, however, to recognize that on occasion, despite significant infection, organisms may not be found in the urine, as, for example, when there is complete obstruction of a ureter or when bacteriuria is masked by antimicrobial therapy.

Urinary tract infection therefore encompasses the clinical entities known as *cystitis*, in which symptoms and evidence of infection are confined to the lower urinary tract (bladder), acute and chronic *pyelonephritis* or disease of the renal parenchyma, and *asymptomatic bacteriuria*, which is an important clue to the presence of infection somewhere within the urinary tract but the significance of which varies in different age and sex groups. Although these clinical categories are useful in orienting our approach to the problem, it should be recognized that symptoms confined to the lower tract do not always give assurance of non-involvement of the kidneys. "Asymptomatic" bacteriuria, furthermore, may in retrospect be associated with a past history of intermittent symptoms or of manifestations not attributed by the patient to the urinary tract.

Pathogenesis

The great majority of microorganisms implicated in urinary tract infections belong to the gram-negative enteric bacilli and consist principally of *Eschericia coli*, Klebsiella-Enterobacter, Proteus species, and Pseudomonas. Other gram-negative species are occasionally involved, usually in chronic, complicated disease. The commonest gram-positive species is the enterococcus, which is also principally implicated in complicated cases while staphylococci, although not infrequent culture contaminants, are relatively rare causes of infection. Perinephric and renal cortical abscesses may occur in association with staphylococcal bacteremia. In fact, over 80 percent of uncomplicated cases are associated with infection by a single species—*E. coli.* Fungi, especially *Candida albicans,* may contaminate urine cultures but may also at times produce serious parenchymal renal disease, especially in patients with underlying renal vascular disease or those on corticosteroids or immunosuppressive therapy.

It is evident that the organisms listed are principally indigenous microflora, and that the patient himself (and especially the colon) is the principal reservoir of the bacteria infecting the urinary tract.

Accumulating clinical and experimental evidence has strengthened the concept that the major pathway by which the kidneys become infected is the "ascending route." Microorganisms enter the bladder via the urethra and ascend to the renal parenchyma where they invade and multiply, predominantly in the renal medullary tissue. The hematogenous route, though clearly important at times, is much less frequently implicated in the pathogenesis of renal infection. Thus, lower urinary tract infection is an important stage in infection of the kidney itself.

Microorganisms introduced into the urethra and bladder tend to be removed in time by the process of micturition and are apparently inhibited directly by antibacterial mechanisms present in the bladder mucosa. Urinary retention due to mechanical or functional obstruction affords an opportunity for organisms to multiply within the bladder urine from whence they may ascend either via the ureteral lumen, probably facilitated by vesico-ureteral reflux or through lymphatics to the renal pelves and calyces. One or both kidneys may be involved. Acute pyelonephritis characteristically begins in the medullary area and spreads in a retrograde fashion from the collecting tubules into the cortex with a resulting wedge-shaped area of involvement with numerous micro-abscesses. Although the glomerulus is often not directly involved, the nephron is rendered functionless by the destructive lesion of the tubule. The inflammatory lesion tends to be confined to the involved segment, which after several weeks undergoes healing, with deposition of fibrous tissue and subsequent contraction to a linear scar. In acute pyelonephritis, because of the focal nature of the lesion, overall renal function usually remains unimpaired.

The resultant effect of persisting and recurrent bacterial infection upon renal parenchymal tissue is a patchy distribution of linear scarring extending out from the medulla into the cortex. Focal areas of mononuclear cell infiltration are also evident and in addition there are often interspersed areas of acute pyelonephritis. The histopathologic entity of "chronic pyelonephritis" is now recognized commonly in patients with chronic renal disease, but it appears likely that a variety of other pathogenetic mechanisms may lead to a similar end result and that in at least some instances bacterial infection is a secondary superimposed process. Thus, vascular disease, chemical agents and drugs (especially analgesics) and immunopathologic disease may produce similar changes. Furthermore, patients with the ultimate diagnosis of chronic pyelonephritis frequently do not give a history of recurrent clinical episodes of urinary tract infection. The common clinical end result in such patients is the insidious development of chronic renal insufficiency.

It is of considerable interest that the medulla has been shown to be much more susceptible to infection than the cortex. A possible explanation for this difference may be the high concentrations of ammonia which occur in the medulla normally in response to an acid load, and which can inhibit the fourth complement component thereby negating this important antibacterial system. In addition, leukocyte phagocytic function may be impaired in the medulla by the high osmolarity of this region. It is the hypertonicity in this area which probably also facilitates the survival of bacterial protoplasts (aberrant forms lacking a rigid cell wall) which may represent the form in which latent infections persist in the urinary tract. A final relative disadvantage for medullary host defense is its considerably smaller blood supply as compared to the cortex.

As indicated, clinical and epidemiologic observations, further clarified by animal experimental models, have identified several key contributory factors of great importance in the pathogenesis of urinary tract infection as follows.

Age and Sex

Urinary tract infections are more common in infancy and among *females,* both in infancy and especially during the child-bearing age. Fecal soiling of the urethral meatus in infants and a high incidence of bladder-neck obstruction and of vesico-ureteral reflux in young females probably account for much of this difference. The shorter female urethra also presumably plays a role in facilitating introduction of bacteria into the bladder. Sexual intercourse appears also to be an important contributing factor in this process. ("Honeymoon cystitis" may be due to traumatic irritation as well as infection.) Another factor contributing to the ten-fold greater incidence of acute pyelonephritis in women of child-bearing age as compared to men in the same age group is the physiologic loss of ureteral tone which usually occurs in the second half of pregnancy. In older men prostatic obstruction becomes an important factor.

Obstruction

Experimentally, it is difficult to produce infection of the normal kidney with coliform bacteria even though these organisms are the commonest cause of human pyelonephritis. Infection is easily accomplished, however, after producing partial or complete obstruction of the ureters. The important role played by obstruction in human disease is clearly confirmed by the 15 to 20 times greater frequency of pyelonephritis observed clinically in patients with obstructive lesions. In males, acute pyelonephritis strongly suggests the likelihood of an obstructive lesion—a congenital anomaly in the younger group, calculi or prostatic lesions in older males.

Vesicoureteral Reflux

Radiologically demonstrable vesicoureteral reflux during micturition has been noted frequently in patients with recurrent episodes of acute pyelonephritis. Such reflux of bladder urine into the ureters may well be an important mechanism by which organisms ascend to the kidney instead of being eliminated by micturition. Reflux may also itself be a consequence of infection.

Neurogenic Bladder Dysfunction

Other conditions in which there is interference with normal bladder function are associated with a high incidence of pyelonephritis. Autonomic disturbances of bladder function occur in patients with a variety of spinal cord lesions and in a significant percentage of diabetics. Organisms are introduced into the bladder during catheterization, which is frequently required in such patients because of urinary retention, and which in turn facilitates microbial multiplication within the bladder urine and subsequent pyelonephritis. An additional hazard in patients immobilized by such conditions is obstruction due to formation of urinary calculi.

Instrumentation

Despite aseptic precautions, persistent bacteriuria results from single bladder catheterizations in 1 to 2 percent of patients, while the establishment of open indwelling catheter drainage leads to bacteriuria in 95 percent or more of patients by the fourth day. In patients in whom prolonged indwelling drainage is necessary, this incidence can be significantly reduced by the use of aseptic closed system drainage or antimicrobial bladder rinses. Other instrumentation procedures including cystoscopy also carry a definite risk of subsequent cystitis and pyelonephritis.

Underlying Disease

Patients with sickle hemoglobin (*sickle-cell trait*) have an increased incidence of pyelonephritis possibly related to thrombosis in the renal vascular system. The apparent increased incidence of urinary tract infections in diabetics appears to be related to two factors: the greater frequency with which catheterization is performed in such patients, and the occurrence of diabetic bladder neuropathy in some. In addition, diabetics along with patients with generalized vascular disease and with analgesic abuse show a particular propensity to develop a severe complication of pyelonephritis—*renal medullary necrosis* (necrotizing papillitis).

Clinical Manifestations

Acute urinary tract infections are customarily divided into two major categories based upon presumed anatomic localization of the process: *lower urinary tract infection* (cystitis and urethritis) in which symptoms include frequency, dysuria or "burning" pain on urination, suprapubic discomfort and the appearance of cloudy, sometimes blood-tinged and foul-smelling urine; and *upper tract infection* (acute pyelonephritis), with sudden onset of fever, chills, aching flank pain and tenderness along with variable signs of lower tract inflammation. In the classic clinical presentations, fever, leukocytosis (and evidence of immunologic response with IgG antibodies to somatic antigens of gram-negative bacteria) are present only in pyelonephritis and absent in simple lower tract infection. Symptoms of cystitis typically subside within a few days even without bacteriologic cure, and pyelonephritis (in the absence of an obstructive lesion) is usually self-limited, symptoms terminating within a week.

As indicated earlier, however, lower tract infection is a stage in infection of the kidneys and may at times be relatively asymptomatic. In addition, predominance of lower tract symptoms, even without fever and leukocytosis, does not give assurance that renal involvement is not present. Accordingly, it has been useful to consider urinary tract infection as part of a continuum of disease, some phases of which may be asymptomatic and which may or may not evolve in a particular patient into a chronic pattern of recurrent symptomatic episodes with potential progressive destruction of renal tissue and deterioration of renal function.

For purposes of estimating prognosis and evaluating the results of therapy, Petersdorf and Turck have suggested classification of patients into four diagnostic categories.

Uncomplicated Acute Urinary Tract Infections

Representative are female patients who present with an initial episode of symptoms, either those of lower or of upper tract infection and who are almost invariably found to have infection with *E. coli*, usually of a serological type present in the patient's own fecal flora. In many of these patients bacteriuria apparently subsides even without treatment, but because of potential evolution into a more serious recurrent form of disease, treatment is recommended. Fortunately, the types of *E. coli* found in such cases are almost invariably sensitive to a wide variety of antibiotics and sulfonamides and they respond quickly to treatment. An initial episode of this sort in a female, especially in the 18 to 40 year age group, is not usually thought to warrant further diagnostic studies. Repeated episodes however should lead to urologic investigation.

Complicated Acute Urinary Tract Infections

Patients with underlying structural abnormalities of the urinary tract are predisposed to infection, the early detection of which is especially important since the abnormalities are often surgically correctable. Since males rarely have simple uncomplicated urinary tract infections, it is recommended that all male patients, following the initial episode of urinary tract infection, undergo urologic investigation with appropriate procedures including cystoscopy and radiographic studies. Also, female patients should have similar studies if they have repeated episodes. In a significant proportion of male patients an underlying lesion, such as a congenital abnormality or stricture in younger men, and prostatic hypertrophy or calculi in older men, will be found. Women will less frequently be found to have underlying lesions, and repeated episodes may be related to sexual intercourse. Organisms implicated in this general category of urinary tract infection are the same as those in the uncomplicated group (*E. coli*) except that occasionally another of the gram-negative organisms or enterococci may be found. The recovery of one of these organisms during an initial episode, in fact, usually indicates the presence of a complicating structural problem. *Proteus mirabilis,* for example, is frequently associated with urinary calculi. Correction of underlying abnormalities is particularly important in this overall group of patients since the presence of uncorrected abnormalities predispose to recurrent infections and ultimate progressive renal damage.

Asymptomatic Bacteriuria

Clinical and epidemiologic studies over the last few years have revealed the fact that a large group of individuals, predominantly females, will be found to have persistent bacteriuria despite few or no definite symptoms of urinary tract infection. Some of these patients will reveal a history suggesting an acute episode of infection at some time in the past, and presumably represent the evolution from acute uncomplicated infection into asymptomatic bacteriuria.

Studies by Kunin and associates revealed a prevalence of bacteriuria among schoolgirls of 1.2 percent in contrast to 0.02 percent in boys of the same age. With a linear incidence of 0.3 percent per year, a cumulative frequency of bacteriuria in schoolgirls at one time or another was calculated to be greater than five percent. With overall frequencies of bacteriuria in adult females on the order of five percent, increasing with age and parity, and with a fairly constant turnover rate, it has been estimated that 15 to 20 percent of the female population will at some time be infected.

Bacteriuria in pregnant women has been studied by Kass and associates who found evidence that many pregnant women with asymptomatic bacteriuria may have chronic infection which is unmasked during pregnancy. Bacteriuria is often difficult to eradicate in these patients despite the usual finding of antibiotic sensitive organisms (usually *E. coli*) unless treatment is continued throughout pregnancy. The significance of bacteriuria in this group is indicated by the fact that 20 to 40 percent of such women found to have bacteriuria early in pregnancy develop symptoms before or immediately after delivery.

Elderly women, who may have rates of asymptomatic bacteriuria as high as 10 percent, may also develop symptoms of urinary tract infection within a year or two of the discovery of bacteriuria, but the eradication of bacteriuria in elderly patients with normal renal function is often difficult, and treatment is usually recommended only for symptomatic episodes. Asymptomatic bacteriuria in men usually is confined to elderly males with prostatic hypertrophy, which should be surgically corrected.

It can be seen that asymptomatic bacteriuria, rather than comprising a distinct clinical entity, may represent either a stage in the evolution of acute disease into a chronic state or may in turn reflect the presence of an underlying chronic condition. Its significance and the vigor with which eradication should be pursued vary with different age and sex subgroups.

Chronic Bacteriuria

This category is composed of approximately equal numbers of men and women and consists of patients (often elderly) whose persistent bacteriuria is associated with clear-cut, recurrent episodes of symptoms alternating with asymptomatic intervals. The group is in part composed of individuals with underlying obstructive disease or calculi who are either refractory to urologic corrective procedures or in whom surgical intervention is contraindicated by general condition. Organisms recovered in these patients, who have usually received multiple courses of anti-microbials include antibiotic-resistant *E. coli* as well as Klebsiella-Enterobacter, Proteus and Pseudomonas species. Treatment is difficult and the recurrence rate following usual two-week courses of anti-microbials is said to be greater than 80 percent. Turck and Petersdorf have divided recurrences into two groups: *relapses* (the reappearance of the same organism during or shortly after therapy) are due to persistence of the organisms in the kidney, and are more likely to respond to prolonged chemotherapeutic courses of up to six weeks. *Re-infections* are due to different organisms, and prolonged chemotherapy apparently produces no better results than shorter term treatment.

Patients with chronic bacteriuria suffer the greatest likelihood of progressive renal parenchymal destruction and chronic renal insufficiency.

Diagnosis

Typically in acute pyelonephritis the urine sediment contains leukocytes, sometimes in clumps and casts and, less often, erythrocytes. Large, pale neutrophilic leukocytes with granules in brownian motion are termed "glitter cells" and are sometimes prominent but not always diagnostic. Reliance upon the detection of pus cells in the urine, however, as the principal sign of urinary tract infection has important shortcomings. Examination of the stained or unstained uncentrifuged urinary sediment for bacteria is a useful technique, but culture of the urine remains the final determinant. Pyuria without bacteriuria or persistent hematuria should suggest the possibility of renal tuberculosis or tumor.

Two aspects of culturing the urine should be stressed: the method of collecting and the method of culturing. Since the distal urethra is normally colonized by bacteria, a voided or catheterized specimen may contain small numbers of organisms. Suprapubic needle aspiration of the bladder is perhaps the most reliable technique for collection, but less practical for routine use. In female patients a voided specimen can be used if proper cleansing of the vulva is carried out. It is crucial that the urine be cultured promptly (or refrigerated) since multiplication in the urine after voiding will negate the value of the quantitative culture.

It is this technique—that of estimating the concentration of bacteria in the urine—which makes it possible to distinguish between insignificant urethral colonizers and pathogens. A number of studies now indicate that the finding of less than 1,000 organisms per ml. indicates contamination, while more than 100,000 organisms per ml. is regularly associated with significant infection. Counts between 10,000 and 100,000 are of uncertain significance. The confidence limits for "significance" of the quantitative technique are said to be approximately 80 percent for a single voided specimen and 95 percent for two voided specimens or a single catheterized specimen. Significant persistent bacteriuria may occur with counts less than 100,000 organisms per ml., but repeated cultures must be obtained or aseptic techniques such as suprapubic aspiration used to validate the significance of such counts. The quantitative technique can be adapted for routine laboratories by the use of calibrated bacteriologic loops. Other promising tests include miniaturized culture techniques, and the use of chemical tests which act as indicators of bacterial metabolism. Several of these newer tests appear to be especially valuable for the practicing physician.

Antibiotic sensitivity testing of of isolated organisms is especially indicated in patients with recurrent infections. *E. coli* strains isolated from patients with initial acute uncomplicated pyelonephritis are almost always sensitive to many of the commonly used antimicrobials.

Intravenous pyelography, although not usually specifically helpful in acute pyelonephritis, is indicated in the management of patients with recurrent episodes (or the initial episode in males) since structural abnormalities may be detected.

In chronic pyelonephritis, asymmetry between the sizes of the two kidneys is often found and characteristic evidence of distortion of calyces and pelves noted. Needle biopsy of the kidney is unreliable because of the uneven patchy distribution of the lesions in pyelonephritis.

Management

Initial uncomplicated urinary tract infection will respond to one of a number of common antibiotics. It is important to select a relatively nontoxic agent, avoiding initially agents such as kanamycin, colistin, polymyxin B or chloramphenicol—or tetracyclines and sulfonamides during pregnancy. Commonly used agents for uncomplicated infections include sulfonamides, ampicillin, tetracyclines and cephalosporins. It is useful to re-culture the urine 48 to 72 hours after starting therapy since an effective agent almost always produces a response by this time. If the culture is not sterile at this time, another agent should probably be substituted. Despite a sterile culture after 48 to 72 hours of therapy, treatment should be continued for 10 to 14 days. Follow-up cultures to confirm bacteriologic cure should be obtained two weeks after cessation of therapy rather than immediately after completion of the course of treatment when antibacterial activity of the agent usually is still present.

In recurrent infections it is important to search for correctable lesions of the genitourinary tract. Treatment of chronic pyelonephritis in general has been difficult, with failure rates as high as 90 percent. Studies by McCabe and Jackson, however, indicate an approach which may yield better results. With the use of an appropriate antibiotic, after corrective surgery when possible, 80 percent of 252 patients showed initial clearing, although a third of these relapsed with the same organism usually within the first month of treatment. One third of the total group remained clear of infection for up to three years. Of significance was the fact that retreatment of relapses or re-infections resulted in long-term clearing of additional groups, producing progressive increases in the total number attaining a bacteriologic cure. Depending upon antibiotic sensitivities, similar results were achieved with chloramphenicol, nitrofurantoin, naladixic acid, tetracycline, colistin and various combinations, but sulfonamides were relatively ineffective.

Additional antibiotics for potential use in patients with chronic bacteriuria include kanamycin, gentamicin, and carbenicillin. The potential toxicities, and contraindications of the antimicrobial agents are discussed in Chapters 27 and 29.

A rational approach to the management of chronic pyelonephritis appears to include surgical correction of obstructive uropathy when feasible, and treatment with an appropriate antibiotic, with repeat culture and sensitivities at 72 hours. If bacteria are not eradicated, another agent should be substituted based on repeat sensitivity studies; otherwise the drug should be continued for two weeks. Of key importance is a follow-up culture a week after ending therapy, and prompt retreatment of any bacteriological relapse. Chemotherapy for up to six weeks, preferably with a bactericidal agent, is more likely to be effective in relapses. Additional follow-up should include cultures at a month, then perhaps at three-month intervals for a year and finally yearly cultures for several years.

Additional approaches of value appear to include the effort to achieve bactericidal levels of antibiotics in the urine, and the use of synergistic combinations of certain antibiotics—the combination of a penicillinase-resistant penicillin such as methicillin plus benzylpenicillin or ampicillin, for example.

Factors such as pH of the urine may be of great importance. Thus, methenamine mandelate requires a urine pH below 5.5 to be effective. Acidifying agents such as ascorbic acid (4 gm./day) may be helpful, but acidification is often virtually impossible in the presence of infections with urea-splitting bacteria such as *Proteus vulgaris*. On the other hand, drugs such as streptomycin and kanamycin require an alkaline pH for maximum effectiveness. This may often be achieved with sodium bicarbonate.

Prevention

Avoidance of unnecessary catheterization is a major preventive measure. When indwelling bladder catheters must be used, the occurrence of infection may be significantly reduced by strict adherence to aseptic techniques during catheterization, the use of sterile closed-system drainage, and antibacterial bladder rinses such as a mixture of polymyxin B and neomycin or one-fourth percent acetic acid. The use of topical antibiotic lubricants during catheterization and for daily meatal care also appear to be helpful.

SELECTED REFERENCES

Beeson, P. B.: Urinary tract infection and pyelonephritis. In Black, D. A. K. (ed.) *Renal Disease,* 2nd Ed. Oxford, Blackwell Scientific Publications, 1967.

Cohen, S. N., and Kass, E. H.: A simple method for quantitative urine cultures. N. Eng. J. Med., *277*:176, 1967.

Freedman, L. R.: Urinary tract infection, pyelonephritis and other forms of chronic interstitial nephritis. In *Diseases of the Kidney,* 2nd ed., M. B. Strauss and L. G. Welt (eds.), Boston, Little, Brown and Company, 1969.

Kass, E. H., Savage, W. and Samtamarina, B. A. G.: The significance of bacteriuria in preventive medicine. In *Progress of Pyelonephritis,* E. H. Kass (ed.), Philadelphia, F. A. Davis, p. 3, 1965.

Kass, E. H. (ed.): *Progress in Pyelonephritis.* Philadelphia, F. A. Davis, 1965.

Kass, E. H. and Zinner, S. H.: Bacteriuria and renal disease. J. Inf. Dis., *120*:*27*, 1969.

Kunin, C. M.: Epidemiology of bacteriuria and its relation to pyelonephritis. J. Inf. Dis., *120*:1, 1969.

McCabe, W. R. and Jackson, G. C.: Treatment of pyelonephritis: Bacterial, drug and host factors in success or failure among 252 patients. N. Eng. J. Med., *272*:137, 1965.

Norden, C. W. and Kass, E. H.: Bacteriuria of pregnancy—a critical reappraisal. Ann. Rev. Med., *19*:431, 1968.

Petersdorf, R. G. and Turck, M.: Some Current Concepts of Urinary Tract Infection. D-M, December, 1970.

Stamey, T. A., Govan, D. E. and Palmer, J. M.: The localization and treatment of urinary tract infections: serum levels. Medicine, (Balt.) *44*:1, 1965.

Vejlsgaard, R.: Bacteriuria in patients with diabetes mellitus. In *Progress in Pyelonephritis*, E. H. Kass (ed.), Philadelphia, F. A. Davis Co., 1965.

Chapter 25

INFECTIVE ENDOCARDITIS

Infection of the endocardium, particularly the cardiac valves, was a uniformly fatal disease before World War II. The availability of penicillin in the mid-1940's completely changed the prognosis of this infection, and today most patients can be cured. The important problems presented by this infection now include 1) endocarditis caused by antibiotic resistant microorganisms, 2) infections involving prostheses inserted during cardiovascular surgery, and 3) complications such as progressive heart failure and embolism. In addition, the presence of bacterial endocarditis is too often overlooked, and prevention of some of these infections by prophylactic administration of anti-microbial drugs to control transient bacteremia in patients with congenital or acquired heart disease is too often not practiced.

Infective endocarditis usually is separable into two clinical syndromes, which also are attributable to infection by different types of microorganisms. *Acute bacterial endocarditis* (ABE) often is a septic process with high fever, chills, sudden onset, rapidly progressive course with highly destructive endocardial lesions. Virulent microorganisms such as the pneumococcus, gonococcus, staphylococcus, and group A streptococcus frequently are responsible for this syndrome. *Subacute bacterial endocarditis* (SBE) is insidious in onset, with low grade, variable fever, manifestations of chronic disease, such as weight loss and anemia, and usually with evidence of pre-existing heart disease. Less pathogenic or ordinarily avirulent microorganisms such as indigenous streptococci other than group A *(Streptococcus viridans, Streptococcus faecalis,* enterococcus or group D streptococcus) and staphylococci frequently are responsible for this syndrome.

There is no absolute separation of these clinical syndromes from each other, and the microorganisms usually producing acute disease may cause subacute disease, and the reverse also is true. Nevertheless, they are sufficiently distinct that their description is divisible. Subacute bacterial endocarditis is the more common, and therefore deserves first attention.

Subacute Bacterial Endocarditis

The subacute variety of bacterial endocarditis begins insidiously and the patient usually cannot date its onset. Commonly, there is a history of recent dental extraction, and occasionally the illness may have been preceded by urethral or pelvic instrumentation. The patient often will have experienced the gradual development of increasing tiredness, malaise, anorexia, weight loss, and easy fatiguability. There may be no awareness of fever, and, in fact, fever may be insignificant, absent or present periodically. Sweating at night may be experienced. The joints often ache but objective evidence of arthritis usually is absent. Occasionally, the first objective manifestation of disease may be anemia demonstrated on routine medical evaluation for vague symptoms of illness. Similarly, microscopic hematuria with azotemia but without hypertension may suggest subacute endocardial infection. The presence of unexplained persistent fever in any patient with evidence of valvular or congenital heart disease demands investigation for bacterial endocarditis.

The chief clinical manifestations of established subacute bacterial endocarditis may conveniently be divided into three groups: 1) signs of cardiac disease; 2) evidence of infection; and 3) embolism.

Signs of Cardiac Disease

Uncommonly, patients with subacute bacterial endocarditis may have no signs of cardiovascular disease. Diagnosis of the infection then becomes dependent upon other manifestations of the disease, such as those related to the infectious process (e.g., fever, leucocytosis), and embolism, but most particularly *repeatedly positive blood cultures* (see Chapt. 9) for *Streptococcus viridans*, *Streptococcus faecalis* or other similar relatively avirulent bacteria.

Acquired valvular or congenital heart disease is found in the large majority of patients with subacute endocardial infection. Most often, mitral and aortic rheumatic valvular disease, bicuspid aortic valves, ventricular septal defect and patent ductus arterious are the underlying cardiovascular abnormalities predisposing to infection. Arteriosclerotic and syphilitic valves are rarely infected.

Aortic insufficiency and mitral stenosis are the common rheumatic valvular lesions affected. The more severe the mitral stenosis, particularly if associated with atrial fibrillation, the less likely is endocarditis. In addition, congestive cardiac failure, although a not uncommon complication of bacterial endocarditis, may reduce predisposition to endocardial infection.

The cardiac signs detected during bacterial endocarditis, of course, may also be produced by deformity of the cardiac valves caused by the infection. The degree to which these signs can be attributed to pre-existing heart disease, therefore, can be estimated only if the cardiac status before onset of the infection is known. Changes in quality of cardiac murmurs during subacute bacterial endocarditis may be related to the degree of anemia or fever and may not result from progressive infection of the valves. Major changes in murmurs, however, such as appearance of a murmur previously unheard, or marked change in quality of a murmur, as with the sudden appearance of a "cooing" sound, may result from perforation of a valve cusp or rupture of a chorda tendinae due to the infection. When this occurs, heart failure may evolve rapidly and severely.

When there are no signs pointing definitely to valvular disease, cardiac enlargement will usually be found and indicate the presence of cardiovascular disease. At times, infection may develop on systemic or pulmonary vascular abnormalities such as arteriovenous fistula. Then, cardiac murmurs may not be found. When bacterial endocarditis is suspected, therefore, in patients without cardiac murmurs, attention to possible peripheral vascular abnormalities is important.

Signs of Infection

Fever is the rule in subacute bacterial endocarditis but may be inconspicuous. The temperature elevation, when present, often is only 1° to 3°F, and the patient may be afebrile for days or weeks at a time. It is not uncommon for the temperature to be normal when taken sporadically during the daytime in patients who are up and about. The temperature may be elevated only in the evening or upon retiring. High remittent, intermittent, or continuous fever is rare except terminally, and in acute bacterial endocarditis.

Leucocytosis is present in most cases of subacute bacterial endocarditis but usually is not above 15000 per mm.[3] Occasionally, however, the white blood cell count is normal. Many other acute phase reactions commonly associated with inflammatory disease also are positive, including an increased erythrocyte sedimentation rate, postive C-reactive protein, and increased serum gamma globulin. A positive rheumatoid factor (latex fixation test) is often found, may be in high titer; and the magnitude of this, as with other acute phase reactions, is closely related to activity of the disease. Peripheral blood, particularly from the earlobe, has been shown to reveal increased numbers of macrophages on smear and stain.

Splenomegaly is almost uniformly detectable, and the spleen is firm and readily palpable a few centimeters below the left cortal margin. Embolic infarction of the spleen may lead to an audible friction rub over the left lower rib cage on deep breathing.

Clubbed fingers are more often present than recognized. The swelling of the distal phalanges usually is not as severe as in chronic suppurative or neoplastic lung disease, and the finger tips are not bulbous. The toes may be similarly affected but less readily detectable. The clubbed fingers in cyanotic congenital heart disease, of course, cannot be differentiated clinically from that which may arise because of endocarditis.

Petechiae are often misinterpreted as embolic lesions, but are attributable to vasculitis which accompanies endocarditis. These lesions are most prevalent on the arms, chest, abdomen, and in the axillae. They do not blanch on pressure and are not pulsatile. As they resolve, the petechiae lose their reddish hue and may be temporarily brownish colored. Petechiae also can be readily detected in the palpebral conjunctivae as small, flame-like hemorrhages, often with a white center. Similar lesions may be present in nasal and buccal mucous membranes and in the retina. Linear-appearing red streaks under the fingernails—splinter hemorrhages, cannot be distinguished easily from traumatic lesions and should not be given any significance. Application of a tourniquet or blood pressure cuff to the arm may result in clusters of petechiae distally—but these also may be observed in some normal persons—particularly women. Petechiae may continue to occur for a short time after termination of the infection with antibiotic.

Urticaria, purpura, and forms of erythema have been described in bacterial endocarditis but are rare.

Congestive heart failure may develop insidiously in patients with bacterial endocarditis and may be related to focal myocardial inflammation (Bracht-Wachter lesions), complicating a marginally compromised cardiac function caused by the underlying cardiovascular disease. Cardiac failure also may occur abruptly and progress rapidly because of ruptured chorda tendinae or valve cusps. Progressive, intractable heart failure is the most common cause of death in bacterial endocarditis; and when it is attributable to mechanical disruption of a valve by the infection, surgical treatment may be urgently required to save a life.

Embolic Manifestations

Systemic emboli are the ones which almost invariably occur in subacute bacterial endocarditis where infection on the left side of the heart predominates. These emboli arise from bacterial and fibrin vegetations on the endocardium and may affect any systemic artery. The severity of the resulting vascular occlusion is related to the organ involved and size of the embolus. When a small embolus affects the middle cerebral arterial branches, an acute cerebrovascular accident (hemiplegia) may result. If an embolus terminates in a retinal artery, blindness, temporary or permanent, may follow. A large embolus may occlude the arteries of leg, arm or mesenteries causing major vascular insufficiency, infarction and gangrene.

Embolism of a coronary artery may cause acute myocardial infarction or angina pectoris. In contrast to embolic disease resulting from intravascular uninfected clots, emboli from infective endocarditis may lead to inflammation of the artery at the site of embolus lodgement, and this may be followed by development of a mycotic aneurysm. Abscesses rarely occur in subacute bacterial endocarditis following embolization. Appearance of a mycotic aneurysum may be identified by tenderness and swelling with increased heat at the site of a peripheral vascular occlusion. When developing in viscera, particularly the brain, however, its presence may first be recognized by bleeding.

Emboli to small arteries of the fingers or hand may result in local nodular lesions which are violaceous in color, may be painful and tender (Osler's nodes and Janeway lesions). These persist for a few days and may be helpful diagnostically.

Acute Bacterial Endocarditis

Bacteremia arising from uncontrolled abscesses as in osteomyelitis, puerperal sepsis, streptoccal cellulitis, or during systemic infection with virulent microorganisms such as the pneumococcus, group A streptococcus, staphylococcus and gonococcus, all may result in acute bacterial endocarditis, even in the absence of underlying cardiac disease. Narcotic addicts are particularly prone to acute endocarditis as a result of injection of material contaminated with these and other virulent microorganisms. The valves of the right side of the heart are much more often affected than in subacute bacterial endocarditis, although the left side still is most frequently involved. One valve, occasionally one cusp, may be infected, whereas in the subacute infection more than one valve often is affected. The infection progresses rapidly, frequently is necrotizing and destroys the heart valve.

The onset of acute bacterial endocarditis may be abrupt, but is commonly preceded by evidence of a severe local or systemic infection. Chills are common, the temperature may be markedly elevated, and the febrile course is often hectic with intermittent or remittent fever. With the more rapid progression of disease, there may be little initial evidence of anemia or weight loss. The diagnosis is often made as a result of sudden development of cardiac murmurs, previously not present, or by detection of continuous bacteremia, as noted in Chapter 9. If cardiac murmurs are inconspicuous, the diagnosis may be overlooked until the sudden onset of cardiac failure, murmurs of valve destruction, ruptured chorda tendinae, or death.

Symptoms and signs of infection may be like those of subacute bacterial endocarditis, but fever, chills, and leucocytosis (20,000 to 30,000 per $mm.^3$) are more severe. Pallor may be inapparent and severe anemia is rare. Clubbing of the fingers is uncommon. The spleen usually is enlarged but may be soft and difficult to palpate. Petechiae may be less common than in the subacute disease, but purpura may occur. Joint pains or arthralgia are less often noted. Valve ring abscesses often occur, characteristically in acute staphylococcal endocarditis, and this may lead to pericarditis. Hematuria and proteinuria usually are found, but nephritis is uncommon.

Embolism to the pulmonary circulation is more common because of the increased frequency of right heart involvement, contrasted with the subacute infection, and pulmonary infarction occurs. The vegetations on the valves usually are large, and major arterial emboli are frequent. The virulent microorganisms responsible for acute bacterial endocarditis often lead to metastatic abscesses, frequently associated with infected emboli. Digital or palmar nodules, as seen in subacute endocarditis, do not occur as commonly.

Patients with acute bacterial endocarditis deteriorate rapidly and may die in a few weeks, often of major emboli or fulminant heart failure due to valve destruction or ulceration. As mentioned before, when this occurs, surgical correction of the defect may be urgently required. These events may evolve even when the infection itself can be controlled with antimicrobial drug treatment.

Pathogenesis of Bacterial Endocarditis

As mentioned in Chapter 9, transient bacteremia commonly occurs following dental manipulation, instrumentation of the urinary tract and pelvis, and incision or squeezing of superficial abscesses. When transient bacteremia with relatively avirulent microorganisms occurs in normal persons, no harm results. This occurrence in patients with valvular or congenital heart disease, however, has the serious implication of possibly being followed by development of bacterial endocarditis. The infection is most frequently localized on the underside of the valve cusp edge, and on the endocardium opposite to the site of valvular insufficiency or the septal defect. These findings and experimental observations suggest that the hemodynamic effects of the valvular disease or the congenital cardiac lesion are important in predisposing to the localization of the infection. The blood jet or site of blood eddying appears to be responsible for endocardial injury, allowing deposition of bacteria, fibrin and platelets.

The vegetations on the endocardium vary in size and may be small or large. The innermost layer of the vegetation is made up of platelets, fibrin, leucocytes, erythrocytes, and there may be necrosis, although usually not extensive in subacute endocarditis. The central area of the vegatation may be composed largely of bacteria, and the outer layer contains fibrin and some bacteria. Healing of the vegetation occurs by fibrosis, calcification of the necrotic area, and further deformity of the involved valve.

The pathology of the underlying acquired valvular or congenital heart disease also is found in subacute bacterial endocarditis, but more frequently is absent in acute endocarditis.

Iatrogenic Bacterial Endocarditis

An important cause of infection of the cardiovascular system has developed with introduction of and increased role of surgical treatment of acquired valvular and congenital heart disease, usually associated with implantation of foreign bodies such as sutures, patches and prostheses. These infections may become evident soon after surgery or after a few weeks or months. The course of these infections may resemble either acute or subacute bacterial endocarditis, and are most often caused by staphylococci, although enteric bacilli, candida and even group A streptococci have been responsible. Most of these infections probably are implanted at the time of surgery and occur at the site of the foreign body. If occurring about a valve prosthesis or septal patch, the prosthesis may become nonfunctional, rupture from its lodging or continue to function adequately despite the infection. If infection occurs about a suture, a stitch abscess may develop and produce septic manifestations without disrupting the corrective surgical procedure.

Effective antimicrobial drugs can terminate the manifestations of the infectious disease, with defervescence, weight gain, disappearance of anemia and improvement in general health, but most of these infections will relapse unless the foreign body responsible for the infection is removed. Even if removed and replaced, recurrent infection is common.

Prophylactic administration of antibiotics immediately prior to and for a few days after cardiac surgery probably should be given to prevent, as much as possible, this post-operative complication. The effectiveness of such prophylactic therapy, however, is disputed. Unfortunately, it is not possible to administer drugs which will prevent infection by all the microorganisms which may be responsible for this iatrogenic cardiac disease, and the administration of an antibiotic will not invariably prevent infection even by a bacterium sensitive to the antimicrobial agent used.

Prolonged (several months) treatment of these infections has been attempted when the surgical procedure performed will not allow re-operation, and some patients in this way have been maintained free of manifestations of infection and some have been cured.

Fortunately, the frequency of iatrogenic cardiac infection is not high, and improvements in surgical technique in experienced hands, has controlled the problem. Careful attention to asepsis and skilled surgery are most important in avoiding this complication.

Prevention of Bacterial Endocarditis

The prevention of acute bacterial endocarditis is dependent upon adequate treatment of the virulent infection which may be complicated by endocarditis. Control of drug abuse by narcotic addicts is a social problem, however; and until this is accomplished, acute endocardial infections among these individuals will continue to occur.

The predisposition of patients with acquired valvular and congenital heart disease to endocardial infection and the frequency of commensal bacteria causing transient bacteremia following dental, urinary tract, and pelvic manipulation, provides the indication for effective prophylaxis. Penicillin should be given prior to and for a short period after dental extraction, and probably following any dental manipulation, in patients with valvular or congenital heart disease. Preceding and following urethral instrumentation and before parturition, these patients should also receive antibiotics prophylactically. The drugs and dosages recommended are outlined in Chapters 9 and 27. It is essential to remember that the prophylactic antibiotics given to patients with rheumatic heart disease to prevent recurrent group A streptococcal infection will not reliably prevent bacterial endocarditis. Furthermore, chronic antibiotic administration to these patients has been associated with increased resistance of commensal oro-pharyngeal streptococci to penicillin, and doses of this drug given prior to dental, urethral or pelvic procedures, therefore, will have to be increased above that usually employed. The effectiveness of this form of prophylaxis in preventing bacterial endocarditis has not been proven but should always be given; as it is the only available method for controlling and possibly preventing endocarditis developing as a complication of induced transient bacteremia. Transient bacteremia will occur under other circumstances, however, and bacterial endocarditis will continue to occur.

Treatment of Bacterial Endocarditis

As discussed in Chapter 27, selection of an effective regimen for antibiotic treatment of any infection is dependent upon knowledge of the microorganisms causing the disease, the antimicrobial drug sensitivity of the infecting bacteria, the doses of drug required to achieve the desired therapeutic effect and the clinical factors affecting the course of infection. Once the infecting microorganism has been identified and its antibiotic sensitivity known, the most effective specific therapy is easily selected. Here, attention will be directed towards 1) when treatment should be initiated, and 2) selection of the antibiotics most likely to be effective before the microorganism and its antibiotic sensitivities are known.

Subacute Bacterial Endocarditis

Once the presence of subacute bacterial endocarditis is suspected, no localized infection possibly responsible for the infection is recognized, and an iatrogenic or self-induced (drug abuse) cause has been eliminated, the necessary blood cultures should have been obtained. As mentioned in Chapter 9, if the blood cultures are to be positive at all, three cultures will detect over 90 percent of the bacteria responsible for bacterial endocarditis. This number is a minimum, and generally four to six cultures should be obtained during the first 24 to 48 hours of observation.

It is controversial in considering patients with subacute bacterial endocarditis whether or not it is best to delay treatment until bacteriological results are available or to initiate therapy before this time. The prolonged course of subacute endocardial infection could be an indication for delay, but the possible risk of valve cusp ulceration, rupture of chorda tendinae and disastrous embolic phenomena could justify prompt treatment before confirmatory bacteriological evidence is available. Furthermore, the treatment required is lengthy; delay will extend the period of hospitalization, and prolongation of illness for an additional time may not be in the patient's best interest. The decision to initiate treatment before bacteriological data is available is dependent upon the certainty of the clinical diagnosis and the ability to select the drugs likely to be effective.

The first requisite in identifying subacute bacterial endocarditis is clear evidence of cardiac disease. Without this the diagnosis will be in doubt and cannot be resolved without signs of embolism and finding continuous bacteremia. With evidence of heart disease, persistent fever raises suspicion of the disease, but alone is inadequate to support strongly the diagnosis. The addition of splenomegaly increases the clinical probability of infective endocarditis but does not readily exclude other causes of fever and splenomegaly unrelated to pre-existing heart disease. Petechiae, particularly in the palpebral conjuctivae, and retinal hemorrhages, will further suggest the diagnosis; and when to this is added microscopic hematuria and anemia, the clinical diagnosis is strongly supported. Even if blood cultures are negative, patients with manifestations of cardiac disease, persistent fever, splenomegaly, petechiae, microscopic hematuria and anemia should be diagnosed as having subacute bacterial endocarditis. Given this clinical setting, treatment may be started without waiting for bacteriological confirmation, as long as blood cultures have been taken properly.

Isolation of a microorganism from a single blood culture cannot reliably be attributable to endocardial infection, but isolation of the same organism from all or almost all blood cultures is the rule if anyone is positive; and about 10 percent of patients with infective endocarditis will never have a positive blood culture. If the patient has received recent antimicrobial treatment for other purposes, or if an inappropriate antibiotic was given for an inadequate time or an inadequate dose before blood cultures were taken, this will either delay growth of the bacteria or nullify temporarily the ability to obtain a positive culture. Under these conditions, it is wise, if clincally possibly, to delay initiation of definitive treatment for two to five days to allow collection of blood cultures which will more likely be positive and provide the bacteriological evidence to reliably continue therapy.

When the decision to begin treatment for subacute bacterial endocarditis is made before bacteriological data is available, a history of recent dental manipulation, urinary tract difficulty or pregnancy is useful in selecting the most appropriate antimicrobial drugs. If there has been dental manipulation, the probability is that the infecting microorganism is a penicillin-sensitive streptococcus (*S. virdans*), not group A or group D streptococci. Aqueous penicillin G in a dose of 6 to 12 million units per day, given intramuscularly or intravenously, will be the treatment of choice. Although the addition of streptomycin intramuscularly in a dose of 0.5 to 1.0 gm. per day may also be given, it adds little to the initial treatment, but may be added if subsequent bacteriological data indicate its use.

If there has been urinary tract difficulty, recent pregnancy, or if the patient is an elderly man, the likelihood of infective endocarditis caused by group D streptococcus (*S. faecalis* or enterococcus) is considerable, and initial treatment should include penicillin G and streptomycin in the doses recommended for endocarditis following dental manipulation. Ampicillin also may be used in these patients in a dose of 4 to 12 gms. per day.

Once bacteriological data become available, these therapeutic regimens may be continued or changed as dictated by the character of the infecting organism and its antibiotic sensitivities. Under either circumstance, treatment should be continued for at least four to six weeks.

Acute Bacterial Endocarditis

As mentioned before, acute bacterial endocarditis most often follows or complicates an uncontrolled infection elsewhere in the body. Characterization of the infection antedating the onset of acute bacterial endocarditis, therefore, is critical in estimating the probable infecting microorganism. Furthermore, this microorganism may have been identified as a result of investigation of the local infection.

The rapid course of acute bacterial endocarditis and the virulence of the infection makes it even more important than in subacute endocardial infection to initiate treatment as soon as the clinical diagnosis is suspected and before bacteriological evidence is available. The septic process of the patient itself will indicate the need for treatment, however, even if acute endocarditis is not initially suspected.

When the inciting extracardiac infection is a cutaneous or subcutaneous abscess, the possibility of acute staphylococcal endocarditis is great. A pencillinase-resistant penicillin analogue such as oxacillin, cloxacillin or methicillin should be given, after blood cultures are obtained, in doses of 4 to 12 gms. per day intramuscularly or intravenously. When bacteriological data are available, the therapeutic regimen may be continued or changed, but treatment should be continued for no less than four to six weeks.

When the inciting extracardiac infection is severe cutaneous and subcutaneous cellulitis without abscess, possibly with bullous formation, and associated with lymphangitis and lymphadenitis, the possibility of group A streptococcal endocarditis is high. After blood cultures are obtained, penicillin G should be given in a dose of 6 to 12 million units daily intramuscularly or intravenously. When bacteriological data are available, this may be revised, but treatment should be continued for four weeks. A similar regimen is desirable if the patient has acute pneumonia like that attributed to pneumococci as discussed in Chapter 14.

Important to recognize is that acute bacterial endocarditis arises from uncontrolled extracardiac infection, and effective management of these infections is the surest way to prevent acute endocardial infection. In addition, local treatment of the extracardiac infection will be necessary while antibiotic treatment of the endocardial infection is underway.

Iatrogenic Bacterial Endocarditis

Most of these infections have been due to penicillin-resistant staphylococci, and treatment as described above in patients with cutaneous-subcutaneous abscesses should be initiated when the diagnosis is made. Generally, in this condition, however, bacteriological data will be necessary before the diagnosis of post-surgical extracardiac infection can be recognized with certainty.

SELECTED REFERENCES

Albrecht, M. and Clowes, G. H. A.: The increase of circulatory requirements in the presence of inflammation. Surgery, *56*:158, 1964.

Angnist, A. A.: Pathogenesis of bacterial endocarditis. J.A.M.A., *183*:249, 1963.

Bashour, E. A. and Winchele, C. P.: Right sided bacterial endocarditis. Am. J. Med. Sci., *240*:411, 1960.

Bennett, I. L., Jr., and Beeson, P. B.: Bacteremia: A consideration of some experimental and clinical aspects. Yale J. Biol. Med., *26*:241, 1954.

Cherubin, C. E., Baden, M., Kavaler F., Lerner, S. and Cline, W.: Infective endocarditis in narcotic addicts. Ann. Int. Med., *69*:1091, 1968.

Dupont, H. L. and Spink, W. W.: Infections due to gram-negative organisms: An analysis of 860 patients with bacteremia at the University of Minnesota Medical Center, 1958–1966. Medicine *48*:307, 1969.

Hodgin, U. G. and Sanford, J. P.: Gram-negative rod bacteremia. Am. J. Med., *39*:952, 1965.

Hook, E. W. and Kaye, D.: Prophylaxis of bacterial endocarditis. J. Chronic Dis., *15*:635, 1962.

Jones, H. R., Jr., Siekert, R. G. and Geraci, J. E.: Neurologic manifestations of bacterial endocarditis. Ann. Int. Med., *7*:21, 1969.

Kerr, A. J., Jr.: *Subacute Bacterial Endocarditis*. Springfield, Ill., Charles C Thomas, Publishers, 1955.

Lerner, P. I. and Weinstein, L.: Infective endocarditis in the antibiotic era. N. Engl. J. Med., *274*:199, 1966.

Martin, C. M., Cuomo, A. J., Geraghty, M. J., Zager, J. R. and Mandes, T. C.: Gram-negative rod bacteremia. J. Infect. Dis., *119*:506, 1969.

Rodbard, S.: Blood velocity and endocarditis. Circulation, *27*:18, 1963.

SECTION FOUR

MANAGEMENT AND PREVENTION OF INFECTIOUS DISEASES

Chapter 26

INTRODUCTION

The treatment and prevention of infectious diseases represent two of the most dramatic and successful accomplishments of modern medical science. Ehrlich's dream of the "magic bullet"—the weapon which would destroy the invading pathogen while remaining innocuous to the host—has been to an important extent realized by the discovery of antimicrobial agents. Jenner's simple efforts to assist nature and in a sense appease her by offering the benign substitute of cowpox in place of the destructive assault of smallpox has had far-reaching consequences leading to modern techniques of immunization. Despite the great advances made possible by these developments, however, infectious diseases have not disappeared.

While contributing to the conquest of many of the epidemic scourges of the past, immunization and antimicrobial therapy must share much of the credit with improvements in sanitation, nutrition, and hygiene. Under the influence of these factors a significant shift has occurred in the types of infectious diseases confronting medical practice. Now much of the problem is a consequence of the microorganisms indigenous to man. Infections produced by these organisms have presented continuing challenges to antimicrobial therapy with the steady emergence of antibiotic resistant bacterial strains. Progress in management of chronic and previously fatal diseases with utilization of complex therapeutic techniques and consequent prolongation of life has exacted the price of increasing the patient's susceptibility to new groups of disease agents. The war is not over; the battlefield is changing.

Prior to the modern antimicrobial era, almost none of the few available effective medicines were actually specific for the disease. To an important degree antibiotics still represent the only major class of therapeutic agents which can effect a complete cure of illness.

However, the multiplicity of new antimicrobials available to the physician has to some extent complicated his treatment. Now he must choose from a long list of agents the single drug or combination most suitable for his patient, requiring not only knowledge of the antibiotic sensitivities of many microorganisms, but also of the toxicities and interactions of the agents with the metabolic and physiologic states of the patient.

Enthusiasm for broad-spectrum "coverage" of the patient with antibiotic therapy has now been replaced with concern about the consequences of disturbing the ecological balance of man's microflora. Eradication of the normal indigenous bacteria is often followed by the substitution of drug-resistant and often potentially pathogenic species. The "ideal" antibiotic in fact would appear to be an agent which is specific for a single species of microorganism without effects on the remaining flora.

In addition to the antibiotic sensitivity of the pathogenic microorganism, it has now become apparent that results of antibiotic therapy are also markedly influenced by a variety of additional factors such as the presence of a foreign body, obstruction of drainage and alteration in microbial form.

While effective antibacterial chemotherapy was evolving, it seemed unlikely that viruses because of their intimate involvement with intracellular metabolism would be susceptible to similar approaches. Already, however, two effective anti-viral agents are available in the United States and a number of other promising agents are under development. The day of anti-viral chemotherapy is just now dawning.

The ideal of the totally innocuous antibiotic has sadly not been realized, and the physician and his patient must now weigh the price of a diverse array of potential adverse effects, toxic and allergic, and of a complex of possible pharmacologic interactions. The very complexity of the problem requires that the physician gain systematic understanding of the basic concepts involved.

As the epidemic diseases are replaced by indigenous and opportunistic infections, and as knowledge of the mechanisms of transmission of infectious agents has developed, the techniques and aims of patient *isolation* have also changed. The hospital is the major focus of isolation technique, and while the capacity to contain the highly pathogenic microbe remains a requisite, emphasis is now shifting toward identification of the susceptible patient so that he can be protected from his own microflora as well as that of other patients and of hospital personnel.

Preventive medicine of the future will increasingly seek to identify susceptible patients before their illnesses become established. Immunization is the keystone by which the patients' own natural defenses can be specifically augmented to avert the serious consequences of infection. Progress as always exacts its price, however, and the advantage to the patient must be weighed against the possible consequences of the procedure. Smallpox for example has not occurred in the United States for over

20 years; yet a number of fatalities as well as other complications of vaccination occur yearly. It is possible to argue that now in the United States the defense is more dangerous than the disease, and re-evaluation of vaccination policy is underway. Nevertheless smallpox is still endemic in many parts of the world and the potential for epidemic introduction of the disease into this country must be weighed. Hospital personnel, for example, are at particular risk of disease during such epidemics.

Presented in this section are the concepts of management and prevention of infectious diseases which are of immediate and practical importance to the physician.

Chapter 27

ANTIMICROBIAL THERAPY

The Dilemma

The judicious selection and use of antimicrobial agents has become an increasingly complex task for most physicians. The reasons for the evolution of this problem are numerous and varied. Historically, only a limited number of pyogenic pathogens accounted for the majority of the morbidity and mortality from acute bacterial infections. The clinical syndromes produced by these commonplace microorganisms were easily recognizable, and laboratory confirmation of bedside diagnoses was relatively uncomplicated. With the advent of the sulfonamide and penicillin antimicrobials (1936 and 1941 respectively), death and disability resultant from these infections was significantly reduced. In addition, there was yet little problem in selection from among the limited number of drugs available to physicians for treatment of acute infections. Shortly thereafter (1944), the discovery of streptomycin led to control of even more acute infections, as well as tuberculosis. An ensuing wave of optimism led to a degree of complacency, epitomized by the epithet—"Infectious Diseases are Dead!" The error of this assertion soon became apparent, almost as an echo.

The optimism of the medical community was first quieted by the emergence of resistance to multiple drugs among pathogenic staphylococci. Epidemic nosocomial infections due to these organisms and increasing drug resistance among other bacterial genera stimulated renewed interest in non-pharmacologic methods of disease control and intensified the search for new chemotherapeutic agents. Concurrently, advances in surgery and pharmacotherapeutics increased survival of many patients with diseases that were formerly rapidly lethal. These diseases and the drugs or devices used in their therapy often resulted in profound decreases in patients' natural resistance to infection. Suddenly, physicians were confronted with an expanding spectrum of hitherto unrecognized or infrequently encountered infectious diseases. Most of the microorganisms responsible for these infections have been shown to be of limited virulence for normal tissues and to originate primarily in the host's indigenous microflora. In addition, many of the bacterial strains have been naturally insusceptible, or rapidly acquired resistance, to a variety of antimicrobial agents.

Thus, the physician is at present confronted with both an expanding and changing spectrum of infectious diseases and a rapidly increasing armamentarium of antimicrobial drugs. The problem has been further compounded by controversies regarding the relative merits of the various drugs and their formulations in both promotional and scientific literature. For example, within the first year of its availability, carbenicillin has been reputed to be additive to, synergistic with, and antagonistic of gentamicin in activity against gram-negative bacilli. Clearly, few among us should be expected to learn and retain all clinically relevant microbiological and pharmacological data for each antimicrobial agent. On the other hand, neither should we attempt to circumvent the problem of drug selection by routine, subjective prescription of broad-spectrum antimicrobial therapy to "cover" all diagnostic possibilities. Our task may be simplified, however, by adherence to a few general principles of choice of antimicrobial therapy. The process of selection, appropriate administration, and management of apparent failures of antimicrobial therapy are the subjects of the following discussions.

The Choice

The selection and administration of antimicrobial agents may be greatly facilitated by rigid and repetitive adherence to a few fundamental microbiological and pharmacologic principles. These principles are elaborated below in the consideration of a series of questions that the physician must pose to himself whenever he faces a choice from among several potentially useful antimicrobial agents. Not always will the answers to these questions be immediately apparent. However, reliable sources of relevant data are usually easily accessible to most physicians. For example, the "package insert" is now a relatively dependable source of prescribing information for specific drugs. Additional pharmacologic data and specific recommendations for therapy of the more common bacterial diseases may be found in this or other standard references. It is hoped that the consideration of these general principles will provide a firm basis for evaluation of the relative merits of currently available drugs, as well as those that may be developed in the future.

Has the Diagnosis Been Made as Objectively as Possible?

One's initial diagnosis is only a clinical impression in most instances. However, it should be based upon as much objective evidence as possible.

A thorough history and careful physical examination are clearly indispensable. Appropriate specimens must be obtained for subsequent laboratory confirmation of the diagnosis and drug-susceptibility testing, which may be a highly valuable aid in drug selection. Blood cultures should be obtained in all serious infections, even though the disease process may appear localized. Infected material from areas usually free of indigenous flora should always be examined microscopically. The nature of the inflammatory cells and infecting bacteria should be recorded. Stains performed by the gram method should always include appropriate material (such as scrapings of one's teeth) on the same slide to verify adequacy of the method. The patient's past hospital or office records should be reviewed immediately to determine results of previous cultures. These may be especially useful in patients with recent or chronic osteomyelitis, endocarditis or urinary tract infections, since recurrences in these diseases are often due to the same microorganisms. For therapeutic purposes, all of the evidence should then by synthesized to achieve a single diagnosis, or as limited a list of differential diagnoses as possible.

In Bacterial Infections, What Class of Drug Should Be Selected—Bactericidal or Bacteriostatic?

The bactericidal and bacteriostatic agents and their mechanisms of activity are shown in Table 27.1. In serious or life-threatening infections, one should attempt to select a bactericidal agent. This is especially true when other factors such as likelihood of toxicity and degree of antibacterial activity of the alternatives are equivalent. Bactericidal agents are clearly preferable in bacterial endocarditis or if there is underlying impairment of the patient's defense mechanisms. In mild infections in otherwise healthy patients, the choice between bactericidal and bacteriostatic drugs may not be critical, and factors such as cost of the drug and ease of administration may be considered.

What Is the Appropriate Route of Drug Administration?

Parenteral therapy should be used in patients with serious or life-threatening infections. Intravenous rather than intramuscular therapy is clearly preferable in patients with the following complications: 1) hypotension; 2) bleeding diatheses; 3) diabetes mellitus or other diseases involving small blood vessels; 4) sepsis; and 5) infections located in sites such as the meninges or humors of the eye where concentrations following intramuscular administration are likely to be suboptimal. Therapy by the oral route may be considered only in less serious infections. One must be cautioned that not all drug preparations for oral use are predictably well absorbed.

The degree of gastrointestinal absorption of most antimicrobial drugs is likely to vary from hour to hour in the same patient, particularly with changes in relation to meals. In addition, there may be considerable variation in absorption from one patient to the next, even under similar circumstances. Nevertheless, the outcome of many mild or moderately severe illnesses, such as sinusitis, otitis, or skin infections, will be favorable even if the patient incompletely absorbs several doses. On the other hand, erratic oral absorption may occasionally defeat one's therapeutic goals. For example, in patients with history of rheumatic fever and recent pharyngitis due to Group A streptococci, it is important that therapeutic levels of penicillin be maintained for 10 days for optimal protection against the rheumatic sequellae. These patients usually should not receive oral penicillin for such episodes.

Will the Drug Achieve Adequate Concentrations or Exert Optimal Activity at the Site of Infection?

Many antimicrobials penetrate poorly into the cerebrospinal fluid or humors of the eyes. Concentrations of drug are usually significantly less in these fluids than in plasma or other soft tissues. Penetration across the "blood-brain barrier" is dependent upon the degree of ionization and lipid solubility of the drug; more highly charged, less lipid soluble molecules are preferentially excluded from these fluids. If necessary, this limitation may be overcome in most instances. Therapeutic concentrations of the penicillins may be achieved by markedly increasing the dosage, so that an adequate concentration gradient is maintained between plasma and cerebrospinal fluid. With other drugs, such as the aminoglycosides or polymyxins, total dosage may seldom be increased with safety. If indicated, these drugs may be instilled directly into the anterior chamber of the eye or cerebrospinal fluid space.

The physiologic conditions at the site of infection may be instrumental in determining the outcome of therapy. Antagonism of the action of the sulfonamides by pus is well recognized. Variations in urinary pH may significantly influence the action of a variety of antimicrobials in the urine. The aminoglycosides and erythromycin may be inactive in acidic urine; whereas mandelamine, tetracycline, nalidixic acid and nitrofurantoin are often less active in alkaline urine. Maintenance of neutral or alkaline pH is especially important to ensure optimal effect of the aminoglycosides in infected urine; while acidic urine is absolutely essential for activity of mandelamine.

For reasons that are yet unclear, other microorganisms may vary in responsiveness according to their location. Meningococci are an example. When present in blood or meninges, susceptible strains are inhibited by a variety of antimicrobial agents such as the penicillins, chloramphenicol, the tetracyclines, erythromycin or the sulfonamides. However, when lo-

TABLE 27.1

Classes of antimicrobial agents and their mechanisms of action

Bactericidal drugs	*Mechanism of action*
1. *The penicillins:* penicillin V and G, ampicillin, phenethicillin, phenbenicillin, methicillin, oxacillin, cloxacillin, nafcillin, carbenicillin	1. Impairs cell wall biosynthesis. Prevents cross-linking of the glycopeptide "backbone" of the cell wall. The defects created expose the bacterial cell to osmotic lysis.
2. *The cephalosporins:* cephalothin, cephaloglycine, cephalexin, cephaloridine, cephapirin	2. Same as penicillin
3. *The aminoglycosides:* streptomycin, kanamycin, neomycin, gentamicin	3. All induce misreading of the genetic code at the ribosomal level. Thus, incorrect amino acids are incorporated into the growing peptide chain. This process of synthesis of defective proteins may be lethal for the cell. Streptomycin may be bactericidal through inhibition of polymerization of amino acids.
4. *The polymyxins:* colistin, polymyxin B	4. Impair function bacterial cell membrane. As cationic detergents with affinity for phosphate radicals, they alter the osmotic barrier function of the cell membrane.
5. Vancomycin, ristocetin, bacitracin	5. Impair cell wall biosynthesis. Inhibit enzyme glycopeptide synthetase—which is responsible for condensation of glycopeptide backbone of cell wall.
6. Cycloserine	6. Structural analogue of D-alanine. Competes for sites on pentapeptide polymer subunits in bacterial cell wall.
Bacteriostatic drugs	*Mechanism of action*
1. Chloramphenicol	1. Inhibits protein biosynthesis. Prevents attachment m-RNA to ribosomes.
2. *The tetracyclines:* tetracycline, minocycline, doxycycline, oxytetracycline, chlortetracycline, demethylortetracycline	2. Inhibit protein biosynthesis by preventing binding of amino acid-activated t-RNA to the 30S subunit of the ribosome.
3. Erythromycin	3. Suppresses protein formation by inhibiting peptide bond synthesis. Binds to 50S subunit of the ribosome.
4. Lincomycin and clindamycin	4. Same as erythromycin.
5. Rifampin	5. Inhibits DNA-dependent RNA-polymerase enzyme activity.

TABLE 27.1—*Continued*

6. Sulfonamides	6. Impairs folic acid biosynthesis by competing with *p*-aminobenzoic acid.
Urinary antiseptics (primarily bacteriostatic)	*Mechanism of action*
1. Methenamine mandelate (mandelamine)	1. Liberates formaldehyde in acid urine.
2. Nalidixic acid	2. Blocks DNA synthesis. Structural analogue to purine nucleotides.
3. Nitrofurantoin	3. Uncertain.

cated in the nasopharynx, susceptible strains may be eliminated only by the sulfonamides. Whether these differences in responsiveness result from failure of many of the drugs to achieve adequate concentrations in the nasopharyngeal milieu, from local physiologic differences that may influence drug action, or in alterations in the physiologic state of the microorganisms (see below) remains to be determined.

Other remedial causes of failure of antimicrobial therapy when infection occurs in certain specific settings or locations are enumerated in the section on therapeutic failures.

What Is the Relative Risk of Each of the Agents That May Be Prescribed?

As with all therapeutic agents or devices, one must first answer the question: is the risk of the disease clearly greater than the risk inherent in its therapy? If the answer is affirmative, only then may one proceed with the process of drug selection.

A careful inquiry into the patient's history of drug allergy and toxicity is imperative before therapy is begun. Patients who respond affirmatively should be questioned regarding the manifestations of their previous reactions, since many tend to equate therapeutic unresponsiveness, past gastrointestinal irritation, or other non-specific symptoms to drug allergy. On the other hand, the absence of a past history of allergy or previous exposure to a given antimicrobial agent by no means precludes the occurrence of an immediate or delayed reaction following its use. Neomycin has been included in deodorants; tetracycline-rinses have been used to prolong shelf-life of poultry products; and penicillin has been detected in milk and other dairy products. In patients with convincing histories of drug allergy, the suspected agent should clearly be avoided if possible. Unfortunately, no safe and reliable diagnostic test is currently available to determine the presence or absence of allergy to penicillin or related drugs.

Toxic reactions to antimicrobial agents have occurred most frequently in the following circumstances: 1) use of excessive dosage; 2) impairment of the primary organ of drug excretion; and 3) antecedent disease of the target organ of drug toxicity. Thus, the physician must be cognizant of the potential toxic reactions of the drugs under consideration and attempt to assess the functional state of the organs likely to be involved in drug elimination and toxicity. The major toxic reactions encountered with commonly used antimicrobials are listed in Table 27.2 and further discussed in Chapter 29. Clearly, one should attempt to select the single drug that is most active and least toxic from among available alternatives.

What Is the Appropriate Dosage to Administer?

Since expense and likelihood of toxicity and superinfection increase in proportion to total dosage, the *least* amount of drug that will produce the desired effect should be administered. Although determined empirically, most recommended dosage schedules will ensure an optimal therapeutic response. Subjective increases in dosage seldom result in more rapid bacterial killing or earlier symptomatic improvement of the patient. If doubt exists regarding adequacy of therapy, precise assays of drug activity against the infecting microorganism and determination of antibacterial activity in the patient's serum at measured intervals following dosing may be performed.

Occasionally, there are few or no alternatives to selection of a potentially nephrotoxic antimicrobial agent for patients with underlying renal disease. In this setting one must first ensure that the clinical microbiology laboratory has exhaustively tested the infecting microorganism for susceptibility to all available, potentially useful antimicrobials. The relative risks of toxicity of most antibacterial agents in patients with renal disease are listed in Table 27.2. Lacking an effective alternative, potentially nephrotoxic drugs may be employed in patients with impaired renal function provided that the dosage of drug or interval of administration, or both, are continually adjusted in an attempt to prevent accumulation of excessive concentrations of the drug. Dosage schedules for use of most antimicrobials in patients with varying degrees of renal impairment have now been established. Unfortunately, these recommendations are insufficiently precise to ensure complete safety. Since the dosage modifications are based upon parameters of renal function (serum creatinine concentration or endogenous creatinine clearance rate) that may vary from day to day, patients should be monitored closely to detect changes in renal function and early signs of drug toxicity. Several promising methods for rapid determination of serum concentrations of the more useful antimicrobial agents have recently been described. Hopefully, these may be adapted for routine use in hospital laboratories to permit more timely and precise adjustments in dosage of potentially hazardous drugs.

TABLE 27.2

Relative risks of antimicrobial agents in patients with impaired renal function

Drug	Toxicity usually associated with excessive accumulation of drug
1. *Relatively safe at normal or slightly reduced dosage*	
Penicillins (Pen G or V, ampicillin, methicillin, oxacillin, cloxacillin, nafcillin, dicloxacillin, carbenicillin)	Convulsions with higher (multimillion unit) doses. Potassium accumulation (1.6 meq/million units) with pen G and V and sodium accumulation with the remainder. Superinfection
Cephalothin	Superinfection. Sodium accumulation in patients with volume overload
Chloramphenicol	Hematopoietic depression of the reversible type. (Irreversible aplasia is not dose-related)
Erythromycin	Little or no effect
Lincomycin	Little or no effect
2. *Potentially toxic, dosage must be reduced*	
Kanamycin, gentamicin	Nephrotoxicity; auditory and/or vestibular impairment; neuromuscular blockade-apnea, especially in association with neuromuscular (N-M) blocking agents such as ether, curare, succinylcholine
Polymyxin B, colistin	Nephrotoxicity; peripheral neuropathy; neuromuscular blockade-apnea, especially with N-M blocking agents
Vancomycin	Auditory and vestibular impairment, nephrotoxicity
3. *Highly toxic, should be avoided except in the most unusual circumstances*	
Tetracycline	Hepatic injury, renal tubular damage, prerenal azotemia
Streptomycin	Vestibular toxicity, possible nephrotoxicity
Cephaloridine	Nephrotoxicity
Sulfonamides	Nephrotoxicity (crystalluria)
Nitrofurans	Peripheral neuritis, hemolytic anemia in patients with G6PD deficiency
Nalidixic acid	Convulsions, hepatotoxicity
Mandelamine	Active only in acidic urine. Attempts to acidify may lead to systemic acidosis

What Is the Appropriate Duration of Therapy?

The antimicrobial agent selected should be administered for the *least* amount of time necessary to achieve the desired results. Most recommendations for dosage and duration of therapy have been based upon the empiric observation of optimal response of the infection and the minimum attainable risk of recurrence or relapse. Subjective prolongation of therapy seldom results in decreases in the rate of relapses or reinfection, and may enhance the likelihood of superinfection or cumulative drug toxicity. Use of long-term suppressive antibacterial therapy to prevent recurrences of urinary tract infections may represent an exception to this general rule.

Most acute pyogenic infections should be treated for 48 to 72 hours after signs and symptoms of infection have abated. Infections that notoriously respond slowly (e.g., bacterial endocarditis) tend to become chronic (e.g., osteomyelitis), are prone to development of metastatic foci (e.g., staphylococcal bacteremia), all should be treated for more prolonged periods. Symptomatic Group A streptococcal infections should be treated for 10 days in an attempt to prevent rheumatic fever.

Tabulation of recommended dosages and duration of antimicrobial drug treatment in different infectious diseases are provided in Table 27.3. These are meant only as a general guide.

The Failures

The failure of seemingly appropriate antimicrobial therapy is a common and often vexing clinical problem. Single causative factors are seldom found. More often, host, microorganism and pharmacologic agents interact to inhibit drug action. Despite the apparent complexity of these interactions, systematic evaluation of the patient and his problem will frequently identify causative factors that may be eliminated or circumvented to permit control of the infectious process. In addition, potentially hazardous, subjective changes in the patient's antibiotic regimen may thus be avoided. The following discussion outlines the remedial causes of failure of "appropriate" antimicrobial therapy. It is predicated on the assumptions that the infecting microorganism has been correctly identified and the prescribed antimicrobial agent(s) have been selected with objectivity.

Pharmacologic Factors

The variabilities in absorption, excretion and tissue distribution of most antimicrobial agents are now well known. Recommended adjustments in dosage or route of administration necessary to compensate for variations in drug absorption, penetration into the cerebrospinal fluid, or excretion in patients with impaired renal function are generally accessible.

Other pharmacologic factors are less often recognized. The list of drugs that may impair the absorption, metabolism or action of antimicrobials is increasing rapidly. Gastrointestinal absorption of most of the tetracyclines may be significantly impaired by oral administration of salts of iron (both ferrous and ferric ions), aluminum, copper, nickel, cobalt, zinc and magnesium. Milk and most antacids act similarly. The action of tetracycline may be impaired by large doses of riboflavin. The oral absorption of oxacillin may be limited by sulfonamides given by the same route. Nalidixic acid absorption may be inhibited by oral administration of nitrofurantoin. The metabolism of griseofulvin may be enhanced by phenobarbital, ophenamide or phenylbutazone. Variations in urinary pH may significantly influence the action of a variety of antimicrobials in the urine as noted above.

Many antimicrobial agents are unstable or are inactivated by other drugs in solutions for intravenous use. The list of drug combinations that are incompatible in this circumstance has become too unwieldy to commit to memory. For this reason, intravenous administration of more than one drug at a time should be avoided. If this is not possible, most pharmacists can provide information regarding the likelihood of incompatibility of a proposed combination.

Although important in specific instances, pharmacologic factors account for the minority of failures of antimicrobial therapy.

Foreign Body

Persistence of infection despite adequate drug therapy frequently results from the presence of a foreign body at the nidus of infection. Suture material, artificial grafts and cardiac or orthopedic prostheses are common sites for persistence of infection. Sequestra in osteomyelitis and calculi in the renal or biliary tracts may act in an analogous fashion. Staphylococci and gram-negative bacilli appear to be especially invulnerable to drug therapy when they are located in proximity to foreign material. In general, a favorable therapeutic response is predictable only when the infected foreign body is removed or spontaneously extruded.

Obstruction to Drainage

Unresponsiveness to drug therapy is frequently encountered when infection is located proximally to an obstruction to natural drainage. Infections behind obstructed renal, biliary, and bronchial drainage are especially likely to respond slowly, if at all. Permanent eradication of infection may be anticipated only when the obstruction is relieved and normal drainage is restored.

Abscess

Similar therapeutic unresponsiveness may be noted in the presence of deep-seated, closed-space infections. Examples are intracranial, intra-ab-

TABLE 27.3
Guide to choice of antimicrobial drugs

Microbes	Diseases	Drugs of choice	Dosages and duration
Gram-positive cocci			
1. Group A streptococcus	a. Pharyngitis	Penicillin G Alt.: Erythromycin	a. 1.2 million u./day for 10 days
	b. Cellulitis, pneumonia, empyema, bacteremia	Cephalothin, Lincomycin	b. 4 to 6 mill. u./day until clinically cured.
2. *Spreptococcus viridans*	Infective endocarditis	Penicillin G Alt.: See 1	10 mil. u./day for 4 wks.
3. Enterococcus (group D streptococcus)	a. Infective endocarditis	1) Penicillin G plus streptomycin or 2) Ampicillin	a. 1) 20 mill. u./day plus 1 gm./day for 4 to 6 wks. 2) 8 gm./day for 4 to 6 wks.
	b. Urinary tract infection		b. 1) 2.4 mill. u./day plus 1 gm./day for 1 or more wks. 2) 2 to 4 gm./day for 1 or more wks.
4. Pneumococcus	a. Pneumonia	Penicillin G Alt.: See 1	a. 600,000 to 1.2 mill. u./day for 5 to 7 days
	b. Meningitis		b. 20 mill. u./day for 10 to 14 days
	c. Empyema, pyoarthritis		c. 6 mill. u./day for 2 wks.
5. *Staphylococus aureus* (penicillin sensitive)	a. Abscess	Penicillin G	a. 1.2 mill. u./day until clinically cured
	b. Infective endocarditis		b. 20 mill. u./day for 4 to 6 wks.
	c. Pneumonia, pyoarthritis		c. 2 to 4 mill. u./day for 4 to 6 wks.

6. *Staphylococcus aureus* (penicillin resistant)	a. Abscess b. Infective endocarditis c. Pneumonia, pyoarthritis	Methicillin, Oxacillin, Cloxacillin Alt.: Cephalothin, Erythromycin Lincomycin, Vancomycin	a. 2 to 4 gm./day until clinically cured b. 4 to 12 gm./day for 4 to 6 wks. c. 4 gm./day for 4 to 6 wks.
		Gram-positive bacilli	
7. *Clostridium perfringens*	Gas gangrene	Penicillin G Alt.: Tetracycline	10 to 20 mill. u./day plus antitoxin (?)
8. *Clostridium tetani*	Tetanus	Penicillin G	2 to 4 mill. u./day for 7 days plus antitoxin
9. *Listeria monocytogenes*	Meningitis	Penicillin G Alt.: Tetracycline or Erythromycin	20 mill. u./day for 7 or more days
10. *Corynebacterium diphtheriae*	Diphtheria	Penicillin G Alt.: Erythromycin	1.2 mill. u./day for 7 or more days plus antitoxin
		Gram-negative cocci	
11. *Neisseria meningitidis*	Meningitis or bacteremia	Penicillin G Alt.: Ampicillin, Chloramphenicol, Erythromycin	10 to 20 mill. u./day for 7 days
12. *Neisseria gonorrheae*	Gonorrhea	Penicillin G Alt.: Tetracycline, Erythromycin, Cephalothin	2.4 to 4.8 mill. u. in a single dose (higher dose in female), or 2 gm. Tetracycline/day for 7 days

TABLE 27.3—*Continued*

Microbes	Diseases	Drugs of choice	Dosages and duration
Gram-negative bacilli			
Sensitivity patterns vary. Antibiotic choice should be based on awareness of sensitivity of isolates.			
13. *Escherichia coli*	a. Urinary tract infection	a. 1) Sulfisoxazole	a. 1) 4 gm. initial dose, 2 gm. qid for 10 days
		2) Trisulfapyrimidines	2) 2 to 4 gm. initial dose, 1 gm. qid for 10 days
		3) Ampicillin	3) 2 to 4 gm./day
	b. Wound infections, pneumonia, bacteremia	a. Gentamicin	a. 0.8 to 5.0 mg./kg./day
		b. Ampicillin	b. 4 to 8 gm./day
		c. Cephalothin	c. 4 to 8 gm./day
		d. Chloramphenicol	d. 2 to 4 gm./day
		e. Kanamycin	e. 15 mg./kg./day (max. 1 to 1.5 gm./day)
		f. Colymycin	f. 2 to 5 mg./kg./day (max. 300 mg./day)
14. Klebsiella-aerobacter	Wound infections, pneumonia, bacteremia	a. Cephalothin	a. 4 to 8 gm./day
		b. Kanamycin	b. 15 mg./kg./day (max 1 to 1.5 gm./day)
		c. Gentamicin	c. 0.8 to 5.0 mg./kg./day
		Alt.: Colymycin, Chloramphenicol	
15. Enterobacter	Wound infections, pneumonia, bacteremia	a. Gentamicin	a. As above
		b. Tetracycline	b. 2 to 4 gm./day
		Alt: Streptomycin, Kanamycin, Colymycin, Chloramphenicol	
16. *Proteus mirabilis*	Urinary tract infection	a. Ampicillin	a. 2 to 4 gm./day for 7 to 10 days
		b. Penicillin G	b. 10 to 20 mill. u./day for 7 to 10 days

17. Proteus (Indole positive)	Urinary tract infection, wound infection, pneumonia, bacteremia	a. Gentamicin b. Chloramphenicol c. Kanamycin	a. As above b. 2 to 4 gm./day c. As above
18. *Pseudomonas aeruginosa*	Urinary tract infection, wound infection, pneumonia, bacteremia	a. Gentamicin b. Colistin c. Polymycin B	a. As above b. As above c. Up to 2.5 mg./kg./day
19. Salmonella	Enteritis, bacteremia	a. Ampicillin b. Chloramphenicol	a. 2 to 4 gm./day b. 2 to 4 gm./day
20. Shigella	Enteritis, bacteremia	As for Salmonella Alt.: Tetracycline	As for Salmonella
21. Bacteroides	Abscesses, bacteremia	Chloramphenicol Alt.: Tetracycline or Penicillin G	2 to 4 gm./day
22. *Hemophilus influenzae*	Pneumonia, meningitis	Ampicillin Alt.: Tetracycline, Chloramphenicol	2 to 4 gm./day for 1 or more wks.
Other microorganisms			
23. *Treponema pallidum*	a. Syphilis—primary, secondary	Penicillin G Alt.: Erythromycin, Tetracycline	a. 1) Benzathine penicillin (Bicillin), 2.4 mill. u. in single dose 2) Procaine penicillin 600,000 u./day for 8 to 10 days
	b. Syphilis—tertiary		b. 1) Bicillin 2.4 mill. u. q. 7 days for 3 doses 2) Procaine penicillin 600,000 u./day for 14 days
24. Rickettsia	Rocky mountain spotted fever, typhus	Chloramphenicol or Tetracycline	2 to 4 gm./day for 7 to 14 days

dominal and poorly drained lung abscesses. Antimicrobial agents alone are seldom effective in eliminating infection. Satisfactory response usually requires adequate surgical drainage or excision of the abscess in conjunction with drug therapy.

The reasons for failure of chemotherapy alone in the presence of foreign body, obstruction and abscess are not clearly understood. A variety of hypotheses have been advanced; however, most have not withstood rigorous testing. It has been suggested that drugs may not penetrate adequately to the nidus of infection, but this has been disproven in most instances. With the possible exception of the sulfonamides, inactivation of the antimicrobial by purulent material does not appear to have occurred. In addition, emergence of genotypic drug resistance has accounted for a minority of therapeutic failures in these circumstances. Clearly, the microorganisms are physiologically or phenotypically unresponsive in these settings. The term "microbial indifference" has been proposed to describe microorganisms in this unresponsive state. These microorganisms presumably subsist at a low level of metabolic activity, analogous to that observed following their rapid multiplication in artificial growth medium. This state of relative inactivity (static phase of growth) may thus render them insusceptible to many antimicrobial agents, particularly those drugs that affect cell-wall biosynthesis, such as the penicillins and cephalosporins. Host and microbial factors that facilitate indifference to antibiotics need to be further elucidated. At present, however, the physician must recognize those remedial situations, such as foreign body, abscess and obstruction, which are known to predispose to the indifferent state.

Emergence of Genotypic Drug Resistance

The tacit assumption that emergence of genotypic drug resistance has accounted for failure of appropriately chosen antimicrobial therapy is one of the commonest errors made in management of patients with infectious diseases. Resultant subjective changes in the therapeutic regimen have frequently exposed patients to unnecessary risks of drug sensitization, toxicity, or superinfection. Emergence of genotypic drug resistance during therapy of most acute infections is a relatively uncommon event and accounts for a minority of therapeutic failures.

What are the circumstances in which emergence of drug resistance might be anticipated? In general, this event is more likely to occur in treatment of infections that are chronic or tend to become so. Examples are bacterial endocarditis, osteomyelitis, pyelonephritis and tuberculosis. Resistance emerges more frequently when other factors predisposing to drug failure, such as abscess, obstruction, or foreign body, are present for prolonged periods. The nature of the infecting microorganism is also a factor; gram negative bacilli, enterococci, and staphylococci appear to acquire resistance more rapidly than other bacteria.

Use of bacteriostatic or aminoglycoside antimicrobials is more frequently associated with appearance of resistance than with other bactericidal drugs. In general, emergence of resistance does not occur until at least 7 to 10 days after institution of drug therapy in optimal doses. Carbenicillin is a possible exception to this general rule, since certain strains of pseudomonas have developed resistance during the first week of therapy. Recognition of predisposing factors and repeated *in vitro* susceptibility testing are essential for detection and rational therapy of resistance-prone infections.

Alterations in Bacterial Form

Certain bacteria, when exposed in hypertonic medium to antimicrobial agents that affect cell wall biosynthesis, have persisted as viable cells lacking a structured wall. These osmotically fragile cells have variously been referred to as spheroplasts, protoplasts, or L-forms, depending in part upon the circumstances of their induction or the parent strain from which they were derived. Since these altered bacteria are resistant to agents that impair cell wall biosynthesis, it has been suggested that their induction in man may account for persistence of infection despite seemingly appropriate therapy. To date, reasonably convincing evidence has been presented to implicate this mechanism of persistence in a few cases of bacterial endocarditis and in urinary tract infections, especially those due to *Proteus mirabilis*. It appears likely that further examples of this mechanism of microbial persistence will be identified when laboratory techniques for detection of altered bacterial forms are improved. Fortunately, most induced cell wall-defective bacteria are susceptible to bacteriostatic drugs, such as the tetracyclines and erythromycin. Thus persistent infections due to altered bacterial forms may be amenable to therapy with these drugs.

Inactivation of Drug by Constituents of the Host Flora

Non-invasive strains of staphylococci, klebsiella, *E. coli* and pseudomonas, resident in the host's indigenous flora, may occasionally produce quantities of penicillinase sufficient to inactivate penicillin on contiguous body surfaces. To date, this phenomenon has been implicated only in persistence of surface infections due to Group A streptococci and gonococci. These persistent infections have usually responded to treatment with alternative, penicillinase-insusceptible antimicrobial drugs. Although protection of other pyogenic microorganisms by penicillinase has not yet been observed, physicians should remain alert to this possibility.

Antagonism Between Antimicrobial Agents

Inhibition of the activity of bactericidal drugs, especially the penicillins, by bacteriostatic agents has been repeatedly demonstrated *in vitro*.

Similar antagonism has been observed in treatment of a variety of experimental infections and in assays of antimicrobial activity in the plasma of human volunteers following simultaneous administration of several drugs. Evidence that antibiotic antagonism has delayed the therapeutic responses of infections in man is meagre. Tetracycline plus penicillin has been shown to be clearly inferior to penicillin alone in treatment of pneumococcal meningitis. Antagonism of lincomycin by erythromycin has been observed *in vitro* and in treatment of pneumococcal pneumonia. On the other hand, combinations of antimicrobial agents have infrequently been demonstrated to be superior to the most active drug used alone. Combined therapy should thus be reserved only for those infections, such as enterococcal endocarditis, brucellosis, and tuberculosis, where superiority of two or more drugs has clearly been demonstrated.

The Enhancement of Infectiousness by Elimination of Competitive Microflora

Prolongation of the asymptomatic carrier state following treatment of acute salmonellosis with sulfonamides, tetracycline and ampicillin has recently been reported. Both the incidence and duration of the carrier state have been increased manyfold following use of these drugs. The phenomenon appears to occur despite continued susceptibility of the salmonellae to these drugs. Results of *in vitro* and *in vivo* studies have suggested that the relatively more susceptible, competing microflora of the intestine is preferentially suppressed so that the salmonellae become established residents of the host's enteric flora. Subsequent elimination of these established strains by antimicrobial agents is exceedingly difficult, if not impossible. Since uncomplicated salmonella gastroenteritis in otherwise healthy adults is a self-limited disease, it may be adviseable not to treat the acute infection, unless extra-gastrointestinal spread of infection occurs or the patient has an underlying disease that predisposes to more severe illness or significant morbidity.

Superinfection

The administration of antimicrobial agents frequently results in temporary qualitative and quantitative alterations in the composition of the patient's indigenous microflora. Often, resistant, or "superinfecting" strains, predominate during therapy, only to recede after discontinuation of the drug. In most instances the induced alterations in the indigenous flora are of little consequence. Occasionally, however, these changes are associated with invasion of the host by the superinfecting strain. Thus, a second infection is superimposed upon one already under treatment. Clinically important superinfections tend to occur more frequently in the following settings: 1) patients of age less than 3 or over 50; 2) initial infection involving the tracheobronchial tree in patients with underlying lung disease, such as emphysema, atelectasis or pulmonary fibrosis; 3) measles; 4) pertussis; 5) use of broad-spectrum antimicrobials; or 6) use of large doses of antibiotics. Recognition and proper management of disease resultant from superinfection depends upon 1) a high index of suspicion; 2) worsening signs and symptoms, often following an initial improvement, in a patient on appropriate drug therapy; 3) demonstration of the absence of other factors predisposing to drug failure, if possible; and 4) laboratory identification and drug-susceptibility testing of the superinfecting microorganism.

Underlying Non-Infectious Disease Process

Impairment of normal host defense mechanisms may significantly alter the response of infection to antimicrobial agents. Examples of underlying diseases that may interfere with host defenses are disseminated malignancies, particularly those involving the reticuloendothelial system, multiple myeloma, uncontrolled diabetes, lymphomas and leukemias, and advanced liver disease. Response of infection to antimicrobial therapy in the presence of these diseases is often unsatisfactory. Bactericidal antibiotics are clearly preferable to bacteriostatic drugs in this setting, but success is not necessarily assured by this choice. Eradication of the infecting microorganisms may be possible only when the underlying disease process is controlled or remits.

Occasionally, the underlying disease may mimic infection, thus obscuring a favorable response of the infectious process to appropriate drug therapy. Drug fever is frequently mistaken for persistence of infection. It may be identified by 1) improvement in other signs and symptoms of infection; 2) sustained nature of the fever, if unaltered by antipyretics; and 3) prompt defervescence of fever (usually within 48 hours) after withdrawal of the suspected drug.

Summary

A variety of remedial factors may account for failure of appropriately chosen and administered antimicrobial therapy. In most instances, factors favoring persistence of infection may be detected by systematic study of the patient. These may then be circumvented or eliminated to permit control of the infectious process.

SELECTED REFERENCES

Carter, W. and McCarty, K. S.: Molecular mechanisms of antibiotic action. Ann. Int. Med., *64*:1087, 1966.

Fekety, F. R., Jr., Allen, J. C., and Cluff, L. E.: Management of infectious diseases. In *The Principles and Practice of Medicine,* 17th Ed., A. M. Harvey, L. E. Cluff, R.

J. Johns, A. H. Owens, Jr., D. Rabinowitz, and R. S. Ross, Eds., Appleton-Century-Crofts, N.Y., 1968, p. 671.

Hartshorn, E. A.: Interactions of antibiotics. In *Handbook of Drug Interactions*, D. E. Francke, Ed., Hamilton Press, Hamilton, 1970, p. 42.

McDermott, W.: Microbial persistence. Yale J. Biol. Med., *30*:257, 1958.

Sanders, E. and Cluff, L. E.: Antimicrobial drugs: Mechanisms and factors influencing their action. In *Antimicrobial Therapy,* B. M. Kagan, Ed., W. B. Saunders, Co., Phila., 1970, p. 3.

Weinstein, L. Superinfection: a complication of antimicrobial therapy and prophylaxis. Am. J. Surg., *107*:704, 1964.

Weinstein, L. and Dalton, A. C.: Host determinants of response to antimicrobial agents. N. Engl. J. Med., *279*:580, 1968.

Weinstein, L. Chemotherapy of microbial diseases. In *The Pharmacological Basis of Therapeutics,* 4th Ed., L. S. Goodman and A. Gilman, Eds., The Macmillan Co., N.Y., 1970, p. 1154.

Chapter 28

VIRUS CHEMOTHERAPY

At present there are two drugs that the Food and Drug Adminstration has approved as safe effective therapy for viral disease. One, idoxuridine (IDU) is used in the treatment of ocular herpes infections, and the other, amantadine (Symmetrel) is used for the prevention of influenza. While these are the only antiviral agents available by prescription in the United States, several other drugs are being clinically tested; and in other countries, a number of additional drugs are used for virus chemotherapy.

The present availability of these drugs and anticipated new developments in the clinical treatment of viral disease merit discussion.

General Problems with Antiviral Drugs

Understanding the Pathogenesis of Disease

Rational treatment of virus disease requires that we first determine what actually causes sickness when virus infection occurs. In mice, for example, lymphocytic choriomeningitis can infect the central nervous system. If animals are rendered unable to respond to this virus with hypersensitivity, they are spared from death in spite of the fact that virus multiplication is not reduced. Similarly, in man, there is evidence that while vaccinia can infect the skin, the lesions we see as the pox are primarily the result of hypersensitivity, rather than virus caused cell death. It appears that vaccinia multiplies within the skin, but that by the time the "disease" appears, most virus multiplication is over. Host reactivity rather than continued viral multiplication is of primary importance in producing the cutaneous lesions. It is likely that hypersensitivity is important in herpetic lesions of the skin, many exanthemata and some types of ocular disease. The treatment of a virus infection by slowing virus multiplication after the disease has appeared may be ineffective unless continuing virus multiplication rather than host reactivity and viral toxins cause the disease. In fact, the therapeutic benefits reported in some cases of hepatitis and deep keratitis after herpes simplex infection (with corticosteroid therapy) may be due to a modification of this host-response mechanism.

Studies of the pathogenesis of disease are similarly important in determining what role previous tissue damage and the consequent, perhaps abnormal, healing process play. In the eye, for example, the epithelium of the cornea rests on its basement membrane and is attached by electron dense hemidesmosomes. If this basement membrane is damaged by an acute infection with herpes simplex virus, this adhesion is destroyed. The ulcer created may persist or heal and then break down again even though virus multiplication does not continue within the tissues. Here, the "disease" is a function of the damaged basement membrane and the inability of the surface epithelium to heal over the damaged area. This situation occurs often after virus infection, can produce severe symptoms, and treatment with agents such as IDU is ineffective. Similarly, in herpes simplex infections of the central nervous system, patients who have positive virus cultures on brain biopsy before treatment and negative cultures after treatment may die from severe brain damage even though no continued virus multiplication is found.

In the treatment of ocular herpes simplex infection, an understanding of the pathogenesis of the different disease phases has been as important as the development of a truly effective antiviral drug. In other types of clinical virus infections, however, our understanding of the actual mechanism by which disease is caused remains rudimentary.

Is Virus Chemotherapy Really Possible?

Less than ten years ago, it appeared that virus took over the cell, and that treatment was impossible since normal cellular mechanisms would be inhibited. It has since become clear that this is incorrect. Virus genetic material induces many virus specific enzymes, and there are a series of unique biochemical steps involved in virus infection. It is possible to interfere with and interrupt these steps at many points with little or no damage to the host (Table 28.1). Some drugs which are being used in man can be shown to *specifically* inhibit virus invasion and multiplication (Fig. 28.1).

How to Recognize a Good Antiviral Agent

A major factor in the slow development of clinically useful virus chemotherapy has been the difficulty in working with laboratory models. For several decades reports on antiviral drugs have appeared throughout the world.

One type antiviral agent (this group includes a variety of heavy metals and protoplasmic poisons) kills virus outside cells. None of these drugs,

TABLE 28.1

Some possible sites of selective antiviral activity

1. Cell penetration
2. Nucleic acid synthesis
   a. Kinase: inhibition
   b. Polymerase: inhibition or incorporation
3. Capsid and specific viral protein synthesis
4. Assembly of genetic material and capsid

however, has any biological utility in treating virus disease in animals or man.

A second type of "antiviral" drug was found active only in tissue culture systems. When this type of substance was placed in the fluid surrounding cells growing in tissue culture, it made these cells more difficult to infect and reduced the amount of live virus produced by the infected cell culture. It was subsequently found that a wide variety of substances which damage cells in a non-specific way could make cells more difficult to infect and reduce the amount of virus produced. This could be accomplished without any direct effect on viral multiplication or selective effect on the metabolism involved with virus reproduction; but again, these substances had no biological effect in treating virus infections in animals or man. New and more sophisticated tissue culture techniques developed by Ernest Herrmann and others have improved the correlation between *in vitro* and *in vivo* antiviral activity, but some consideration of the potential pitfalls of tissue culture selection of antiviral agents is important.

After the initial selection of an antiviral agent, animal testing is usually done, and here too the possibility of error is enormous. In terms of the pathogenesis of disease, the relevance of an animal testing model must be clearly apparent. Perhaps more important, enormous variations in drug effects between species can occur. For example, in the development of interferon inducers, synthetic double stranded RNA molecules such as polyinosine:polycytosine have been used. These are highly effective in preventing infection, and somewhat effective in treating disease in mice and rabbits. In spite of the enormous number of studies documenting this effect in rodents, our present evidence suggests that these substances and other interferon inducers may have little or no significant effect in primates or man. This is not intended to downgrade the importance of animal test systems, which are clearly vital, but rather to emphasize to the clinician the importance of evaluating animal studies with a great degree of caution. Such caution may be even more important in dealing with the antiviral drugs which are so intimately involved with specific host metabolism.

Amantadine (Symmetrel)

This compound is available by prescription for the chemoprophylaxis of influenza A infection. It is a simple (Fig. 28.2) compound which was detected by the routine screening of compounds rather than by an understanding of its biochemical mechanism of action. Most evidence indicates that in the presence of amantadine, influenza virus can adsorb to the surface of the cell but does not penetrate (there is some evidence that with fowl plague virus, the amantadine may prevent removal of the viral coat within the cell and prevent exposure of the cell to viral genetic material). The drug is well absorbed and active orally. It can prevent the emergence of clinical disease in man in natural experimental influenza and prevent family contacts and others exposed to the disease from contracting the illness. The incidence of seroconversion in exposed contacts is also de-

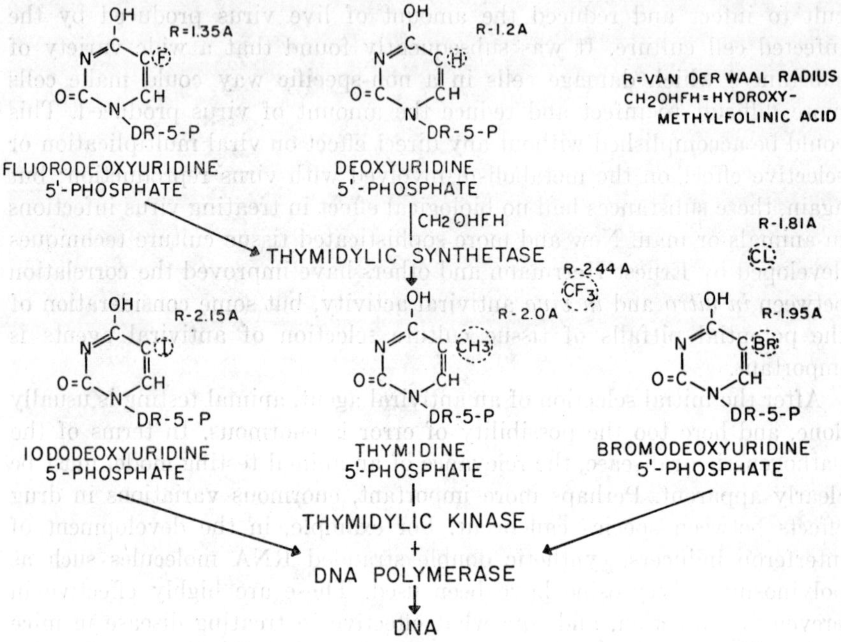

FIG. 28.1. Sites of inhibition of various antiviral agents.

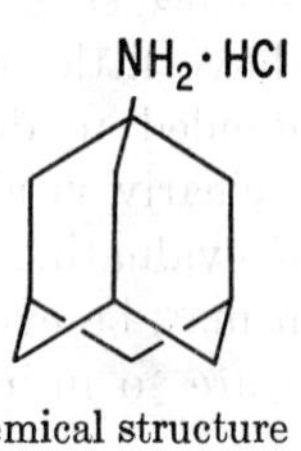

FIG. 28.2. Chemical structure of amantadine.

creased. In spite of this ability to prevent influenza infection, amantadine does not prevent the development of antibodies to inactivated influenza virus vaccine.

Amantadine seems at least as effective against susceptible influenza strains as influenza vaccine. It has the advantage that its spectrum is broader so that it protects against new strains. It is especially useful in situations where exposure to influenza is expected, but vaccination is impossible or impractical.

Amantadine in higher doses is a CNS stimulant, and in very high doses has been used for the treatment of Parkinson's disease. Small doses of 100 or 200 mg. a day were tested in a severe influenza outbreak in Leningrad. In more than 4,559 patients taking the drug, there was a 1.14 percent increase in the number of complaints of various sleep disturbances. This was considered "quite insignificant." A similar study of 3,000 naval recruits in Illinois revealed "no adverse reactions and no evidence that the drug interferes with training." However, with doses greater than 300 mg. a day, the incidence of central nervous system stimulation increases. In general these minor complications are gradual in onset and easily reversible by stopping the drug. If there is not adequate time for immunization, or vaccine is unavailable, or an allergy to vaccine products is present, amantadine is probably superior to vaccination with its limited spectrum and efficacy.

Other derivatives of amantadine have been developed. These include remantadine, which seems more effective than amantadine in some species, but the ultimate value of these derivatives will require further investigation.

Idoxuridine (IDU) and Other Antimetabolites

Just as it is possible to interfere with the penetration of virus into the cell, it is possible to interfere with the synthesis of new viral genetic material and viral reproduction. The first antiviral developed for practical use by man was IDU. This drug was first synthesized as an anticancer compound by Prusoff. Herrmann found that it was active against herpes virus in tissue culture, but it was not evident at that time that the tissue culture systems Herrmann used for detecting this activity had a better correlation with biological activity than the unreliable systems used earlier. In 1962 our laboratory reported that IDU could treat herpes simplex keratitis in rabbits and had a profound therapeutic effect both in rabbits and man.

Herpes simplex keratitis is the most common specific corneal infection in man. When herpes occurs on the lip, the infection is usually transient and short lived; but in the eye it can cause prolonged pain and morbidity, and lead to blindness. IDU was selected for investigation because, although it can compete to some extent with the phosphorylation of thymidine and exert some feedback inhibition on the synthesis of nucleotides, it also has an effect on the polymerase enzymes which assemble nucleotides into new viral genetic material. There is good evidence that both the phosphorylating enzymes and the polymerase enzymes are virus induced, and a drug with activity at these sites offers some hope for biological selectivity.

The testing of this drug in animals was relatively straightforward and its effect was easy to document. The testing of the drug in humans, however, brought great confusion. To a large extent this was because of a lack of knowledge about the pathogenesis of the ocular disease.

In the case of acute epithelial dendritic corneal ulcers, it became clear that virus went from cell to cell killing cells and damaging tissue, and that an antiviral agent could halt this type of epithelial disease. Not infrequently, however, epithelial ulcers recurred. Initially, we treated this type of disease with an antiviral agent. When the ulcers did not respond to treatment, questions of resistance were raised, but it became evident that the pathogenesis of these post-infectious ulcers was different. Most evidence suggests that when tissue is damaged by virus, the damaged basement membrane provides a poor base for adhesion of the newly healing epithelium. The epithelium may not adhere, or may adhere enough to heal, only to be rubbed off by the lids. Virus is not found in the ulcers, and agents which halt virus multiplication are of no value.

Similarly, hypersensitivity seems to play a part in disciform edema (a deep stromal swelling without epithelial ulceration or necrosis) that occurs after herpes simplex infection. Corticosteroids suppress this condition, relieve pain and discomfort, and restore vision. Corticosteroids, however, may reactivate the epithelial ulceration process and cause perforation of the cornea. IDU can competitively antagonize the tendency of corticosteroids to produce this type of corneal ulceration. Although the antiviral agent itself is not of primary therapeutic value in this phase of disease which is presumably due to hypersensitivity, it permits greater safety in the use of corticosteroid drugs.

The exact mechanism of action of IDU remains unclear. It may inhibit enzymes at several sites and may also be incorporated into DNA, providing a false code for future virus multiplication and the synthesies of late proteins and other components required for virus replication. Although its primary site of activity is on enzymes which are induced by virus infection, it is not clear from *in vitro* studies how selective the inhibition and binding are to virus induced enzymes as opposed to normal cellular enzymes. Evidence for such selectivity in tissue culture is not compelling. When large artificial stromal wounds are made, however, it can prevent virus multiplication in the cornea with virtually no inhibition of epithelial healing and only slight inhibition of stromal healing. In all the double blind studies reported, IDU has proven to be generally nontoxic, and clearly effective against dendritic keratitis (Table 28.2). IDU penetrates the tissues poorly and is rather rapidly broken down by enzymes in vascularized tissue.

Incorporation into host DNA appears to be of no significance when the drug is used topically. When systemic use is contemplated, this should be considered, and its use restricted to the treatment of very serious disease. Systemic IDU has been used for the treatment of herpes simplex encephalitis in a relatively large number of cases and appears beneficial. In this disease one of the primary problems is making the diagnosis early enough to prevent extensive (fatal) brain damage. Our limited experience suggests that fluorescent antibody examination of spinal fluid cells may (at least in some cases) permit an early diagnosis. Spinal fluid cultures are often negative, however, and brain biopsy has been the mechanism most used for establishing a diagnosis.

The use of IDU on skin has been a controversial topic. Some studies have indicated that its early use, when lesions are just beginning, may be beneficial; other studies have not shown this. The work of McCollum and Juel-Jensen indicates that this may be due to the relative insolubility and rapid breakdown of the drug. When IDU is dissolved in DMSO, it can be obtained in high concentrations; and when applied to the skin in this form, is clearly effective against early herpes simplex, chicken pox, and herpes zoster infections. A soaked bandage of IDU prevents chicken pox

TABLE 28.2

Double blind human studies; acute dendritic keratitis

Study		IDU	Placebo
Patterson, *et al.*	Healed 5 days Rx	74% 24/33	7% 2/29
Burns	Good and Excellent	65% 15/23	33% 5/15
Laibson and Leopold	Good 8 days Rx	68% 15/22	27% 7/26
Jepson	Improved 7 days Rx	92% 11/12	58% 7/12
Hart *et al.*	Healed 7 days Rx	73.7% 14/19	15.4% 2/13
Total cases studied		109	95

from developing in the bandaged area, and when the bandage is removed, new crops of lesions are seen in the previously bandaged area.

A large number of newer antimetabolites have been developed for clinical study. Cytosine arabinoside is used in cancer chemotherapy, and reports indicate it is effective systemically in the treatment of herpes simplex encephalitis. While it is effective and not rapidly degraded, it appears to be more toxic than IDU.

Adenine arabinoside appears quite different from many of the antimetabolites. It is effective orally, relatively non-toxic, and highly effective systemically. Evidence indicates that it is not incorporated into DNA and its potential seems great. These, and many other substances remain experimental, however, and their future uncertain.

N-Methylisatin-β-thiosemicarbazone (*Methisazone*)

Methisazone has been used extensively throughout the world and proven effective in the prophylaxis of smallpox in man. In a smallpox epidemic in Madrid, 2,227 persons in contact with smallpox cases were vaccinated and of these 1,101 received methisazone. In the group that did not receive the drug, 78 developed smallpox of whom 12 died; whereas the group on methisazone therapy had only three mild cases of smallpox and no deaths. Bauer extended these studies and reported that among 2,297 contacts, only 6 developed smallpox and 2 died; whereas among 2,842 untreated contacts, 114 developed smallpox and 20 died. Similarly, in an epidemic of alastrim in Brazil, 42 cases developed among 520 contacts who were untreated, but among 384 treated contacts only 8 developed the disease.

Therapeutic effects have been observed in patients with *vaccinia gangrenosum* treated with methisazone, as well as in those with *eczema vaccinatum*. This drug has been so effective in the prevention of smallpox that Kempe, struck by the significant incidence of complications with smallpox vaccination (in the United States over a hundred children a year die due to this vaccination), suggested that the drug might well replace vaccination. Epidemics in the United States have not occurred during recent years, and it would be possible to treat contacts of any known cases to minimize disease spread. Regardless of the validity of this rather controversial point of view, it is clear that drugs like this must force us to think about complications of previous prophylaxis which we have taken for granted for many years. It is not clear that the repeated injection of microbiological antigens and tissue culture or animal products is as harmless as was previously thought.

The major toxicity of methisazone is its gastrointestinal intolerance. It produces a high incidence of nausea and a significant incidence of vomiting which varies with the dose being used in the population under study.

This can, under some circumstances, limit the value of the drug, but no other significant toxicity has been observed in man.

Rifampicin

Rifampicin is a new valuable antiviral agent. It markedly inhibits the multiplication of vaccinia virus, but experience with its use in man is too limited for definite conclusions at present.

Interferon

Interferon is a protein made by virus infected cells that imparts to other cells a broad spectrum of resistance against virus infection. Although evidence is not totally conclusive, it appears that the natural production of interferon by the body may be correlated with recovery from virus disease and that interferon production may be an important natural defense. This high molecular weight protein is rather species specific—human interferon seems to work better in human tissues than in tissue of other species, etc. Because of this, the artificial production of large amounts of interferon for the prevention of disease is difficult.

Recently, the finding of synthetic chemicals which can induce the cells to make interferon has caused excitement. Most evidence indicates that interferon is made by the infected cell because the viral RNA undergoes a double stranded phase in its multiplication which the cell recognizes as foreign. When this occurs, the cell produces interferon, which can then enter other cells probably permitting the synthesis of a protein which prevents foreign viral genetic material from attaching to a cell's ribosomes and causing alterations in the infected cell's metabolism. Although double stranded RNA's may be the most effective interferon inducers, single stranded RNA's, and various long chain high polymers may also stimulate interferon induction.

Synthetic double stranded RNA is relatively simple to make in the laboratory. It is possible to make a long strand of the polymerized base inosine, one of the complementary base cytosine, and have these strands bind to each other producing a polyinosine:polycytosine double stranded chain. It is not clear whether such synthetic molecules induce the synthesis of interferon *de novo* or stimulate cells to liberate interferon molecules which have already been partially synthesized; nevertheless, there is no question about their capacity to induce interferon production in many cell lines.

Studies with the synthetic double stranded RNA's show that they are highly effective in provoking interferon induction in tissue culture and many animal systems. In mice and rabbits they prevent infection by a variety of viruses and have some relatively weak therapeutic activity.

In spite of the promise of such compounds, they are relatively toxic drugs which may have significant immediate toxicity in terms of brain damage, hematopoietic inhibition, and ocular damage, and they may have long term genetic effects. Perhaps equally important is the accumulating evidence from our laboratory and others that there is an enormous species difference in response to these agents. Our own work, as well as the work of Hill *et al.*, suggests that whereas rodents may respond with significant production of interferon for a relatively long period of time, the response in humans is relatively slight and very brief. Similarly, our work would suggest that even a small molecular weight interferon inducer (tilorone) which chemically is totally unrelated to the long chain polymers, and highly effective in rodents, is neither safe nor effective in monkeys and man.

This recent knowledge of the systemic toxicity of interferon inducers and the apparent difficulty in artificially stimulating the human interferon system has brought a renewed interest in the possibility of using pre-synthesized interferon. Human leukocyte cultures and other tissue cultures are being employed to produce adequate human interferon for study, but the value of this substance remains to be proven.

Summary and Conclusion

There are specific biochemical steps involved in viral invasion and viral synthesis which can be selectively inhibited. The three drugs widely used in man exemplify some of these principles. Amantadine, approved for general use in the United States, prevents infection with influenza A, and appears to impede the entrance of virus into the cell. IDU is effective in the treatment of herpes simplex keratitis, and interferes with final synthesis of viral genetic material. Methisazone, (N-Methylisatin-β-thiosemicarbazone) effectively prevents smallpox and alastrim, and appears to have some beneficial effect in *vaccinia gangrenosum*. It inhibits the final synthesis of the protein coat which envelopes the viral genetic material. Many other substances (interferon inducers as well as interferon itself) now under active investigation show great promise in the area of virus chemotherapy. Toxicity and species differences in response to these agents, however, may limit their use.

Although the development of the first practical antiviral for use in man (IDU) was only 10 years ago, progress in this field has been relatively rapid, and antiviral agents may soon become a common part of each physician's armamentarium.

SELECTED REFERENCES

Goz, B. and Prusoff, W. H.: Pharmacology of viruses. Ann. Rev. of Pharmacology, *10*:143, 1970.

Herrmann, Jr., E. C.: Plague inhibition test for detection of specific inhibitors of DNA-containing viruses Proc. Soc. Exp. Biol. Med., *107*:142, 1961.

Kaufman, H. E., Nesburn, A. B. and Maloney, E. D.: IDU therapy of herpes simplex. Arch. Ophth., *67*:583, 1962.

Kaufman, H. E. and Maloney, E. D.: IDU and hydrocortisone in experimental herpes simplex keratitis. Arch. Ophth., *68*:396, 1962.

Kaufman, H. E.: *In vivo* studies with antiviral agents. Ann. N.Y. Acad. Sci., *130*:168, 1965.

Kaufman, H. E.: Herpes simplex keratitis. Intn'l. Ophth. Clinic, *4*:269, 1964.

Kempe, C. H.: Discussions in Proc. First Intn'l. Conferences on Vaccines against Viral and Rickettsial Diseases of Man. W.H.O. Scientific Pub., *147*:476, 1967.

Partridge, J. W. and Millis, R. R.: Systemic herpes simplex infection in a newborn treated with intravenous idoxuridine. Arch. Dis. Childh., *43*:377, 1968.

Prusoff, W. H.: Recent advances in chemotherapy of viral disease Pharmacol. Rev., *19*:209, 1967.

Wingfield, W. L., Pollack, D., and Brunet, R. R.: Therapeutic efficacy of amantadine HCl and rimantadine HCl in naturally occurring influenza A2 respiratory illness in man. N. Eng. J. Med., *281*:579, 1969.

Chapter 29

UNTOWARD EFFECTS OF ANTIMICROBIAL DRUGS

The benefits of antimicrobial drug therapy are considerable and undisputed. Nonetheless most physicians are uncomfortable with the knowledge that significant harm can also derive from their therapeutic maneuvres. Unfortunately, this conflict is often side-stepped, probably because of a sense of helplessness in preventing such adverse reactions. The purpose of this essay is to explore what can reasonably be done to avoid adverse effects, or failing that, to reduce their frequency and severity. Only two principles need be observed.

The *first*, and most important, is to accept that adverse reactions do, in fact, occur—"there are no roses without thorns"! The axiom that physicians *must do no harm* is totally irrelevant to modern therapeutics. Acceptance of this principle by both public and profession is basic to the maintenance of trust between patient and physician. The best therapeutic result cannot be guaranteed for the individual even with the exercise of supreme knowledge and diligence, qualities which vary, not only from doctor to doctor but also in the same doctor under different conditions of stress. Errors of judgment resulting in misuse of drugs are also inevitable. Therefore, only by anticipating that adverse effects will occur can we be well placed to prevent or rectify them. For example, this means that on a hospital ward round one should look for and find untoward reactions in approximately one patient in seven. Of these, one in seven will be due to antimicrobial drugs.

The *second* step is the acquisition of pertinent *information*. In theory, the best possible results can only be achieved by the application of policy decisions based on quantitative information about the relative merits and demerits of each drug, singly and in combination with others, in each and every disease. Clearly, this sophisticated type of information is available

TABLE 29.1
Classification of adverse effects of antimicrobial drugs

INDIRECT	Effects on environmental flora		Increased chance of infection with drug resistant pathogen or opportunist
	Effects on commensal flora	Animal	
		Human	
DIRECT	No effect—i.e., therapeutic failure		
	Patient allergy		
	Drug toxicity—often related to dose and underlying disease		

only for a few simple situations. For example, we do not even know the true incidence and natural history of many common diseases such as acute urinary infection; far less the effects of antimicrobial therapy. Nonetheless the central problem is clear and a considerable body of relevant, albeit fragmentary, information is available to us.

Antimicrobial drugs are unique because not only can they be allergenic and toxic to the patient but they also affect the normal commensal and environmental microbial flora. It follows that those adverse effects on the individual which are "undesired and unintended by the prescribing physician" can arise in two ways, i.e., *direct* and *indirect* (Table 29.1).

Indirect Effects

The Environmental Flora

Antimicrobial drugs are among the most dangerous environmental pollutants. Unfortunately the full impact of this is seldom felt by the prescribing physician who is not only a prime polluter but also in a key position to minimize the dangers. Failing some dramatic, and usually serious, event, only epidemiologic surveys can reveal what is happening to the environmental flora and its antibiotic sensitivity pattern (the antibiogram) in both community and hospital. From these, the message is clear, with 70 percent of *Shigella sonnei* resistant to three or more antibiotics in the City of London. Similarly two thirds of coagulase-positive staphylococci are now resistant to penicillin in hospital. It is well established that the percentage of sensitive strains can be increased by rational restriction of antibiotic usage. At the University of Florida, 96 percent of *Staphylococcus aureus* strains are sensitive to erythromycin, reflecting the fact that only two prescriptions were written for this drug in three years (1967–70) on the medical service of that hospital!

The opposite is observed when antibiotics are used routinely or indiscriminately, especially for prophylaxis. A striking example of this was reported recently when an outbreak of Klebsiella infections in a neurosurgical unit was *terminated* by prohibiting the use of prophylactic ampicillin and cloxacillin. This practice had been introduced in response to a previous outbreak of wound infections with staphylococci and antibiotic sensitive coliforms. In addition, ampicillin had been used routinely to treat all unconscious patients with purulent sputum while awaiting the bacteriology report. The sequelae were predictable from earlier related observations: "Those who do not read (or believe) history must needs relive it." A concise statement of those situations where antimicrobial prophylaxis *is* justified can be found in Medical Letter, 1969 (p. 42).

Commensal Flora

Antimicrobial drugs affect the commensal flora in two distinct ways which are often synergistic in producing disease. Firstly, the normal commensal flora can be reduced or eradicated, leaving a dangerous microbial vacuum. It can never be sufficiently emphasized that the commensal flora form a protective insulating layer over our mucous membranes with which any potential pathogen must compete for survival. This "commensal carpet" is physiologic and is as much a part of our anatomy as the mucous membranes themselves. Removal is tantamount to an extensive burn! For example, it is difficult to implant a staphylococcus in the anterior nares unless the normal flora is suppressed by an antimicrobial (e.g., tetracycline). The clinical counterpart of this is staphylococcal enterocolitis following attempts to "sterilize" the bowel preoperatively with broad spectrum antibiotics such as neomycin. This entity is entirely avoidable and should never occur. Again, antibiotics given for mild and non-septicemic salmonella enteritis often *prolong* the period of excretion of the pathogen without shortening the clinical course. This paradoxical effect is presumably due to interference with the normal flora and its interaction with the pathogen.

Secondly, exhibition of an antibiotic while suppressing sensitive flora will also selectively allow the emergence of resistant organisms. Examples are the emergence of Pseudomonas and Klebsiella species in patients treated with broad spectrum antibiotics. Although these do not always cause clinical infections, the dangers are clear. An important example of this is the development of relatively resistant *Streptococcus viridans* in the mouth, following oral penicillin prophylaxis for rheumatic fever. Dental surgery in such patients necessitates cover with a large dose of penicillin G with the addition of streptomycin. Alternatives such as cephaloridine or erythromycin estolate have also been advocated in these circumstances. Endocarditis due to penicillin-resistant streptococci has been reported in patients with heart disease whose prophylactic penicillin was begun only several days before their dental procedure. Therefore, in patients not already on penicillin, this drug should not be given until half an hour prior to the procedure. (Brit. M. J. *2:* 63, 1971.)

Another facet of this problem is the use of antibiotics in animal husbandry to promote growth. This practice evokes large numbers of resistant organisms which may be transferred to man, occasionally with the production of disease. In one instance, 500 cases of human salmonellosis with resistant organisms were traced to an animal source. The existence of resistance transfer factors (RTF's), which enable drug resistance (often multiple) to be transferred from one coliform to another, adds another dangerous dimension to the general problem. The large (52 percent) numbers of multiply resistant *E. coli* in some communities, many (60 percent) of which possess RTF's, illustrates the magnitude of this potential threat.

Direct Effects

An adverse drug reaction (ADR.) has already been defined as a therapeutic result "undesired and unintended by the prescribing physician." For this essay it is justifiable to include under this definition not only positive ADR.'s (e.g., toxicity) but also an important group of negative ones, i.e., avoidable therapeutic failure resulting from incorrect choice or use of antibiotics. Clearly an antimicrobial drug to which the organism is resistant "in vitro" is unlikely to succeed "in vivo." However, despite the high incidence of resistant strains, tetracyclines are still commonly employed in the treatment of streptococcal pharyngitis, sulphonamides, ampicillin and tetracyclines for Sonne dysentery, and sulphonamides for the prophylaxis of meningococcal meningitis. Only knowledge of the local antibiogram can now best guide the use of these drugs. The bi-annual production and distribution of a current antibiogram, describing the antibiotic sensitivity pattern of all the common pathogens, is within the scope of most diagnostic laboratories. A general statement on the choice and use of systemic antimicrobial drugs is contained in Medical Letter (p. 77, 1968).

Incorrect administration of a drug is also avoidable. For example, tetracycline is bound by some divalent and trivalent cations and its absorbtion is therefore reduced by the presence of calcium in milk, dairy products and antacids. This group of drugs should therefore be taken between meals. Similarly the tetracyclines are bound by ferrous sulphate, which taken concomitantly reduce plasma levels of the antibiotic by 50 to 90 percent. Again, erythromycin lactobionate, oxacillin sodium and oxytetracycline lose potency (12 to 21 percent) in some fluids over 12 hours. Similarly, penicillin G, methicillin and erythromycin lose potency in an acid solution. Also, most penicillins are even less stable in alkaline sucrose solutions with ampicillin, oxacillin, cloxacillin, dicloxacillin and nafcillin all losing 75 percent potency in 6 hours and penicillin G losing 90 percent in 24 hours. Consequently, when intravenous administration of an antimicrobial is indicated, it is best to give it as a bolus and not by slow infusion, *providing* there is no toxic danger from high peak blood levels as with the aminoglycosides, e.g., streptomycin, kanamycin and gentamicin. There are also an infinite number of drug interactions which occur when drugs are mixed in the one bottle for simultaneous infusion, e.g., tetracyclines and cephalothin with calcium gluconate. If at all possible, drugs should therefore be infused separately by a T-tube arrangement and never mixed.

Adverse Effects of Individual Drugs

In preface, it is worth pointing out that, as with most other drugs, allergic reactions to antimicrobials, as a group, *are much less common* than toxic and pharmacologic effects. For all drugs, allergic reactions account for less than 15 percent of all ADR's. The outstanding toxicological safety of the penicillins and the newer sulphonamides should not be allowed to obscure the high incidence of purely toxic effects of other antibiotics.

The following account is abbreviated, and only includes the most important reactions to the more commonly used agents. For fuller accounts, reference should be made to publications such as Medical Letter (1968) and *Side Effects of Drugs* (1968). The latter should be accessible to every practising physician.

Aminoglycosides (Streptomycin, Kanamycin, Neomycin, Gentamicin)

The most important ADR's of this group of drugs are ototoxicity and nephrotoxicity. Ototoxicity of the vestibular portion of the 8th cranial nerve is manifest in order of frequency by streptomycin, gentamicin, kanamycin, and neomycin. Toxicity of the auditory portion occurs, again in order of frequency of production, with neomycin, kanamycin, gentamicin and streptomycin. Nephrotoxicity frequently occurs with neomycin and kanamycin (in that order) but is less common with streptomycin and gentamicin (2 percent). It should be noted that deafness from neomycin has also been reported following inhalation and irrigation of the colon and wounds, and that ototoxicity of both streptomycin and kanamycin is increased in the elderly. All these effects are made more likely by high blood levels resulting from high prolonged dosage or renal impairment.

With the exception of gentamicin, all the aminoglycosides share with the polymyxins the ability to produce paralysis from neuromuscular block. This occurs especially when given in large doses into the peritoneal or pleural cavities (e.g., following perforation of the gut) and may complicate anesthetic procedures by producing prolonged apnea. The danger of staphylococcal enterocolitis following "sterilization" of the bowel with neomycin cannot be overemphasized.

Neomycin and kanamycin can also produce malabsorbtion. The use of topical neomycin for skin infection produces allergic dermatitis of variable severity in approximately 15 percent of patients, even months after the last exposure. This can also occur in nurses dispensing and administering streptomycin. Apart from this, all drugs in this group can produce a wide variety of allergic reactions including rashes, drug fever, purpura and also marrow depression.

Paromomycin has the same toxic effects as neomycin. Its sole place is in the treatment of neomycin resistant Sonne dysentery. With these dangers in mind the aminoglycoside antibiotics should have a restricted therapeutic application.

Neomycin—skin infections and Sonne dysentery. It should *never* be given parenterally.

Kanamycin—severe gram-negative infections. Dose—usually no greater than 1 G each day best given in divided doses as 250 mg. qid. and never more than 40 G total in a lifetime or 20 G in a single course of treatment. Urine output, blood urea, serum creatinine and urinalysis should be performed twice weekly and audiometry weekly if treatment goes beyond 10 days.

Streptomycin—tuberculosis therapy, always in combination with other anti-tuberculous drugs to prevent the emergence of drug resistant organisms. It is also used to treat enterococcal endocarditis along with penicillin, tularemia and plague and as an alternative to neomycin in Sonne dysentery.

Gentamicin—serious gram-negative infections (including pseudomonas). Probably drug of choice for initial therapy of gram-negative septicemia before bacteriology report is available. It should be noted that slow intravenous infusion may result in low blood levels and possibly therapeutic failure. It is also useful in prophylaxis of extensive burns. For other situations this drug should probably only be used when no alternative is available. Its dose should be monitored to keep blood levels at less than 10 μg/ml., especially in patients with renal impairment. Only in extremity should the daily dose exceed 3 mg./kg./day. An approximate scheme of dosage for gentamicin in relation to renal function can be found in Table 29.2.

Amphotericin B frequently causes renal damage with or without renal tubular acidosis and hypokalemia. Consequently this drug should only be given in hospital with frequent monitoring of blood urea and electrolytes. Other common adverse effects include fever, rigors, anorexia, nausea and vomiting, and abdominal pain. Thrombophlebitis at the successive sites of infusion is a practical obstacle during the course of treatment. Allergic reactions including rash, optic and peripheral neuropathies have also been observed. The initial dose is 0.25 mg./kg. in a concentration of 10 mg. percent in 5 percent dextrose (pH >5) given over a period of 6 hours. The dose is gradually raised to an optimum, usually 1 mg./kg./day, never

TABLE 29.2
Gentamicin: approximate scheme of dosage for initiating therapy (Gingell and Waterworth, 1968)

Blood Urea mg./100 ml.	Creatinine clearance	Dose and frequency of administration
<35	>70	80 mg. 8 hourly (60 mg. if body weight <60 kg.)
50–100	30–50	80 mg. 12 hourly (60 mg. if body weight <60 kg.)
>200	5–10	80 mg. every 48 hrs (60 mg. if body weight <60 kg.)
Twice weekly intermittent haemodialysis	<3	80 mg. after dialysis (gentamicin is a dialysable antibiotic and further dosage may be required during and immediately after dialysis)

exceeding 1.5 mg./kg./day. Initially the drug is given daily and then alternate days after optimal dosage has been determined. Rapid administration has been associated with convulsions, hypotension, anaphylaxis and cardiac arrest. A rise in blood urea nitrogen above 40 mg. percent is an indication for cessation of therapy until the level returns to normal, restarting at 0.25 mg./kg./day. Significant reduction in creatinine clearance (50 percent) indicates greater renal damage and may necessitate withdrawal of therapy for several weeks.

Cephalosporins—cephaloridine may cause renal damage, especially when doses greater than 4 G daily are employed. The probability of nephrotoxicity is enhanced if cephaloridine is given along with a diuretic such as furosemide, in the presence of dehydration or in the post-operative period. Allergic reactions may be less common than with the penicillins although some cross-reactivity between the two groups does occur. Although thousands of patients with previous penicillin allergy have now been treated, caution is nonetheless indicated when giving a cephalosporin to patients with a history of penicillin allergy. Other adverse reactions include blood dyscrasias, Coomb's positive reactions not so far associated with hemolytic anaemia, and thrombophlebitis at the site of intravenous administration.

Cephalothin has the same allergic reactions as cephaloridine including cross reactivity with the penicillins. In contrast to cephaloridine, nephrotoxicity has only been reported with very high doses (greater than 8 G/day) in patients with severely impaired renal function. This may be related to the lower serum half life of cephalothin (40 minutes) compared with cephaloridine (90 minutes). Therefore, in serious infections and in patients with renal impairment, cephalothin is probably to be preferred to cephaloridine. Intramuscular injection is painful, and thrombophlebitis at sequential sites of intravenous administration can be a serious inconvenience during the course of therapy. Blood dyscrasias have rarely been observed.

Cephalexin shares its allergic reactions with the other cephalosporins but, being an oral preparation, it has a significant (9 to 35 percent) incidence of gastrointestinal effects such as candida infections, pruritis ani and vulvovaginitis, nausea, vomiting and diarrhea. Significant changes in bowel flora also occur, especially the emergence of Pseudomonas species. It may be that the rather high incidence of these side effects will limit the application of this drug. Conversely, ease of administration may result in increased usage and subsequent diminished usefulness of all related cephalosporins due to the emergence of resistant organisms.

Chloramphenicol can produce a variety of extremely serious ADR.'s, the true frequency of which is unknown. The gray baby syndrome may occur when chloramphenicol is given (usually in high doses) to mothers near term or to neonates. The baby collapses and assumes a gray cyanosis to which the syndrome owes its name.

Chloramphenicol induced anemia assumes two forms. The first, which is reversible and dose related, consists of depression of red cell synthesis with reticulopenia and raised serum iron. The other, a pancytopenia which may be genetically determined, is fortunately rare but can develop after the course of treatment has been completed. The incidence of this event has recently been calculated at 1 in 22,000–36,000. Allergic and febrile reactions may also occur as can optic and peripheral neuropathies. Gastrointestinal upsets include nausea, diarrhea, pruritis ani and superinfections.

Colistimethate (polymyxin E, colymycin) and **Polymyxin B** have similar toxic effects when given in doses yielding similar antibacterial activity. High blood levels (>20 μg/ml.) may cause apnea, and Polymyxin B should therefore be given slowly intravenously and not as a bolus. Neurotoxic effects such as dizziness, ataxia and sensory neuropathy with paresthesiae are both reversible and related to factors influencing blood levels, such as dose and rate of excretion. Intrathecal polymyxin B (polymyxin E cannot be given intrathecally) may increase the clinical features of meningeal irritation with increase in cerebrospinal fluid (CSF) protein and cell counts and fever when given for gram-negative meningitis (especially pseudomonas). Nephrotoxicity is commonly observed during treatment with the polymyxins.

Proteinuria and hematuria alone do not necessitate dosage reduction. If high doses are employed (>2 mg./kg./day polymyxin B *or* >1 mg./kg./day polymyxin E), urea retention may also occur but is reversible if the dose is reduced. In the presence of pre-existing renal failure the daily dose should be reduced with titration of blood levels by the laboratory. Thus, nephrotoxicity is usually avoidable or reversible in the normal patient and manageable (with care) in those with diminished renal function. Colistimethate is given by intramuscular injection and cannot be given intravenously or intrathecally. It contains an anesthetic (dibucaine) which may also give rise to allergic phenomena, and previous allergic reactions to other " 'caine" anesthetics should be asked for. Polymyxin B is usually given intravenously because of the considerable pain of intramuscular administration.

Cycloserine has the disadvantage of causing CNS effects such as confusion and occasionally coma. Convulsions are rare. Peripheral neuropathy, liver damage, folate deficiency and the malabsorbtion syndrome have also been observed. These effects are mainly observed with doses of 1 g to 1.5 g daily. When doses of 250 mg. twice daily are employed for urinary infections, or the blood levels kept below 25 μg/ml. in patients with renal failure, these toxic effects are rarely observed.

Erythromycins are, in general, a very safe group of drugs (Medical Letter, 1970, Vol. 12, no. 8). With the exception of intrahepatic cholestasis due to erythromycin estolate, other allergic reactions are uncommon. This reaction usually appears after 10 days of therapy or on repeated courses. Hence the justification for its brief employment in the prophylaxis of bacterial endocarditis (vide supra). It can take a period of weeks to resolve. Oral preparations may sometimes cause gastrointestinal upsets such as stomatitis, abdominal pain, vomiting and diarrhea. Phlebitis is a problem with intravenous preparations. The intramuscular route (ethyl succinate preparation) is painful and carries the additional risk of an allergic reaction to the incorporated butylaminobenzoate, a local anesthetic, which may cross react with other "caine" local anesthetics. Antagonism occurs between the erythromycins and lincomycins and they should not be used together.

Ethambutol is a useful second line antituberculous drug. It is given in doses of 25 mg./kg./day for four to six weeks then 15 mg./kg./day for the remainder of this course. Higher doses have been reported to cause visual loss due to an optic neuritis. All patients should have regular (monthly) tests of visual activity and green color vision. Deterioration necessitates discontinuance of the drug. Peripheral neuropathy, nephropathy and allergic reactions have rarely been observed.

Ethionamide commonly results in anorexia, nausea, vomiting, epigastric pain and a bad taste in the mouth. There is a significant (2 percent) incidence of clinical jaundice (9 percent incidence of abnormal liver function tests). As with pyrazinamide, all patients on this drug should have regular monitoring of liver function and an alternative regime considered should these become abnormal. There is also a low incidence of optic neuropathy, peripheral neuritis with paresthesiae and burning sensations, allergic reactions, and difficulty in controlling diabetes mellitus with fluctuations in blood sugar levels. Psychic disturbances of varying degree have also been reported. In one series there was a 30 percent incidence of congenital malformations in the children of 22 mothers treated with ethionamide either before or during pregnancy!

Griseofulvin is a drug of low toxicity with the important exception of an interaction with coumarin anticoagulants which, by *reducing* their effect, makes control difficult. This may cause serious hypocoagulability when the course of griseofulvin is ended if a compensatory increase in anticoagulants has been introduced. Griseofulvin can occasionally raise blood porphyrins and induce photosensitivity, urticaria and gastrointestinal upsets.

Isoniazid is an extremely safe drug when used in doses up to 5 mg./kg./day. Occasionally it causes a peripheral neuropathy or pellagra-like syndrome, probably reversible by pyridoxine. Glossitis, gastrointestinal disturbance and hepatic dysfunction occasionally occur. Rarely, CNS effects such as psychosis or an exacerbation of occult or previously well-controlled epilepsy can arise. Allergic reactions, lupus-like syndrome, optic neuritis and hyperglycemia with glycosuria have also been observed.

Lincomycin. Apart from chronic staphylococcal osteomyelitis or erythromycin allergy, the therapeutic role of this drug remains to be seen. Like erythromycin it can cause stomatitis, gastrointestinal upset (including an enterocolitis with blood, mucus and pus) allergic reactions and blood dyscrasias. One important difference between the drugs is that lincomycin is not effective against the Neisseriae or enterococci. Clindamycin has the same spectrum of activity and toxic effects as lincomycin. It is better absorbed and is several times more active against staphylococci and pneumococci and is probably to be preferred for these reasons.

Methenamine Mandelate (Mandelamine) requires an acid urinary pH (<5) to be effective. The mandelic acid portion encourages but does not always achieve this and ascorbic acid 100 to 200 mg. qid may need to be added. The urinary pH must be checked several times daily to assure acidity and to avoid futile therapy. Side effects include GI upset and crystalluria.

Nalidixic Acid (Negram) is a drug of low toxicity. It is not effective against pseudomonas. GI upsets and pruritis, allergic reactions including drug fever and eosinophilia, blood dyscrasias, photosensitivity, nitrogen retention and cholestatic jaundice have all been reported. CNS effects are rare but important. They include dizziness, vertigo, visual disturbance, psychosis and convulsions. This drug should be avoided or used with care in epileptics.

Nitrofurantoin frequently causes nausea and vomiting. Allergic pneumonitis and other allergic reactions such as fever, rigors and anaphylaxis may occur. Peripheral neuropathies occur especially in patients with renal impairment in whom the drug should be avoided or used with caution. Alopecia, blood dyscrasias and rarely a cholestatic jaundice are other rare effects. A hemolytic anemia may be precipitated in patients with G6PD deficiency.

Nystatin is an antifungal drug used especially in superficial candida infections of the skin, mouth, GI and respiratory tracts. It is not absorbed from the gut and is of no value in systemic fungal infections. It cannot be given parenterally. It has no place in the treatment of dermatophyte infections. Used as prophylaxis it has not been shown to diminish the incidence of clinical candida superinfections when given along with tetracyclines. Allergic reactions and GI upsets occasionally occur.

Para Amino Salicylic Acid (PAS). The majority of patients receiving PAS experience some nausea and epigastric discomfort. Taking the drug with meals or an enteric coated preparation may reduce these troublesome symptoms of which the patient should be forewarned. Allergic reactions such as fever and rashes are common and an infectious mononucleosis syndrome (Paul-Bunnell negative) has also been observed. Liver damage with jaundice carrying a high (10 percent) mortality, megaloblastic anemia and goitrous hypothyroidism can also occur.

Penicillins. These are among the safest drugs we have. Although 2 to 5 percent of the general public are allergic to penicillin G (5 to 10 percent to ampicillin), serious immediate reactions such as anaphylaxis or angioneurotic edema are rare, occurring in less than one percent of all reactors. Nonetheless, because of the massive consumption of penicillins, most physicians see these reactions not infrequently. They can also be produced by oral preparations which carry the additional risk of superinfections with Candida, resistant coliforms and staphylococci which may result in stomatitis, enterocolitis, etc. Delayed allergic reactions (incidence five percent) include fever, eosinophilia, serum sickness, dermatitides ranging from rash to exfoliative dermatitis, vasculitis and Coombs' positive hemolytic anemia. Ampicillin skin rash is almost a "diagnostic test" for infectious mononucleosis, appearing in nearly all cases when this drug is used!

Serious penicillin allergy can be detected in 50 percent of susceptible patients with a small (100 μg or units) dose by intracutaneous injection. If positive, another drug should be used. In cases where the use of a penicillin is mandatory (e.g., septicemia or SBE) treatment can be begun with small amounts (1000 units), progressively increasing the dose till full therapeutic levels are achieved. This procedure and all skin tests should, of course, be attended by great caution, with intubation equipment and oxygen at hand and epinephrine already drawn into the syringe. If a mild reaction does occur, antihistamines and perhaps steroids can sometimes control its expression sufficiently well to enable the course to be continued.

Other ADR's occur which are significant but less common. Hyperkalemia can come about when high doses of potassium penicillin G are employed in patients with renal failure (16 mega units $\equiv$ 10 G $\equiv$ 25 meq K^+). Similarly, sodium retention can occur when massive doses of sodium penicillin G are given to patients in heart failure with subacute bacterial endocarditis. Doses of penicillin G in excess of 20,000 units intrathecally or 50 mega units intramuscularly may precipitate convulsions. Methicillin is painful intramuscularly and may rarely cause marrow depression and renal irritation with hematuria and nitrogen retention. Oxacillin has rarely produced a cholestatic jaundice not observed, to date, with any other penicillins. A bleeding diathesis due to interference with platelet function has been reported with carbenicillin used for Pseudomonas infections.

Pyrazinamide. This second line anti-tuberculous drug can cause liver damage. Liver function should be monitored during therapy; and if the SGOT rises above 100 units, the drug should be discontinued. It should be avoided in patients with pre-existing liver disease. Skin rashes, photosensitivity reactions, raised serum urate and gout have also been recorded.

Sulphonamides. The true percentage incidence of adverse reactions to this group of drugs is unknown but, like the penicillins, because of massive usage, ADR's are commonly observed. The most prominent of these are allergic reactions such as rashes, drug fever and photosensitivity. They decrease the protein binding of bilirubin and so raise the level of free circulating bilirubin. This can give rise to kernicterus if given to the newborn or to the mother near term. This risk is especially great in the presence of rhesus incompatibility. The sulphonamides should therefore be avoided late in pregnancy and in the neonate. Because of this effect on protein binding, the sulphonamides also potentiate the effects of coumarin anticoagulants and the sulphonylureas and may render treatment with these drugs difficult.

Other adverse reactions include liver damage with jaundice, blood dyscrasias, methemoglobinaemia, cutaneous and systemic vasculitis, and Heinz body hemolytic anemia in patients with G6PD deficiency. The Stevens-Johnson syndrome, due to sulphonamides, has received a great deal of publicity, particularly in regard to the long-acting preparations. The true incidence of this occurrence is probably very low and has been estimated by the FDA at around one case per "10 million doses." Crystalluria (with hematuria and oliguria) was a common problem with the older preparations. It can still occur with less soluble preparations such as sulphadiazine and sulphamethoxazole with which alkalinization of the urine is still advisable. All sulphonamides should, in any event, be avoided in cases of dehydration or in patients with significantly impaired renal function.

Tetracyclines frequently give rise to nausea, vomiting, diarrhea and pruritis, the last two possibly associated with superinfection with staphylococci or Candida. Superinfections of the respiratory tract also occur and may be particularly dangerous if it occurs in the hospital environment. Systemic moniliasis has also been observed following tetracycline therapy.

Given after the fourth month of pregnancy and to children under eight years of age, enamel dysplasia and yellow staining of the teeth can occur. Given to premature infants, tetracyclines may possibly interfere with growth of the tibia. Given intravenously in large doses (>2 G/day) to pregnant women, it can also cause hepatic necrosis. Staphylococcal enterocolitis is a serious hazard and can be produced by both oral and intravenous administration presumably because of excretion in the bile. For this reason prolonged courses of high doses of these drugs should be avoided. Photosensitivity reactions occur with all tetracyclines but more cases have been reported following demethylchlortetracycline than other preparations.

Nephrotoxic effects can come about in several ways. Firstly, tetracyclines can cause deterioration of pre-existing renal failure and should be avoided or used with caution and reduced dosage in this group of patients with monitoring of the BUN. Secondly, a Fanconi-type of nephropathy with proteinuria, glycosuria and amino aciduria has been reported with degraded tetracycline. The responsible toxic degradation product was probably epianhydrotetracycline which only forms in the presence of moisture and acid. Citric acid therefore is no longer used as a preservative for tetracycline capsules, which should in any event be kept in a dry atmosphere. There is no evidence that pure tetracycline is toxic in this way. Finally, a diabetes insipidus type syndrome has been reported with demethylchlortetracycline.

As mentioned previously, the simultaneous oral administration of milk and dairy products containing calcium, or oral ferrous sulphate, can reduce blood levels by binding tetracycline in the gut.

Trimethoprim. This drug has recently been combined with sulphamethoxazole (Septrin, Bactrim) as a broad spectrum combination for the treatment of urinary and respiratory tract infections. It has also been used in combination with sulfametopyrazine in drug resistant falciparum malaria, Proteus septicemia and in one case of nocardiasis. Like the sulphonamides, with which it is synergistic, it interferes with folate metabolism. It is not surprising that it reduces serum folate levels in man although no actual hematological abnormality has yet been noted. Pruritis and skin rash have been reported with the combination of sulphamethoxazole and trimethoprim (Septrin, Bactrim). However, it is to be expected that this combination will share all the side effects of the sulphonamides and it is therefore difficult to assess any unique ADR's due to trimethoprim at this time.

Large doses of trimethoprim are teratogenic in rats. Although it has been used to treat urinary tract infection in each trimester with no abnormality in the infants, its safey in human pregnancy cannot be taken as established.

Vancomycin often causes eighth nerve (especially auditory) damage, particularly if given in large doses for more than 10 days in patients with renal impairment. In such patients blood levels should be monitored and kept between 5 and 25 μg/ml. In this regard it should be noted that vancomycin is not dialysable. It can also produce nephropathy (usually reversible), fever, urticaria, and other allergic reactions. Peripheral neuropathy may also occur. It is too painful to be given intramuscularly but produces phlebitis at the site of intravenous injection. It should be reserved for patients with serious staphylococcal infections resistant to other antibiotics.

Conclusions

Contemporary compilations of the adverse effects of drugs are encyclopedic. The avoidance of such adverse effects in clinical practice, however, does not rest on comprehensive knowledge but rather on an attitude of mind. Clearly one should restrict one's prescribing to a few well-known and trusted agents. Most importantly, adverse effects should be anticipated and looked for as a routine part of patient management. Because of the high (10 to 15 percent) incidence of adverse effects, it now seems justified to say that all hospitals should have some kind of monitoring system which examines not only drug usage but also untoward effects. This would give early warning of any epidemic of adverse reactions and is akin to the procedure employed in most hospitals for detecting and preventing hospital cross infection.

SELECTED REFERENCES

Allison, M. E., Kennedy, A. C., McGeachie, J., McDonald, G. A.: Sulphamethorazole-trimelhoprim therapy in urinary tract infection with reference to its haematological effects. Scot. Med. J., *14*:355, 1969.

Anderson, E. S.: Drug resistance in salmonella typhimurium and its implications. Brit. Med. J., *3*:339, 1968.

Atuk, M. O., Mosca, A., Kunin, C.: The use of potentially nephrotoxic antibiotics in the treatment of gram-negative infections in uremic patients. Ann. Intern. Med., *60*:28, 1964.

Baikie, A. G., MacDonald, C. B., Mundy, G. R.: Systematic nocardiosis treated with trimethoprim and sulphamethoxazole. Lancet, *2*:261, 1970.

Barber, M., Dutton, A. A. C., Beard, M. A., Elmes, P. C., Williams, R.: Reversal of antibiotic resistance in hospital staphylococcal infection. Brit. Med. J., No. 5165:11-7, 1960.

Barr, J. N., Carew, D. P.: Bull. Parenteral Drug Ass., *19*:153, 1965.

Benner, E. J.: Renal damage associated with prolonged administration of ampicillin, cephaloradine, and cephalothin. Antimicrobial Agents Chemotherap., *9*:417, 1969.

Brown, J. J., Gleadle, R. I., Lawson, D. H., Lever, A. F., Linton, A. L., Macadam, R. F., Prentice, E., Robertson, J. I. S., Tree M.: Renin and acute renal failure: Studies in man. Brit. Med. J., *1*:253, 1970.

Brunner, F. P., Frick, P. G.: Hypokalaemia, metabolic alkalosis, and hypernatraemia due to "massive" sodium penicillin therapy. Brit. Med. J., *4*:550, 1968.

Bulger, R. J., Sherris, J. C.: Decrease incidence of antibiotic resistance among *Staphylococcus aureus*. A study in a university hospital over a 9-year period. Ann. Int. Med., *69*:1099, 1968.

Cluff, L. E., Thornton, G. F., Seidl, L. G.: Studies on the epidemology of adverse drug reactions. I. Methods of surveillance. J. Amer. Med. Ass., *188*:976, 1964.

Cohlan, S. Q., Bevelander, G., Tiamsic, T.: Growth inhibition of prematures receiving tetracycline. A clinical and laboratory investigation of tetracycline induced bone fluorescence. Amer. J. Dis. Child., *105*:453, 1963.

Datta, N.: Drug resistance and R factors in the bowel bacteria before and after admission to the hospital. Brit. Med. J., *2*:407, 1969.

Davies, J. R., Farrant, W. N., Uttley, A. H.: Antibiotic resistance of *Shigella sonnei*. Lancet, *2*:1157, 1970.

Dowling, H. F., Lepper, M. H.: Hepatic reactions to tetracycline. J. Amer. Med. Ass., *188*:207, 1964.

Doyle, E. F., Spagnulo, M. J., Taranta, A., Kuttnan, A. G., Markowitz, M.: The risk of bacterial endocarditis during antirheumatic prophylaxis. J. Amer. Med. Ass., *201*:807, 1967.

Editorial, Brit. Med. J., *2*:181, 1969.

Editorial, Brit. Med. J., *2*:571, 1970.

Editorial, Lancet, *2*:993, 1969.

Editorial, Lancet, *2*:1296, 1970.

Ekyn, S., Editorial, Lancet, *2*:1231, 1970.

Falco, F. G., Smith, H. M., Arcieri, G. M.: Nephrotoxicity of aminoglycosides and gentamicin. J. Inf. Dis., *119*:406, 1969.

Foord, R. D., Dash, C. H., Johnson, Susan E., 1970: Progr. Antimicrob. Anticancer Chemother. Proc. Sixth Internat. Congr. Chemother., p. 705 Univ. Tokyo Press.

Gardner, P., Cluff, L. E.: The epidemology of adverse drug reactions. A review and perspective. John Hopkins Med. J., *126*:77, 1970.

Garrod, L. P., Waterworth, P. M.: The risks of dental extraction during penicillin treatment. Brit. Heart J., *24*:39, 1962.

Gaya, H., Adnitt, P. I., Turner, P.: Changes in gut flora after cephalexin treatment. Brit. Med. J., *3*:624, 1970.

Gingell, J. C., Waterworth, P. M.: Brit. Med. J., *2*:19, 1968.

Green, G. R., Peters, G. A., Geraci, J. E.: Treatment of bacterial endocarditis, in patients with penicillin hypersensitivity. Ann. Intern. Med., *67*:235, 1967.

Grüneberg, R. N., Kolbe, R.: Trimethoprim in the treatment of urinary infections in hospital. Brit. Med. J., *1*:545, 1969.

Kass, E. H.: Symposium on newer aspects of antibiotics: Chemotherapeutic and antibiotic drugs in management of infections of urinary tract. Amer. Med. J., *18*:764, 1955.

Kunin, C. M., Atuk, N.: Excretion of cephaloridine and cephalothin in patients with renal impairment. N. Eng. J. Med., *274*:654, 1966.

Kutscher, E., Southern, P. M., Sanford, J. P.: Clinical significance of lincomycin-resistant *Neisseria gonorrhoeae*. Antimicrobial Agents and Chemother., *8*:331, 1968.

Lawson, D. H., Macadam, R. F., Singh, H., Gavras, H., Linton, A. L.: The nephrotoxicity of cephaloridine. Postgrad. Med. J., Suppl. 36–39, 1970.

Last, P. M., Sherlock, S.: Systematic absorption of orally administered neomycin in liver disease. N. Eng. J. Med., *262*:385, 1960.

Leading Article, Brit. Med. J., *2*:509, 1970.

Leading Article, Brit. Med. J., *2*:571, 1970.

Leading Article, Brit. Med. J., *1*:63, 1971.

Leigh, D. A., Faiers, M. C., Brumfitt, W.: Bacteriology, pharmacology, and clinic studies with trimethoprim-sulphonamide combinations with particular reference to the study of urinary infections. Postgrad. Med. J., *45:*Suppl. 56–61, 1969.

Lindholm, D. D., Murray, J. S.: Persistance of vancomycin in the blood during renal failure and its treatment by hemodialysis. N. Eng. J. Med., *274:*1047, 1966.

MacKay, D. N., Kaye, D.: Serum concentrations of colistin in patients with normal and impaired renal function. N. Eng. J. Med., *270:*394, 1964.

McLure, B. D., Casserly, J. G., Charney, M., Crozir, D.: Lancet, *2:*1307, 1970.

MacMillan, B. G.: Gentamicin in the management of thermal injuries. J. Inf. Dis., *119:*493, 1969.

Medical Letter, *9:*68, 1967.

Medical Letter, *10:*no. 15, 56, 1968.

Medical Letter, *10:*no. 20, 77, 1968.

Medical Letter, *11:*42, 1969.

Medical Letter, *11:*58, 1969.

Medical Letter, *12:*no. 8, 1970.

Montgomerie, J. Z., Doak, P. B., Taylor, D. E. M., North, J. D. K., Martin, W. J.: Klebsiella in faecal flora of renal-transplant patients. *2:*787, 1970.

Murdoch, J., in The Therapeutic Use of Antibiotics in Hospital Practice, Ed. Ridley M., Phillips J., Publ. E. & S. Livingstone, Edin. and London.

Neuvonen, P. J., Gothoni, G., Hacknan, R., Bjorksten, K.: Interference of iron with the absorption of tetracyclines in man. Brit. Med. J., *4:*532, 1970.

Petersdorf, R. G., Curtin, J. A., Hoeprich, P. D., Peeler, R. N., Bennet, I. L.: A study of antibiotic prophylaxis in unconscious patients, N. Eng. J. Med., *257:*1001, 1957.

Pickering, M. J., Spooner, G. R., Quesada, A.: Declining renal function associated with administration of cephalothin. Southern Med. J., *63:*426, 1970.

Pohlman, G.: Respiratory arrest associated with intravenous administration of polymyxin B sulfate. J. Amer. Med. Ass. *196:*181, 1966.

Potworowska, E.: Leczewie etionamidem a ciaza. Gruzlica, *34:*341, 1966.

Price, D. J. E., Sleigh, J. D.: Control of infection due to *Klebsiella aerogenes* in a neurosurgical unit by withdrawal of all antibiotics. Lancet, *2:*1213, 1970.

Report, Brit. Med. J., *2:*411, 1968.

Report, Lancet, *2:*1159, 1970.

Robertson, M. H.: Tetracycline resistant streptococci in southwest Essex: A continuing survey. Brit. Med. J., *3:*349, 1968.

Sanders, W. E.: A challenge of salmonellosis. Clinical Med., *72:*45, 1965.

Sanders, W. E.: Erythomycin vs. lincomycin: A choice or an echo. Ann. Int. Med., *70:*585, 1969.

Satter, E. J.: J. Urol., *96:*86, 1966.

Shils, J. E.: Renal disease and the metabolic effects of tetracycline. Ann. Int. Med., *58:*399, 1963.

Side Effects of Drugs. Meyler, L., Herxheimer, A. (editors), Excerpta Medica Foundation, Amsterdam, Vol. VI, 1968.

Simberkoff, M. S., Thomas, L., McGregor, D., Shenkein, I., Leveine, B. B.: Inactivations of penicillins by carbohydrate solutions at alkaline pH. N. Engl. J. Med., *283:*116, 1970.

Stewart, G. T., Boyd, J. F., Butcher, B. T.: The place of cephalosporins in medicine. Postgrad. Med. J., Suppl 133–7, 1970.

Tozer, R. A., Boutflower, S., Gillespie, W. A.: Antibiotics for prevention of bacterial endocarditis during dental treatment. Lancet, *1:*686, 1966.

Wallerstein, R. O., Condit, P. K., Casper, C. K., Brown, J. W., Morrison, R.:

Statewide study of chloramphenicol therapy and fatal aplastic anemia. J. Amer. Med. Ass., *208*:2045, 1969.

Wersall, J., Lundquist, R. G., Bjorkroth, B.: Ototoxicity of gentamycin. J. Inf. Dis., *119*:410, 1969.

Westenfelder, G. O., Paterson, P. Y.: Life-threatening infection. Choice of alternate drugs when penicillin cannot be given. J. Amer. Med. Ass., *210*:845, 1969.

Williams, J. D., Brumfitt, W., Condie, A. P., Reeves, D. S.: The treatment of bacteriuria in pregnant women with sulphamethoxazole and trimethoprim. Postgrad. Med. J., *45*: Suppl. 71–6, 1969.

Chapter 30

ISOLATION OF THE HOSPITALIZED PATIENT

Reports of sporadic outbreaks of hospital based infections constantly remind us that the acquisition of infection within the hospital persists as a serious hazard. The magnitude of the problem is indicated by the fact that about five percent of all hospitalized patients will develop an infection prior to discharge. The control of the microbial agents responsible for these infections depends upon many factors. Among these are 1) the presence of an active surveillance program guided by individuals that are capable of detecting clusters of infections before they can spread; 2) the activities of an aggressive infections committee that recognizes and corrects the defects in infection control indigenous to the particular institution; 3) the availability of a laboratory capable of identifying pathogens with a span of time brief enough to be clinically useful; 4) the effects of an educational program that imbues all employees with the awareness that infections are a problem and instructs them in the techniques of asepsis and isolation; and 5) the cooperation of an administration that enforces a written code of infection control. Each of these is important in minimizing the dangers of infection.

Isolation of patients with infections constitutes a small segment of the entire infection control program. Unfortunately as practiced in most hospitals today, the principles of isolation have been reduced to an arcane, confused and contradictory list of policies that have been relegated to the custody of some member of the nursing hierachy. Isolation procedures vary not only from hospital to hospital, but even among services within the same institution. The policies seldom heed the epidemiology of an individual microbial agent or the effectiveness of a procedure in preventing its spread. Furthermore, the isolation regulations that have been established for a patient are frequently ignored by the patient's physician, rendering the precautions useless.

Isolation may be disadvantageous to the hospital and to the patient. The isolation requirements are expensive. When a separate room is required, valuable space is eliminated that could be used by additional patients. The requirements for gowns and masks for all individuals ministering to a patient is a drain on the linen and laundry resources of the hospital. The procedures themselves are time consuming. As a result, they discourage floor staff from giving optimal care to the isolated individual. Very importantly, isolation can severely deprive the patient of normal social contacts and become psychologically injurious.

The purpose of this chapter is to present a rational, simplified system of isolation which is based upon sound epidemiological principles and which balances the disadvantages of isolation with the potential risk of spreading a given infectious agent. To enable one to understand the individual specifications for a given type of isolation, the epidemiology of the microorganisms involved in hospital infections will be briefly reviewed. The individual specifications of isolation will then be discussed. Finally, the several categories of isolation will be described.

Epidemiology of Hospital Infections

The presence of an infection implies the successful interaction of three essential elements: 1) a *source* of the infectious agent; 2) a means by which the agent spreads; and 3) a host susceptible to it. Absence of any single factor aborts the infectious process.

In the hospital, infectious agents arise from two sources—the human population and the inanimate environment. The human reservoirs are patients or personnel with clinically apparent illness or individuals who carry the microorganism without signs of disease. Thus a staphylococcus may originate from a patient with a staphylococcal wound infection, or from an employee with a boil, or from a physician who is asymptomatically carrying an epidemiologically virulent strain of the microorganism in his anterior nares. Disease-producing bacteria frequently come from the patient himself. For instance, the *E. coli* which cause the overwhelming majority of urinary tract infections most frequently originate in the gastrointestinal tract of the patient with the infection. In the GI tract the bacteria do not cause illness; however, when the patient contaminates the urethra with fecal flora, an ascending infection of the urinary tract may result.

The hospital environment is another, but a far less important, source of disease-producing microorganisms. Intermittent positive pressure breathing (IPPB) equipment, anesthesia machines, and suction appliances are commonly contaminated with *Pseudomonas aeruginosa* or *Serratia marsescens*. These organisms can cause tracheitis or bronchitis and occasionally pneumonia. A thermometer rinse solution which contained Proteus once led to an outbreak of Proteus urinary tract infections on a urology ward.

Cases of tetanus have been traced to hospital dust, or to Plaster of Paris, which contained large numbers of the *Clostridium tetanus* spores. One can cite multiple instances in which the environmental pathogens ultimately cause human disease; however, the importance of the environment has been overemphasized in the past and the environmental bacteria play a minor role in the overall hospital infection problem.

Microorganisms are transmitted in three ways within the hospital: by the airborne route, by contact spread, and by means of a common vehicle. The airborne route is unusual. It depends upon dust particles or droplet nuclei (dehydrated particles of droplets that have been coughed or sneezed into the air) which are capable of remaining suspended in the air for prolonged periods of time. For a pathogen to be transmitted by air it must become attached to one of these particles and maintain its viability and virulence while suspended in air. Additionally, they must be deposited on the appropriate site of the host in sufficient numbers to produce disease. Few pathogens—such as the tubercle bacillus, and the viruses that produce smallpox or rubella—are capable of satisfying these criteria.

Contact transmission is the most common means by which infectious agents are spread within the hospital. It is often subdivided into three types: 1) direct contact implies physical apposition between the reservoir of the agent and the susceptible host; 2) indirect contact involves the intermediation of some article, such as clothing, contaminated linen, etc., between the reservoir and susceptible individual; 3) droplet spread occurs when infections are coughed, breathed or sneezed from one individual into the nose, mouth or eyes of the susceptible person. The pyogenic bacteria, staphylococci, pneumococci, streptococci, and many common viruses are spread by contact.

Common vehicle spread is unusual in the hospital environment. It has occurred when Salmonellae are transmitted within contaminated food, when hepatitis is spread by transfusion of contaminated blood, or when gram-negative bacteria are spread by contaminated drugs.

The third element in the infectious process is the susceptible host—that individual whose natural defenses have been compromised in such a manner as to allow colonization and invasion by some microorganism. Disease entities such as diabetes, uremia, malignancy, or agranulocytosis, therapeutic measures such as antibiotics, steroids or immunosuppressive drugs, and host factors such as age, debilitation or trauma, all decrease a person's resistance and render him much more susceptible to infection.

The purpose of isolation is to interrupt the infectious process by preventing the second of these three elements of the infectious process—the mode of transmission. Different microorganisms are spread in different fashions and the risk of spreading varies greatly among the different agents. To account for these differences, several categories of isolation have been devised: 1) strict isolation; 2) respiratory isolation; 3) protective isolation; 4) enteric isolation; and 5) wound and skin isolation. The isolation specifications within each category become less stringent. Some specifications are common to more than one category. These will be discussed presently.

Isolation Specifications

Private Room. Some institutions have reserved a suite of rooms in a particular part of the hospital for isolation purposes. Others have a separate room on each floor or service. Most community hospitals convert a private room into an isolation area when the need arises. The isolation unit should contain its own handwashing, bathing and toilet facilities. It should be constructed to allow a minimum of six changes of air every hour to prevent cross circulation with other sections of the hospital. Many older hospitals are not designed to allow control of air flow; this makes difficult the control of particles upon which microorganisms become airborne. In the absence of engineering facilities that filter and regulate air movement, the door to the isolation room should be kept closed except for truly necessary entrances and exits. The creation of aerosols by carelessly rough handling of linen must be avoided. Additionally, exhaust fans can be set up in the window of the room to direct air away from the corridor. Ultraviolet radiation of the upper levels of air of the room may reduce the number of airborne tubercle bacilli in the rooms of patients with active pulmonary tuberculosis.

Gowns. The requirement for gowns dictates individual gown technique, i.e., the gown is used once and then discarded into a soiled linen receptacle within the isolated area. Adequate supplies must be available at all times outside the patient's room. Sterile gowns should be used for patients in protective isolation.

Masks. Masks are to be used once and then discarded into a plastic-lined wastebasket within the isolation unit. They must not be allowed to dangle around the neck of the wearer after leaving the isolation area. The disposable synthetic fiber masks are most efficient in controlling droplets and smaller particles. All masks become inefficient when moist and so should be changed if they become damp. They must cover both the nose and the mouth.

Gloves. Gloves should be worn once and then discarded before leaving the contaminated area. Their use does not abolish the necessity of good handwashing both before and after contact with the patient or any object in his room. When removing a contaminated dressing from a purulent draining wound, gloves should be changed before applying fresh dressings.

Handwashing. Handwashing before and after contact with any patient remains the most important means of preventing the spread of microorganisms. Additionally, if the hands contact excreta or secretions, handwashing should be repeated while ministering to the patient. Sinks must be conveniently available to the patient's bedside. Preferably, water spigots and soap dispensers are operable by knee or foot pedals. Adequate supplies of antimicrobial detergent or soap must always be available.

Articles. Articles such as sphygmomanometers and stethoscopes should be kept within the isolation unit. Thermometers should be stored in a disinfectant solution containing 70 to 90 percent ethyl or isopropyl alcohol which contains 0.2 percent iodine. This solution must be changed every three days. Linen should be handled cautiously to avoid aerosolization of pathogens. It should be removed from the patient's room by double bag technique; i.e., the linen should be placed in a clean bag within the isolation unit; this bag is then inserted into a second clean bag situated on a hamper or held by someone outside the isolation area. The second bag is labelled "contaminated" so the laundry personnel may take appropriate precautions. Soiled dressings and tissues must be placed in an impervious bag made of plastic or paper that can be securely closed; this bag should be placed in a wastebasket lined with impervious plastic within the room. The plastic liner should be removed from the room using doublebag technique. All bags should be transferred to the incinerator without opening.

Visitors. Visitors should be limited to the immediate family and preferably only two people should see the patient at any one time. All visitors must check in at the nursing station before entering the patient's room and receive instructions concerning the purposes of isolation and the use of gowns, masks, or gloves.

Categories of Isolation

Strict Isolation. (Table 30.1). The purpose of strict isolation is to prevent the transmission of highly communicable bacteria and viruses that are spread by both the contact and airborne routes. Diseases in this category are rarely seen in the average community hospital and strict isolation therefore will be rarely necessary. The patient should be kept in a private room at all times. Gown and mask must be worn by every individual entering the room. Gloves should be worn by all persons coming in contact with the patient or any article touched by him. Individuals administering to patients with diphtheria, rubella or smallpox should be immune either by having previously experienced the disease or by immunization. Visitors, equipment and furniture should be kept to a minimum. Articles necessary for tending to the patient (as thermometers, stethoscopes) must remain in the room. Mattresses and pillows should be covered with impervious plastic which can be cleaned with a germicidal detergent solution. The patient's clothing should be laundered or sterilized with ethylene oxide prior to being sent home.

Respiratory Isolation (Table 30.2). This category has been designed to prevent transmission by means of droplets and droplet nuclei that are coughed, sneezed or breathed into the environment. The patient should be

TABLE 30.1

Strict Isolation: Diseases and Duration of Isolation

1. Burns, extensive (infected with staphylocci or streptococci for duration of open skin lesions).
2. Diphtheria—until 2 cultures taken from both the nose and throat after discontinuation of antibiotics are negative for *C. diphtheriae.*
3. Eczema vaccinatum—for duration of illness.
4. Melioidosis, pulmonary, or extrapulmonary with draining sinuses—for duration of illness.
5. Neonatal vesicular disease (Herpes simplex)—for duration of illness.
6. Plague—until culture negative.
7. Rabies—for duration of illness.
8. Rubella, congenital syndrome—for duration of hospitalization. Infants born with this syndrome should be isolated during any subsequent hospitalizations during the first year of life.
9. Smallpox—until all crusts are shed.
10. Staphyloccal enterocolitis—for duration of illness.
11. Staphylococcal pneumonia—for duration of illness.
12. Streptococcal pneumonia—for duration of illness.
13. Vaccinia, generalized and progressive—for duration of illness.

Strict Isolation: Specifications

1. Room: Private room is necessary.
2. Gowns: All persons entering isolation room must wear a gown.
3. Masks: To be worn by all persons entering the room.
4. Gloves: To be worn by all personnel before entering the room and discarded into an appropriate receptacle before leaving the room.
5. Handwashing: Imperative for all persons before entering and after leaving the room.

placed in a private room. All susceptible individuals entering the room must wear face masks. Gowns and gloves are not required.

Patients with tuberculosis should be isolated until a clinical response (as indicated by decreased coughing, sputum production and fever) is noted. The patient should be instructed to cover his nose and mouth with a handkerchief when coughing or sneezing; he should learn to cough or spit into a disposable handkerchief that can be discarded into an impervious bag which is situated at the bedside. When out of his room he must wear a face mask at all times.

Protective Isolation (Table 30.3). This category has been established to minimize contact between pathogens and patients whose resistance has been seriously impaired due to some underlying disease or condition. A few institutions have experimented with specialized patient isolation units in which the bed is enclosed within a plastic tent. Air is pumped into the unit through high efficiency filters and bacterial contamination is diminished with an efficiency greater than 99 percent. Food and equipment are passed in and out of the tents through special locks bathed in ultraviolet light.

TABLE 30.2

Respiratory Isolation: Diseases and Duration of Isolation

1. Chickenpox—for 7 days after eruption appears.
2. Herpes zoster (shingles)—for duration of infection.
3. Measles: Rubeola—for 7 days after appearance of rash.
4. Meningococcal meningitis—for 24 hours after the initiation of appropriate therapy.
5. Meningococcemia—for 24 hours after the initiation of appropriate therapy.
6. Mumps—for 9 days after the onset of the parotid swelling.
7. Pertussis (whooping cough)—for duration of hospitalization.
8. Rubella (German measles)—for 5 days after appearance of rash. Strict isolation for patients with congenital rubella.
9. Tuberculosis—pulmonary or respiratory tract. Sputum positive or suspect cases—until patient shows response to therapy—usually 2 to 3 weeks after initiation of drug administration.
10. Venezuelan equine encephalomyelitis—for duration of illness.

Respiratory Isolation: Specifications

1. Private room: Necessary.
2. Gowns: Not necessary.
3. Masks: To be worn by all persons entering the room who are susceptible to the specific disease.
4. Gloves: Not necessary.
5. Handwashing: Imperative for all persons before entering and after leaving room.

TABLE 30.3

Protective Isolation: Diseases and Duration of Isolation

1. Agranulocytosis—until remission
2. Dermatitis—severe and extensive which is non-infected—until substantial healing of skin surface occurs.
3. Immunosuppressive therapy: For certain patients whose immune response is thought to be severely compromised—until therapy discontinued.
4. Lymphoma or leukemia—for those patients whose immune response or blood granulocyte is severely compromised—until clinical improvement is demonstrated.

Protective Isolation: Specifications

1. Private room: Necessary.
2. Gowns: Sterile gowns should be worn by all persons entering room.
3. Masks: Should be worn by all persons entering the room.
4. Gloves: To be worn by all persons having direct contact with the patient.
5. Handwashing: Imperative for all persons before entering and after leaving the room.

Such systems, though probably effective in reducing the incidence of infections in patients enclosed within, are too costly for most community hospitals. Furthermore, they make excessive demands upon nursing and maintenance staff. For the vast majority of community hospitals a private room can be utilized for protective isolation that is designed so that air flows from the room to the corridor at all times.

Patients with illnesses requiring this type of isolation should not be subjected to many "routine" hospital procedures such as urethral or intravenous catheterization. Such procedures can lead to a fatal infection in patients who have been treated with immunosuppressive drugs, who have received large doses of x-ray therapy, or who have widespread malignancy.

Persons entering the isolation area must wear masks and sterile gowns. In some cases, caps and shoe booties may be indicated if the patient's resistance is so low as to warrant these extreme precautions. Handwashing is, of course, of paramount importance in preventing contact transmission. Gloves should be worn by all personnel having direct contact with the patient.

The length of time that a patient is maintained within protective isolation will depend upon the clinical judgment of the attending physician who must rely upon such indicators as the white cell count, the stage of the patient's illness and so forth.

Enteric Isolation (Table 30.4). Diseases in this category can be transmitted by the fecal-oral route through indirect or direct contact with feces or heavily contaminated articles. A private room is necessary only for children. Gloves and gowns should be worn by all persons having direct contact with the patient or with articles contaminated with fecal material. Handwashing is most important, not only for individuals coming in contact with patient or articles soiled by his excreta, but also for the patient

TABLE 30.4

Enteric Isolation: Diseases and Duration of Isolation

1. Cholera—for duration of illness.
2. Enteropathogenic *E. coli* gastroenteritis—for duration of illness.
3. Hepatitis, viral infectious or serum—for duration of hospitalization.
4. Salmonellosis—for duration of illness.
5. Shigellosis—for duration of illness.
6. Typhoid fever—until patient has had 3 consecutive negative cultures—taken 24 hours apart.

Enteric Isolation: Specifications

1. Private room: Necessary for pediatric patients: Children infected with the same microorganism may be housed in the same room. Adults capable of maintaining routine practices of personal hygiene may be housed with other patients.
2. Gowns: To be worn by all persons having direct contact with the patient.
3. Masks: Not necessary.
4. Gloves: To be worn by all individuals who have direct contact with either the patient or potentially contaminated articles such as bedpans or urinals.
5. Handwashing: Imperative for all persons before and after entering patient care area.

himself. He should be instructed in careful handwashing technique, particularly after defecation. Bedclothes and linens should be changed at least daily and immediately if they become soiled.

Infants with gastroenteritis caused by Salmonella, Shigella, or *E. coli* are particularly hazardous to uninfected infants within a nursery. Infants with active disease should be removed from the nursery if at all possible or geographically separated in a manner which will prevent cross infection.

Recent epidemiological data suggests that the two types of hepatitis virus can be transmitted by both the fecal-oral and injection routes. All cases of hepatitis, therefore, should be considered as potentially communicable by fecal-oral spread and all patients with hepatitis should be subjected to enteric isolation precautions.

Wound and Skin Precautions (Table 30.5). Bacteria-producing purulent drainage in wounds can be spread by direct contact with the infected wound or with heavily contaminated dressings, tissues and instruments. All major wounds draining purulent material are included here—not just those caused by Proteus, Pseudomonas, *E. coli*, etc.

It is desirable that the patient be placed in a private room. Gowns and gloves should be worn by all persons having direct contact with the patient or articles contaminated by wound drainage.

The person performing dressing changes must wear a mask and wash his hands and put on gloves before lifting the soiled dressing away with sterile instruments. Following removal of a dressing he removes his gloves, washes his hands again and puts on a second set of sterile gloves before applying the fresh dressing. All soiled dressings should be placed in an impervious plastic bag that can be sealed, double-bagged, and transferred, unopened, to the incinerator.

TABLE 30.5

Wound and Skin Precautions: Diseases and Duration of Isolation

1. Burns Extensive—for duration of illness.
2. Gas gangrene (due to *C. perfringens*)—for duration of illness.
3. Impetigo—for duration of illness.
4. Staphylococcal skin and wound infection—for duration of illness.
5. Streptococcal skin infection—for duration of illness.
6. Wound infection, extensive—for duration of illness.

Wound and Skin Precautions: Specifications

1. Private room: Not necessary but desirable.
2. Gowns: Must be worn by all persons having direct contact with the patient.
3. Masks: Necessary for individual changing dressing.
4. Gloves: To be worn by all persons having direct contact with the patient, the articles in his immediate vicinity, or dressing material.
5. Handwashing: Imperative for all persons before and after administering to the patient.

Discussion

A code of isolation should be adopted by the Infections Committee of every hospital. The decision to place a patient in isolation rests with the attending physician. He has the obligation to protect the hospital personnel and other patients from the risk of infection. If he neglects his responsibility, then this obligation must be fulfilled by the head nurse. When disagreement arises between a physician and a nurse over the need for isolation or for the implementation of isolation procedures, a member of the Infections Committee—preferably its chairman—must arbitrate the dispute. The regulations must be uniformly applied to the patients of every physician on every service within the hospital and the hospital administration must enforce the code.

A card listing the type of isolation and the specification it requires should be prominently displayed on the door of the isolation unit or above the patient's bed so that all persons within the vicinity will be instantly apprised of the patient's infectious status.

The decision to institute isolation commits everyone—physicians, nurses, paramedical personnel and visitors—to a policy of strict adherence to the isolation regulation. Failure to follow the procedures negates their effectiveness and sharply increases the risks of spreading the patient's infection.

Summary

A simplified, rational system of isolation has been presented. It is grounded in current epidemiologic data regarding the transmission of infectious agents within the hospital. Five categories of isolation have been proposed. The diseases and specifications of each consider the potential risk of spread of a given infectious agent and the effectiveness of different techniques in minimizing that risk. Isolation can be a truly effective tool in reducing transmission of infectious agents. Each hospital should develop a system suited to its needs and resources and strictly enforce the regulations throughout the institution.

Note: The concepts of isolation contained herein were developed by a committee of interested professionals at the National Center for Disease Control.

SELECTED REFERENCES

Brachman, P. S. (Ed.). Isolation techniques for use in hospitals. Public Health Service Publication No. 2054, 1970.

Kunin, C. M., Henley, R. H., Jr.: Isolation procedures for the community hospital. JAMA *200*:295, 1967.

Levitan, A. A. and Perry S.: Use of an isolation system in cancer chemotherapy. Am. J. Med., *44*:234, 1968.

Chapter 31

IMMUNIZATION PROCEDURES

Immunization is derived from the Latin "immunis," meaning "exempt from public burden." The purpose of immunization is to reduce morbidity and mortality from infectious agents or their toxic products. Immunization procedures can be conveniently divided into two types, passive and active. Most of this chapter will be involved with a description of active immunization procedures; however, a brief description of passive immunization is worthwhile. Passive immunization is the administration of antibody made in another human or animal and passively administered, usually by subcutaneous or intravenous injection.

Situations in which passive immunization is useful are:

1) Insufficient time for active immunization; i.e., insufficient time for antigens administered to the patient to stimulate the recipient's own immunologic system. Prime examples of this are the bacterial toxins, for example, tetanus or botulinus; however, this same line of reasoning might also be used in epidemic situations where a vaccine is not generally available.

2) No vaccine is available. The prime example of this is infectious hepatitis. This will hopefully soon change as a result of the isolation of the virus(es) responsible for the hepatitides.

These two situations differ in the type of passively administered antibody. In both instances the immunoglobulin fraction of serum is administered. In the first instance this immunoglobulin fraction has a very high titer of a specific antibody as a result of hyperimmunization of a person or animal or because the serum is obtained from convalescent patients. In the case of tetanus, although people have had routine immunization, gamma globulin prepared from a random group does not have a high enough titer to use as prophylaxis against tetanus. In the second instance, antigen is not available for hyperimmunization of man or animals, and it is unsafe to use serum from patients who have recovered from the infection since there is no way to insure that the infectious agent, in this case the presumed hepatitis virus, is no longer circulating.

3) Immunologic deficiency states. Passive administration of human gamma globulin has been shown to be beneficial to some extent in alleviating the chronic infectious processes these patients suffer, particularly chronic skin infections.

There are also instances where *specific* passive immunization is carried out in persons with immunologic deficiency diseases. For example, if such a patient *must* travel to an endemic area, smallpox immune serum would be necessary since smallpox vaccine is dangerous in these patients. A hypogammaglobulinemic would be more likely to need human tetanus immune globulin following a fairly innocuous injury than would a normal individual. If a pregnant woman must travel to an endemic area, passive immunization rather than active immunization with a live attenuated vaccine should be performed since it is possible, although not proven, that any attenuated virus vaccine could infect the placenta and cause fetal deformities, *a la* rubella infection.

4) "Non-specific" use of gamma globulin might be effective where a wide range of infectious agents are involved, making active immunization with each agent impractical. With regards to respiratory infections, gamma globulin injections have not been shown to be efficacious in the normal individual. This is not unexpected, since significant amounts of injected immunoglobulins and antibodies do not reach secretory surfaces. (See Chapter 4, "Secretory Immunologic System.") However, it is conceivable that direct application of gamma globulin to a mucosal surface might protect against a wide range of infectious agents. This has not been adequately tested.

5) Inhibition of antibody production by the patient. Administering gamma globulin to inhibit the host's own defense mechanisms is generally considered undesirable. However, in certain conditions, excellent use of this basic immunologic principle has been made. Rh disease is caused by maternal anti-Rh antibody crossing the placenta and hemolysing fetal Rh positive red cells. As prophylaxis against the disorder, anti-Rh antibody is administered to the mother. This procedure inhibits production of her own anti-Rh antibody; therefore, she is not sensitized and does not make antibody during subsequent pregnancies. The passive administration of the anti-Rh antibody is done immediately following parturition, since at this time the passively administered antibody would not affect the baby, and it is at birth that the fetal Rh positive red cells gain access to maternal circulation and sensitize the mother.

The disadvantages of passive immunization are:

1) Protection is of short duration. The half-life of passively administered IgG is about three weeks. However, under field conditions, it has

been shown that protection against infectious hepatitis persists much longer than this. The recommended dosage interval for gamma globulin is four to six months in highly endemic areas.

2) Immunoglobulins are themselves immunogens, especially serum from other species. Horse serum, which was the predominant source of antitetanus antiserum for many years, is highly immunogenic and frequently caused serum sickness. Human immunoglobulins are also immunogenic but this is rarely of clinical importance. However, there have been a few reported cases of hypersensitivity reactions to human gamma globulin, so this must be kept in mind when repeated doses are used. Related to this is the recent observation that a frequent cause of transfusion reactions are antibodies to IgA in IgA deficient individuals. IgA deficiency has a frequency of about one in 700 people; and in these individuals, IgA is a foreign protein. With repeated administration of plasma or whole blood, antibodies against IgA develop. The clinical picture is an urticarial or erythematous skin rash, flushing, anaphylactoid symptoms and respiratory distress.

3) Gamma globulin injections are painful and expensive.

The rest of the chapter will be devoted to active immunization, the purpose of which is to stimulate the individual's own protective mechanisms. In order to do this in a rational manner, the protective mechanisms must be known. Unfortunately, there are few instances in infectious diseases where the protective mechanisms have been elucidated. One of the few examples is tetanus, where serum antibody to the toxin is known to be protective. The various host defense mechanisms have been discussed in the opening section of this book.

Despite the fact that little is known about the mechanism of protection in most infectious diseases, from a practical point of view the central question is whether a vaccine works or not. Thus, the most important aspect with regard to a vaccine development is to assess its efficacy. Some vaccines were introduced into general use before they were critically assessed, and at about the same time that great advances were being made in other general public health measures. When the diseases for which some vaccines were given decreased in incidence, the vaccines were widely accepted as being efficacious, although the improvement in hygienic conditions in this country in the early part of this century may have been responsible.

Vaccines can be evaluated indirectly by measuring the immune mechanism thought to play a role in protection. These are not often known. The measurement of serum antibody has been assumed too often to correlate with vaccine efficacy. This is the easiest parameter to measure, but serum antibody has not been shown to play a protective role in very many infectious diseases. Thus, a potent and prolonged serum antibody response when vaccines with adjuvants are used, is not necessarily a good indication of vaccine effectiveness. The lack of evidence that serum antibody rises are directly related to protective mechanisms cannot be over-emphasized.

A second indirect measure of vaccine efficacy is the development of secretory antibody. But once again, it must be emphasized that there are even fewer infectious diseases in which secretory antibody has been proven to play an important role.

A third indirect measure of vaccine effectiveness is the development of cell-mediated immunity, almost always as determined by the development of the delayed hypersensitivity skin test. This is not a commonly used indicator; however, it may be more commonly used in the future, and in particular with respect to *in vitro* correlates of cellular immunity such as lymphocyte transformation, macrophage migration inhibition and cytolytic effects of sensitized lymphocytes. Cellular immunity plays a more important role in protection than has been generally appreciated, particularly with respect to viral infections. It has been noted that patients with agammaglobulinemia, but with intact cellular immune mechanisms, are adequately protected against most viral infections. On the other hand, patients with deficiency of the cellular immune mechanism are particularly susceptible to viral infections.

Finally, immunity to infections could be a result of some immune mechanism that has not yet been identified, or to some non-specific mechanism, for example, stimulation of interferon.

Although indirect measurements of vaccine efficacy are much easier and less expensive, the only definite way to define vaccine effectiveness is its ability to protect against illness. This is most accurately done in a field trial. Obviously, to be worthwhile, the field trial must have an adequate control group with assurance that it is identical to the vaccine group in all respects. Vaccine field trials where one community receives a vaccine and the control group is another community which receives nothing, while possibly yielding some important information, is inadequately controlled. Different communities may vary in several important parameters, most importantly subtle environmental differences, and possibly not-so-subtle socio-economic differences. The placebo effect is also important to consider in such studies.

While field trials are valuable in indicating protective efficacy, they are difficult to carry out and are expensive. A second direct means of assessing the vaccine's effectiveness is the use of challenge studies. A challenge study has the advantage of being more convenient, since much smaller populations need to be involved. For example, it has been calculated that a cholera field trial in an endemic area requires approximately one million individuals for each vaccine to be tested. A challenge study might be carried out with only fifteen individuals in each group.

The disadvantages of challenge studies are two: one scientific, the other ethical. The scientific disadvantage is that the dose of the challenge organism used in a study may not be equivalent to that which occurs naturally. In challenge studies with influenza virus, for example, most investigators try to infect 50 percent of the control group. During an epidemic, however, only 10 to 20 percent of susceptibles become infected. Thus it would appear that in many challenge studies, volunteers receive a much higher dose and therefore the results might erroneously indicate that a vaccine is ineffective.

The ethical question regards the sources of the volunteers. Most challenge studies in the United States use prisoner volunteers. Another source is draftees into the Armed Forces. It is questionable whether either of these groups can ever be true volunteers.

A recent area of interest with respect to immunization is the route of vaccine administration. The commonest method of vaccine administration has been the parenteral route, although alternate routes have been used for many years. In the Middle Ages, the Turks used intranasal immunization with crusts from smallpox lesions, believed to be the first example of immunization. Since the most common method for assessing a vaccine's effectiveness has been the measurement of serum antibody, the most common route for immunization has been the parenteral one.

However, one recent highly successful immunization has been given by an alternate route, i.e., the oral attenuated polio vaccine. The route of immunization should depend upon the immune host defense mechanism that is responsible or is thought to be responsible for protection. If the stimulation of serum antibody is the aim of immunization, then subcutaneous, intramuscular, or intradermal immunization would be most efficient. However, if secretory antibody or cellular immunity on secretory surfaces are the aim of the immunization, then local application of the antigen such as by nose drops, aerosol, oral ingestion, intravaginal or eye drops would be most efficient. This is covered in detail in Chapter 4.

There are also other considerations with respect to alternate routes of immunization. In general, oral or aerosol administration of a vaccine is more pleasant for the recipient. In some under-developed areas this is even more important, since certain cultures refuse to receive an injection. Another consideration is that mass immunization is easier with non-parenteral immunization. With regards to aerosol immunization, it is conceivable that mass immunization of whole populations could be carried out with a minimum of professional personnel and equipment.

The final consideration is the side effects which result from various routes of vaccine administration. In general, local side effects are nil with aerosol, intranasal or oral administration of vaccines. With influenza vaccine administration, there are significant local and general side effects following subcutaneous administration; for example, heat, redness and tenderness at the site of injection, fever, generalized malaise, etc. When the same vaccine is given by aerosol, there are no significant side effects.

Another important consideration in evaluating vaccines is the duration of protection. In most instances, it would be very desirable to give a vaccine once and obtain lifelong immunity. This is not an unrealistic aim, since many infectious diseases, i.e., measles infection, render the individual immune for life.

It is generally felt that live attenuated organisms give longer immunity than do killed organisms. The evidence for this is not good. There have been no controlled studies in which a live attenuated vaccine has been compared with the comparable killed vaccine. The evidence brought forth supporting live attenuated vaccines compares, for example, the protection afforded by the smallpox vaccine versus the typhoid vaccine, which is obviously an invalid comparison. Live attenuated oral polio vaccine as compared with the killed injected vaccine, again is an invalid comparison since more than one variable has been changed; i.e., in addition to the difference in live versus killed organisms, the route of administration of vaccine is different.

Although there have been no direct studies comparing the two, the general results with the live attenuated measles vaccine have been superior to that of the killed measles vaccine. However, this is probably not due to a difference in the duration of protection but due to the poorly understood hypersensitivity reaction which is induced by the killed measles vaccine.

In some studies, higher titers of antibody result from live vaccines as compared to killed vaccines. This is probably due to a larger antigenic mass, since the organisms replicate, and also due to longer contact with immunocompetent cells, since again, with replication, the antigens are present in the body for a longer period of time. Theoretically, the same result would be obtained by administering killed organisms repeatedly and in larger doses. This may be impractical in many cases, and thus a real advantage of live vaccines is that fewer doses may be given and less material must be prepared. The disadvantages of live vaccines are that they necessitate more care in handling since, if the organisms die from lack of refrigerated conditions or if lyophylized vaccines become moist, the result is a killed vaccine with very little antigenic mass. This is, of course, more important in underdeveloped areas of the world than in North America or Europe. Killed vaccines are in general more resistant to changes in environmental conditions.

The second disadvantage of live vaccines is the ever present danger of administration of an adventitious agent along with the live organism. This is especially important with respect to viral vaccines in which viruses are grown in a living cellular milieu, and it is virtually impossible to rule out the presence of another agent. With killed vaccines this is still a consideration, but less important since when the vaccine virus is killed, adventitious agents are likely to be killed also. Of course, there is still a danger with any vaccine, since the killing process may not inactivate all viral agents and "killing" a virus does not guarantee that it is non-oncogenic.

Another consideration with respect to duration of protection is the question of booster immunization. There is very little data on the timing, number, or necessity of booster immunizations. The only well documented use for immediate "booster" immunizations, that is, those given two to four weeks following the primary, is "insurance." If there is a 90 percent "take" with a particular vaccine, with two doses the susceptibles decrease from 10 percent to 1 percent. With the third dose of a vaccine, one lowers this to less than 1 percent. Boosters give added insurance when the primary immunization is given early in life, since maternal IgG antibody may still be present and inhibit the infant's antibody response. A second type of booster immunization is given at a much later date; i.e., one to five years later. There are more data indicating that this type of booster is useful. When immunity is waning, the booster immunization leads to a secondary antibody response with respect to serum IgG antibody, and immunity may be greatly prolonged. For example, with tetanus toxoid, a booster immunization every 10 years results in virtually 100 percent immunity.

Specific immunization suggestions are shown in Table 31.1 These recommendations reflect only minor modifications of those established by the Public Health Service.

In ending a discussion of immunizations, it is imperative that the dangers and potential dangers of immunizations be emphasized. Obviously one must always balance the risks of the procedure with the benefit. This is nowhere better exemplified than with the smallpox immunization. There are well-documented dangers associated with vaccination. This must be balanced with the danger of introduction of smallpox into the United States. It would appear at the present time that the balance is swinging towards the side of a greater danger from immunization than the risk of disease. One must still consider, however, that the highest incidence of side effects from smallpox immunization is in adults. If people were not immunized as children, and then travel to an endemic area either by choice or as members of our Armed Forces, the risk of vaccination becomes greater.

Another example of the dangers of immunization is the polio virus vaccine. The danger of immunization is less clear cut but it would appear that there have been cases of polio occurring as a result of the vaccine virus becoming more virulent on passage through the gut. At the present time, most of the workers in the area would agree that the dangers of polio immunization are far less than the danger of the disease.

There are many potential dangers with respect to the rubella virus

TABLE 31.1

Vaccine	Presently available			Possibilities within next 5 to 10 years
	Type of vaccine	Suggested use	Comment	
Cholera	Killed whole organism	For travel to South and Southeast Asia and Middle East. Dose #1 0.5 ml. SQ or IM; dose #2 1.0 ml., about 1 mo later.	High incidence of local and general reactions of "nuisance" type. Effectiveness marginal and of short duration. Because of rarity of cholera in westerners, vaccine not recommended except for fulfilling requirements of Int'l Certificate of Vaccination.	1. Toxoid vaccine: possibly analogous to diphtheria vaccine, to be tested in field trial in 1972. 2. Oral attenuated: Mukherjee strain being tested by W.H.O. 3. Oral killed.
Diphtheria, tetanus Pertussis	Toxoid-adsorbed Toxoid-adsorbed Killed bacteria or bacterial fraction	DTP, Td or T. alone. DTP at 6 wks–3 mos. 3× at 4–6 wk intervals, booster 1 yr later. Booster at time of entrance to school. Td. thereafter and 10 yr, unless used as part of wound management. Wound: previous dose 1 yr before, give Td booster. No previous, give Td × 2 4–6 wks interval, booster 1 yr later.	Tetanus is almost an ideal immunizing agent: sensitization a slight problem. Pertussis difficult to document that the vaccine is responsible for the decline in incidence of the disease. Why is the disease most common in infants 3 mos old? Rare side-effects of severe CNS reaction occasionally leading to permanent sequelae and death.	Tetanus and diphtheria toxoids have been effectively used via the respiratory tract for booster immunization.
Tetanus	Passive TIG	250 units IM in separate syringe, separate site from tetanus toxoid.	Indications: 1) location of wound; 2) type and severity; 3) contamination; and 4) time since injury.	
Viral hepatitis	Passive ISG	0.01 ml./pd body weight; extended residence 0.02 ml./lb every 6 mos.	Indications: definite exposure or anticipated continuous or intermittent exposure. Not enough data to recommend ISG for recipients of transfusion of blood or blood products.	Killed or attenuated viral vaccine(s)
Influenza	Egg-grown virus, formalin inactivated; also highly purified (zonal ultracentrifugation)	2 doses subcutaneously 6–8 wks apart in "high risk" groups, completed by early Dec.	1) High incidence of local and general reactions of "nuisance" type, but much less with highly purified preparation. 2) Immunize late Oct. or Nov., booster early to mid-Dec. 3) No evidence that ID is effective. 4) Some indication that everyone should be immunized every year.	1. Live attenuated vaccine 2. Aerosol killed vaccine—good protection, absence of side effects 3. Tissue culture grown virus 4. "Split" virus (purified hemagglutinin) vaccine.

Other respiratory viruses				1. Killed vaccines for rhinovirus, parainfluenza and respiratory syncytial virus by aerosol. 2. Live attenuated respiratory syncytial virus vaccine intranasally 3. Live attenuated adenovirus vaccine orally.
Rubella	Live attenuated vaccine, prepared in a variety of cell cultures	All children 1 yr to puberty. *Routine* immunization of adolescent girls *not* indicated because of danger of inadvertently administering vaccine during pregnancy. Each case considered individually.	Purpose: preventing infection of fetus; accomplished by eliminating transmission among source of infection for pregnant women, i.e., among children. Risk of vaccine virus for fetus is unknown. Side effects: arthritis 2–4 wks after vaccination with HPV77 strain, less so with Cendehill. Duration of protection unknown.	1. Killed vaccine for women of child-bearing age potentially exposed to infection. 2. Live vaccine by aerosol has been shown to be effective in stimulating seroconversions; theoretical advantage of stimulating respiratory secretion antibody.
Plague	Formaldehyde inactivated *Pasteurella pestis*	Persons travelling to Indochina, persons in contact with wild rodents in endemic areas and lab. personnel working with the disease. 0.5 ml. × 2–4 wks. apart then 0.2 ml. 4–12 wks later, 0.2 ml. booster at 6–12 mos.	Unknown effectiveness. Local and systemic reactions mild, but tend to become more severe with repeated doses.	
Polio	Inactivated virus	Beginning at any age from 6 wks—3× at 1 mo intervals, 4th dose 12 mos later. Booster at 2–3 yrs.		
	Attenuated virus-monovalent or trivalent	Dose 1 at 6 wks, dose 2 at 14 wks, dose 3 at 1 yr, dose 4 on entering school.	Not suggested for adults not immunized previously. Duration of protection not known. Easier to give, stimulates local immunity thereby decreasing circulation of virus, immunity may be longer duration.	

TABLE 31.1—*Continued*

Vaccine	Presently available			Possibilities within next 5 to 10 years
	Type of vaccine	Suggested use	Comment	
Measles (rubeola)	Live attenuated virus, chick embryo or canine tissue culture grown	At one yr; susceptibles any time thereafter.	Very common febrile reaction day 6–11, but more severe reactions very rare. Use should be postponed in children with acute febrile illness. Should not be used in children with severe underlying diseases that are associated with lowered resistance or in pregnant women. All children who have received prior immunization with inactivated measles virus vaccine should receive live attenuated measles vaccine despite risk of local reaction. Duration of protection unknown.	Simultaneous use of live attenuated measles, mumps and rubella, either subcutaneously or by aerosol.
Mumps	Live attenuated virus, chick embryo cell culture	At 1 yr or later	Untoward reactions very rare. Duration of protection unknown. Only warranted use probably in males approaching puberty who have not had mumps parotitis, either unilateral or bilateral (mumps skin test too unreliable to warrant use as test for immunity).	
Rabies	Active: 1) Beta-propiolactone inactivated virus grown in embryonated duck eggs.	Post-exposure: DEX suggested; 14 daily doses subcutaneously 21 doses in cases of severe exposure. Boosters given 10 and 20 days after completion of primary course. Pre-exposure: in high risk groups (e.g., vets.): 3 doses for primary immunization; booster at 2 yr.	Effectiveness of post-exposure prophylaxis unproved. Local and systemic reactions common, especially late in course of immunization.	Live attenuated vaccine
	2) phenol inactivated virus grown in rabbit brain.		Same plus neuro-paralytic reactions. Rationale of treatment: 1) species of animal; 2) circumstances of biting incident; 3) extent and location of bite wound; 4) vaccination status of biting animal; 5) presence of rabies in area. Local therapy probably the most effective means of preventing rabies.	

	Passive equine hyperimmune serum	Use only in severe exposure, all bites by documented rabid animals, unprovoked bites by wild carnivores: 1000 units per 40 lbs. body weight.		
Smallpox	Live vaccinia virus: glycerenated or lyophilized; latter more stable.	Active: between 1st and 2nd birthdays, or at any time of exposure or foreign travel; boosters on entering school, at 3 yr intervals for exposed persons, at 10 yr intervals for all others. Primary vaccination must be examined for presence of Jennerian vesicle.	Difficult problem of balance of risk of the disease against efficacy and risk associated with vaccination. Is routine vaccination warranted? Although controlled trials have never been performed, it would appear that protection is almost complete for 3 yrs, substantial for 10, and protects against fatal outcome for decades. Complications: $1/10^6$ encephalitis, $1/10^6$ vaccinia necrosum, $1/10^5$ eczema vaccinatum, $1/10^6$ deaths (11 in 1968). All deaths and nearly all complications in primary vaccinees. High risk: 1^0 in 1 yr old and after puberty. Contraindications: skin disorders in potential vaccinee or in a household contact; (if vaccination essential, Vaccinia Immune Globulin should be used); pregnancy; altered immune states.	1. More attenuated live virus vaccine 2. Killed virus vaccine
	Passive: Vaccinia Immune Glоublin	Prophylaxis: 0.3 ml./kg. IM Therapy: 0.6 ml./kg. IM for eczema vaccination, progressive vaccinia or autoinoculation of the eye, generalized vaccinia. No benefit in postvaccinial encephalitis	See above under contraindications of vaccination.	

TABLE 31.1—*Continued*

Vaccine	Presently available			Possibilities within next 5 to 10 years
	Type of vaccine	Suggested use	Comment	
Typhoid	Whole organism killed by several different techniques	Intimate exposure to carrier or case or travel to endemic area. 0.5 ml. subcutaneously ×2, 4 wks apart.	Immunization: has probably played no role in the decline of typhoid fever in the U.S. in the last 60 yrs. Recent field trials have demonstrated slight, but definite, protective effect of vaccine, for short period of time; however, best prophylaxis is careful selection of food and water in endemic area. Immunization for foreign travel, when balanced against side-effects and tendency to relax hygiene, probably not worthwhile.	Oral killed or attenuated vaccines have been tested and seem to be more effective with fewer side-effects.
Paratyphoid A and B	TAB Vaccine combined with typhoid	Not suggested—TAB should not be used.	Not effective	
Shigella	—	—	—	Same
Typhus	Formaldehyde inactivated *Rickettsia prowazekii* grown in embryonated eggs.	May be used prior to travel to remote highland areas of Ethiopia, Rwanda, Burundi, Mexico, Ecuador, Chile, Bolivia, Peru and mountainous areas of Asia. Suggested for field workers in close contact with natives, medical personnel providing pt. care and lab workers. 2 subcutaneous doses 4 wks apart followed by a 6–12 mos booster.	Effective in North Africa during World War II. Local reactions common—general reactions uncommon.	
Yellow fever	Live attenuated virus prepared in chick embryo-Dakar strain or 17D strain	Persons traveling to or living in area where the infection exists (Africa and S. America); lab personnel, revaccination at 10 yrs.	Dakar strain—0.5% incidence of meningoencephalitic reactions—not recommended. For international travel, vaccination must be certified on Int'l Certificate of Vaccination (yellow card) at a Yellow Fever Vaccination Center listed with WHO. Mild systemic reactions 5–10 days after vaccination.	

Dental caries				Local or systemic immunization against the streptococci known to cause the plaques which lead to caries, or against the dextranase which is necessary for plaque formation—encouraging results *in vitro* and in experimental animals.
Trachoma and other eye infections				Vaccines are being tested which will be administered onto the conjunctival surface. Trachoma agent given parenterally gave no protection.
Venereal diseases				Vaccines are being tested to be administered intravaginally.
Passive administration of antibody into secretory surfaces.				1. HGG by aerosol being tested. 2. Hyperimmune cow's milk being tested for therapy of enteropathic *E. coli* infections in infants.

vaccine, particularly the danger of the vaccine being administered or being transmitted to a pregnant woman. With some of the vaccines currently in use, it has been shown that the vaccine strain, although attenuated, can infect the placenta. Thus, there is a real danger that fetal abnormalities could be induced by the vaccine. The second potential danger of the rubella vaccine is that if duration of protection is not life-long, and we continue the procedure of immunizing young children, we could be producing an adult population which is completely unprotected 20 years from now.

The injected killed respiratory syncytial virus vaccine has been used experimentally, and in a field trial the vaccine group had an increased illness severity as compared to the control group. The cause of this is not definitely known but has been postulated as due to an "imbalance" in the systemic and secretory systems; i.e., by injecting the RSV vaccine, only serum antibody was stimulated with no stimulation of secretory antibody. Conceivably, when the individual was then exposed to the wild virus, an Arthus-like reaction, possibly involving complement fixation by serum IgM and IgG antibody, was set up in the lung leading to increased tissue damage. Similarly, as mentioned above, the killed measles vaccine has led to severe reactions when the individuals were exposed to wild measles virus.

With the widespread use of a vaccine, the disease often becomes much less prevalent. When the prevalence decreases, the population very rapidly becomes lax about obtaining the immunization. This can lead to a very large adult susceptible population. Many diseases, which are fairly benign in childhood, become much more virulent when they affect adult populations. Two examples are measles and polio, which, while certainly not considered benign in childhood, are known to be much less virulent in this age group.

A final theoretical danger of immunizations is the development of new strains of the organism. It has been postulated that immunization simply hastens the evolution of new strains, as, for example, with influenza virus, in which new strains develop periodically, possibly as a result of population immunity.

SELECTED REFERENCES

Benenson, A. S., Mosley, W. H., Fahimuddin, M. and Oseasohn, R. O.: Cholera vaccine field trials in East Pakistan. Bull. Wld. Hlth. Org., *38*:359, 1968.

Cluff, L. E. and Allen, J. C.: Principles of active immunization for prevention of infection. J. Chron. Disc., *15*:575, 1962.

Finn, R.: Rh haemolytic disease. Recent advances in Rh isoimmunization prevention. Brit. Med. J., *2*:219, 1970.

Hornick, R. B., Woodward, T. E., McCrumb, F. R., Snyder, M. J., Dawkins, A. T., Bulkeley, J. T., de la Macorra, F. and Corozza, F. A.: Typhoid fever vaccine—yes or no? Med. Clin. N.A., *51*:617, 1967.

Janeway, C. A. and Rosen, F. S.: The gamma globulins, IV. Therapeutic uses of gamma globulin. N. Eng. J. Med., *275:*826, 1966.

Meyer, H. M. and Parkman, P. D.: Rubella vaccination, a review of practical experience. J. Amer. Med. Assoc., *215:*613, 1971.

Perkins, J. C., Tucker, D. N., Knopf, H. L. S., Wenzel, R. P., Hornick, R. B., Kapikian, A. Z., and Chanock, R. M.: Evidence for the protective effect of an inactivated rhinovirus vaccine administered by the nasal route. Amer. J. Epidem., *90:*319, 1969.

Pollock, T. M.: Assessing immunization procedures. Proc. Roy. Soc. Med., *63:*811, 1970.

Smith, C. B., Purcell, R. H., Bellanti, J. A. and Chanock, R. M.: Protective effect of antibody to parainfluenza type 1 virus. N. Eng. J. Med., *275:*1145, 1966.

Stollerman, G. H.: Prospects for a vaccine against group A streptococci: The problem of the immunology of M proteins. Arth. Rheumat., *10:*245, 1967.

Von Magnus, P., Engbaek, H. C. and Jespersen, A.: Tuberculosis and BCG. Med. Clinics of N. Amer., *51:*753, 1967.

Waldman, R. H., Mann, J. J., and Small, P. A., Jr.: Immunization against influenza: Prevention of illness in man by aerosolized inactivated vaccine. J. Amer. Med. Assoc., *207:*520, 1969.

Yamamoto, K., Anacker, R. L. and Ribi, E.: Macrophage migration inhibition studies with cells from mice vaccinated with cell walls of *Mycobacterium bovis:* Relationship between inhibitory activity of lung cells and resistance to airborne challenge with *Mycobacterium Tuberculosis* H37Rv. *Infect. Immun., 1:*595, 1970.

SECTION FIVE

TABULATION AND OTHER REFERENCES OF INFECTIOUS DISEASES

Chapter
32

INTRODUCTION TO TABULATION AND REFERENCES

Attention has been directed heretofore to selected essays on infectious diseases to emphasize clinically important pathogenetic mechanisms, general and specific problems, and principles of management and prevention. No effort has been made to be encyclopedic or comprehensive. Approaches and perspectives have been the objective.

Patients with infectious diseases usually present with manifestations affecting one or more regions or systems of the body. These regional or system manifestations often are distinctive for infections caused by different microorganisms. Furthermore, the microorganisms usually responsible for particular manifestations are limited in number and familiarity with them often may assist in identifying the infecting agent and initiating the appropriate treatment.

Tabulation of important clinical syndromes or manifestations of infectious disease, the etiologic agents often responsible for the manifestations, and comments about some distinguishing characteristics of the diseases caused by different microorganisms, was considered useful in orienting an approach to diagnosis. Certainly, this tabulation could be more complete or comprehensive, but we believe it will prove useful. Subsequently, the table might be expanded, or could serve to structure a more fully developed text on infectious diseases.

Once the microorganisms possibly responsible for a disease are identified, the list of selected references provided can serve as a source of detailed information and as an entré to the literature on the subject. Certainly, important references have been left out; these can be added in subsequent editions or the reader may add his own.

Problems on microorganisms covered in the text are identified by reference to specific chapters. Learning to use this table and selected reference list could provide a means for increasing familiarity with infectious diseases.

Chapter
33

TABULATION OF INFECTIOUS DISEASES BY SYNDROMES OR MAJOR MANIFESTATIONS

I. Cutaneous Infections

Syndromes	Etiologic agents or disease	Clinical characteristics
Pustules	1. *Corynebacteriium acnes*	1. Acne
	2. Cryptococcosis	2. Usually with meningitis or lung lesions
	3. Group A streptococcus	3. *Chapt. 20*
	4. Pseudomonas	4. Also necrotizing
	5. Sporotrichosis	5. Also nodular lymphangitis
	6. Staphylococcus	6. *Chapt. 19*
	7. Orf	7. On hands in sheep herders, abattoir workers
Vesicular—bullous	1. Dermatophytosis	1. Athletes foot. Tinea
	2. Erysipeloid	2. Hands, violaceous lesions
	3. Group A streptococcus	3. Bullous with cellulitis. *Chapt. 20*
	4. Herpes simplex	4. Mouth, fingers, genitalia
	5. Herpes zoster	5. Dermatome lesions (shingles)
	6. Lymphograumloma venereum	6. Venereal
	7. Pseudomonas	7. Bullae with necrosis and hemorrhage
	8. Rickettsialpox	8. May resemble varicella
	9. Sporotrichosis	9. Nodular lymphangitis
	10. Varicella	10. Chickenpox—lesions differing stages
	11. Variola-vaccinia	11. Lesions same stage
Ulceronecrotic	1. Anthrax	1. Eschar, edema, contact with goat hair products, wool or hides
	2. Blastomycosis	2. Sharply demarcated—Eastern U.S.
	3. Catscratch disease	3. Regional lymphadenopathy. Cat scratch or contact
	4. Chancroid	4. Venereal
	5. *Clostridium welchii*	5. Gas gangrene
	6. Cryptococcosis	6. Usually with meningitis or lung lesions
	7. Diphtheria	7. Tropical ulcer on legs
	8. Granuloma inguinale	8. Venereal
	9. Pseudomonas	9. Ecthyma gangrenosa
	10. Sporotrichosis	10. Nodular lymphangitis
	11. *Staphylococcus aureus*	11. Scalded skin syndrome in infants. *Chapt. 19*
	12. *Treponema pallidum*	12. Secondary syphilis
	13. Tularemia	13. Eschar with regional adenopathy. Contact with wild rabbits
	14. Variola-vaccinia	14. Smallpox
Hemorrhagic	1. Bacteremia	1. With consumptive coagulopathy. *Chapts. 9, 10*
	2. Bacterial endocarditis	2. Petechiae or purpura. *Chapt. 25*
	3. *Clostridium welchii*	3. Gas gangrene
	4. Hemorrhagic fever (viral)	4. Fever, myalgia, leukopenia neurologic manifestations, petechiae, purpura

I. Cutaneous Infections—*Continued*

Syndromes	Etiologic agents or disease	Clinical characteristics
Hemorrhage—*Continued*		
	5. Meningococcus	5. Petechiae, purpura
	6. Pseudomonas	6. Ecthyma gangrenosa
	7. Rocky Mountain Spotted Fever (*Rickettsia rickettsiae*)	7. Petechiae peripherally. Tick borne
	8. Rubeola	8. Measles
	9. Typhus (*Rickettsia prowazeki*)	9. Petechiae on trunk. Louse-borne
Cellulitis and lymphangitis	1. Group A streptococcus	1. *Chapt. 20*
	2. *Staphylococcus aureus*	2. *Chapt. 19*
	3. Erysipeloid	3. Burning, tingling, violaceous lesions of hands. No fever. Contact with animal products
	4. Rat bite fever (*Spirillum minus*)	4. Nodular lymphangitis; relapsing
Regional lymphadenitis	1. Atypical mycobacteria	1. Cervical adenitis—chronic. *Chapt. 16*
	2. Cat scratch disease	2. Cat scratch or contact. Eschar often
	3. Group A streptococcal infection	3. *Chapt. 20*
	4. Lymphogranuloma venereum	4. Venereal disease
	5. *Pasteurella pestis*	5. Bubonic plague-Louse borne
	6. Primary syphilis	6. Rubbery, firm, painless inguinal nodes
	7. Tuberculosis	7. Cervical adenitis—chronic. *Chapt. 16*
	8. Tularemia	8. Skin ulcer or eschar. Exposure to wild rabbits
Nodular		
1. Erythema	1. Tuberculosis Coccidioidomycosis Histoplasmosis Group A streptococcus	1. Violaceous, painful, nodules on extensor surfaces. *Chapts. 16, 17, 20*
2. Osler's nodes	2. Subacute bacterial endocarditis	2. Painful nodules, toes and fingers *Chapt. 25*
3. Papulo-nodular	3. Tuberculosis Blastomycosis Cryptococcosis Leprosy Secondary syphilis	3. Leprosy-anesthetic, depigmented, thickened peripheral nerves
Exanthemata and erythema	1. Echo viruses	1. Erythematous rash, rhinitis, pharyngitis
	2. Group A streptococcus	2. Scarlet fever. *Chapt. 20*
	3. Leprosy	3. Erythematous or depigmented anesthetic area of skin
	4. Meningococcus	4. Petechial and erythematous rash

I. Cutaneous Infections—*Continued*

Syndromes	Etiologic agents or disease	Clinical characteristics
Exanthemata and erythema—*Continued*		
	5. Rocky Mountain Spotted fever	5. Petechial and erythematous rash on extremities
	6. Rubella	6. Erythematous rash, posterior cervical adenopathy
	7. Rubeola (measles)	7. Erythematous rash, conjunctivitis, Koplik's spots, rhinitis
	8. Tinea (dermatophytosis)	8. Pruritic erythematous rash, vesicles or fissures of moist skin regions
	9. Tularemia	9. Transient erythematous trunkal rash
	10. Typhoid fever	10. Abdominal erythematous rash. Rose spots
	11. Typhus	11. Petechial and erythematous rash on trunk
Nails		
1. Splinter hemorrhages	1. Bacterial endocarditis	1. *Chapt. 25*
2. Onychomycosis	2. Dermatophytosis (*Tinea rubrum*) *Candida albicans*	2. Thickened, scaly, deformed nail and nail bed

II. Ocular Infections

Conjunctivitis	1. Adenovirus	1. Common cold, pharyngitis. Also epidemic keratoconjunctivitis
	2. Cat scratch disease	2. Similar to tularemia. Cat exposure
	3. Gonorrhea	3. Purulent exudate in newborn
	4. *Hemophilus influenzae*	4. Particularly in children
	5. Herpesvirus hominis	5. Often with corneal ulceration
	6. Herpes zoster	6. Always with periorbital vesicular, dermatome lesions
	7. Leptospirosis	7. Common manifestation in Weil's disease and other leptospiral infections
	8. Newcastle disease virus	8. Exposure to chickens
	9. Pseudomonas	9. Purulent discharge, usually following trauma or complicating ulcerative disease of eye
	10. Rubeola	10. Measles rash, Koplick spots
	11. Trachoma and inclusion conjunctivitis	11. Follicular hypertrophy, mucopurulent discharge, keratitis, pannus, blindness
	12. Tularemia	12. Ulcerative, purulent lesion with regional adenitis. Wild rabbit exposure
	13. Mumps	13. Inflammation with involvement parotid glands

II. Ocular Infections—*Continued*

Syndromes	Etiologic agents or disease	Clinical characteristics
Conjunctival petechiae	1. Bacterial endocarditis	1. *Chapt. 25*
Corneal ulceration	1. Herpesvirus hominis 2. Herpes zoster 3. Listeriosis	
Hypopyon and panophthalmitis	1. Pyogenic bacteria	1. Following traumatic lesions to eye
	2. Pneumococcus and meningococcus	2. With disseminated infection
Chorioretinitis	1. Histoplasmosis	1. Granulomatous uveitis. *Chapt. 17*
	2. Syphilis	2. Tertiary or congenital syphilis
	3. Toxoplasmosis	3. Usually congenital infection. Rarely acquired
	4. Tuberculosis	4. Choroidal tubercles. *Chapt. 16*
Optic atrophy-neuritis	1. Mumps and other acute viral infections	1. May be post-infectious
	2. Syphilis	2. Late CNS manifestations
Retinal hemorrhage	1. Bacterial endocarditis	1. Also Roth spots. *Chapt. 25*
Ocular nerve paralysis	1. Botulism	1. Ingestion of spoiled canned food. Generalized weakness and paralysis
	2. Encephalitis	2. *Chapt. 22*
	3. Meningitis	3. *Chapt. 21*
	4. Poliomyelitis	4. Usually epidemic and seasonal

III. Ear Infections

Otitis externa	1. Candida 2. Pseudomonas 3. Staphylococci 4. Trichophyton	Mucopurulent discharge. Pain on moving pinna of ear
Otitis media	1. Acute pyogenic bacteria—e.g., pneumococcus, staphylococcus, group A streptococcus	1. Painful, loss of hearing, fever, purulent
	2. Chronic pyogens e.g. Proteus, Pseudomonas, staphylococcus	2. Chronic mucopurulent discharge, loss of hearing, may be recurrent
	3. *Mycoplasma pneumoniae*	3. Bullous myringitis. Respiratory infection
	4. Respiratory viruses	4. Serous, nonpurulent otitis, often no fever
	5. Tuberculosis	5. *Chapt. 16*

III. Ear Infections—*Continued*

Syndromes	Etiologic agents or disease	Clinical characteristics
Deafness		
1. VIII Nerve	a. Maternal rubella	a. Deafness in newborn infant with congenital rubella
	b. Mumps	b. Usually a late complication
	c. Post meningitis	c. *Chapt. 21*
	d. Syphilis	d. Usually congenital infection
2. Middle ear	a. Otitis media b. Respiratory viruses	

IV. Respiratory System Infections

Common cold	1. Adenoviruses 2. Coxsackie A viruses 3. Coxsackie B viruses 4. Echo viruses 5. Influenza virus A, B, C 6. Parainfluenza viruses 7. Polioviruses 8. Respiratory syncytial virus 9. Rhinoviruses	Rhinitis, pharyngitis, conjunctivitis, tracheitis, cough may each be present, with or without fever. *Chapt. 15*
Acute bronchitis	1. *C. diphtheriae* 2. *Hemophilus influenzae* 3. *Hemophilus pertussis* (whooping cough) 4. Influenza A, B, C 5. Mycoplasma 6. Parainfluenza viruses 7. Respiratory syncytial virus	Cough usually productive of mucopurulent sputum if bacterial, non-productive and harassing if viral or mycoplasmal
Chronic bronchitis	1. *Hemophilus influenzae* 2. Pneumococcus	Dyspnea, emphysema, exacerbations with purulent sputum.
Laryngotracheo-bronchitis	1. Parainfluenza viruses 2. Influenza virus *A*, *B*, *C* 3. Respiratory syncytial virus 4. *C. diphtheriae*	Croup and respiratory difficulty, usually in children
Pharyngitis	1. Adenoviruses 2. Coxsackie A viruses 3. Polioviruses 4. Group A streptococcus 5. *Staphylococcus aureus* 6. Infectious mononucleosis 7. Pneumococcus 8. *Mycoplasma hominis* 9. *C. diphtheriae* 10. *Candida albicans*	(1–8) May be exudative (especially if bacterial) or non exudative 9, 10. Membranous pharyngitis in diphtheria and candidiasis (thrush)
Vesicular stomatitis	1. Coxsackie A viruses 2. Herpesvirus hominis	1. Herpangina 2. Fever blisters

IV. Respiratory System Infections—*Continued*

Syndromes	Etiologic agents or disease	Clinical characteristics
Ulcerative stomatitis	1. Fusiform bacilli and *Borrelia vincenti*	1. Vincent's angina—painful
	2. *Treponema pallidum*	2. Syphilitic chancre—painless
	3. Herpesvirus hominis	3. Aphthous stomatitis
Parotitis	1. Myxovirus parotitis	1. Mumps
	2. *Staphylococcus aureus*	2. Suppurative parotitis
	3. Coxsackie A viruses	3. Non-suppurative parotitis
Interstitial pneumonia	1. Adenoviruses	1–10. *Chapt. 14*
	2. Cytomegalovirus	2. In patients with immune deficiency
	3. Herpesvirus varicella	3. Chickenpox
	4. Influenza A viruses	4. *Chapt. 15*
	5. *Mycoplasma pneumoniae*	
	6. Parainfluenza viruses	
	7. *Pneumocystis carinii*	7. In patients with immune deficiency
	8. Psittacosis	8. Exposure to birds
	9. Respiratory syncytial virus	
	10. Rubeola	10. With rash
Acute lobular or lobar pneumonia		1–9. *Chapt. 14*
	1. Aspergillus fumigatus	1. With immune deficiency disease
	2. Histoplasmosis	2. Exposure to starlings, bats, chickens. *Chapt. 17*
	3. Klebsiella-aerobacter	
	4. Plague (*Pasteurella pestis*)	4. During bubonic epidemic
	5. Pneumococci	
	6. *Coxiella burneti* (Q fever)	6. Exposure to cattle
	7. *Staphylococcus aureus*	7. *Chapt. 19*
	8. Tuberculosis	8. *Chapt. 16*
	9. Tularemia (*Pasteurella tularensis*)	9. Hilar adenopathy
Eosinophilic pneumonia	1. Aspergillus	1. Eosinophilia in blood and sputum. *Chapt. 6*
	2. Ascaris lumbricoides	2. Eosinophilia, worm in sputum
	3. Dirofilaria	3. Transient eosinophilic granuloma
	4. Visceral larva migrans	4. Dog tapeworm
Chronic granulomatous and cavitary lung disease	1. Actinomycosis	1. Pyogenic empyema. Sinus tracts
	2. Aspergillus	2. Fungus ball in cavity
	3. Blastomycosis	3. Usually skin lesions
	4. Coccidioidomycosis	4. Southwest U.S.
	5. Cryptococcosis	5. Often meningitis
	6. Histoplasmosis	6. *Chapt. 17*

IV. Respiratory System Infections—*Continued*

Syndromes	Etiologic agents or disease	Clinical characteristics
Chronic granulomatous and cavitary lung disease—*Continued*	7. *Maleomyces pseudomallei* (glanders)	7. Exposure to horses
	8. Nocardiosis	8. Like actinomycosis
	9. Paragonimiasis	9. Asia—lung fluke
	10. Pyogenic lung abscess	10. Aspiration, staphylococcus, Klebsiella and others
	11. Tuberculosis	11. *Chapt. 16*
Hemorrhagic mediastinitis	1. Anthrax	1. May or may not be pneumonia. Exposure to infected animal products (wool)

V. Cardiovascular Infections

Syndromes	Etiologic agents or disease	Clinical characteristics
Pericarditis	1. Pyogenic bacteria (staphylococci, pneumococci, meningococci, salmonella, etc.)	1. Usually with bacteremia. May complicate cardiac surgery
	2. Rheumatic fever—post streptococcal	2. *Chapt. 20*
	3. Tuberculosis	3. Effusion or constrictive pericardial disease. May be pericardial calcification. *Chapt. 16*
	4. Viral—acute benign (Coxsackie B viruses)	4. May be recurrent, marked effusion
Myocarditis	1. Bacterial endocarditis	1. *Chapt. 25*
	2. Rheumatic fever—post streptococcal	2. *Chapt. 20*
	3. Viral (Coxsackie B viruses, influenza and other respiratory viruses or viral exanthemata)	3. Usually benign
	4. Many fulminant infections	4. Probably "toxic"
Endocarditis and endarteritis	1. Bacterial endocarditis	1. *Chapt. 25*
	2. Rheumatic fever	2. *Chapt. 20*
Septic thrombophlebitis and emboli	1. Group A streptococci, staphylococci, other pyogenic bacteria and Candida	
	a. Pelvic veins	1a. May follow abortion
	b. Peripheral veins	1b. Complicates intravenous catheterization
	c. Cavernous sinus	1c. Complicates facial infection
	d. Lateral sinus	1d. Complicates otitis media or mastoiditis
	e. Superior sagittal sinus	1e. Spreads from cavernous sinus or from pelvis via vertebral veins
	f. Cortical veins	1f. Complicates pyogenic meningitis

Cardiovascular Infections—*Continued*

Syndromes	Etiologic agents or disease	Clinical characteristics
Aortic aneurysm	1. *Treponema pallidum*	1. Tertiary syphilis
Mycotic aneurysm	1. Usually complicates bacterial endocarditis	1. *Chapt. 25*

VI. Gastrointestinal Infections

Diarrhea and vomiting	1. Cholera vibrio	1. Fulminant, devastating, diarrhea—Asia
	2. *Clostridium welchii*	2. Diarrhea, of short duration, no vomiting or fever.
	3. *Entameba histolytica*	3. Gradual onset diarrhea, blood and mucus, asymptomatic carriers.
	4. Enteropathogenic *Escherichia coli*	4. Fulminant diarrhea, particularly in infants
	5. Enteroviruses Coxsackie B viruses Polio viruses	5. Acute diarrhea, little or no fever, lasting 1–2 days, may be epidemic
	6. *Giardia lamblia*	6. Acute diarrhea, may be chronic, asymptomatic carriers
	7. *Leptospira interrogans*	7. Diarrhea, water-borne
	8. Salmonella (not typhoid)	8. Diarrhea, abdominal pain, tenesmus, fever-chills, blood and mucus in feces lasting 2–7 days. Often food-borne
	9. Schistosomiasis	9. Diarrhea, fever, urticaria, eosinophilia, blood and mucus in feces. Not in U.S.
	10. Shigella	10. Similar to Salmonella, fever less common, lasting 7–15 days.
	11. Staphylococcal food poisoning	11. Severe diarrhea, acute vomiting, no fever, may be common source outbreak. Onset 4 hours after eating. *Chapt. 19*
	12. Typhoid fever	12. Constipation more common; perforation, hemorrhages
Hepatic disease	1. Amebic abscess or hepatitis	1. May be no jaundice or fever. Amebae in feces. Fecal—oral spread.
	2. Cholangitis—coliforms	2. Obstructive jaundice, hectic fever, chills
	3. Infectious mononucleosis	3. Hepatitis—Jaundice, abnormal lymphocytes, positive heterophile test
	4. Leptospirosis (Weil's disease)	4. Jaundice, conjunctivitis, leukocytosis, CSF pleocytosis. Rat-borne
	5. Pylephlebitis and pyogenic liver abscess-coliforms, bacteroides, and others.	5. Fever, chills. Bacteremia, jaundice may be absent

Syndromes	Etiologic agents or disease	Clinical characteristics
Hepatic disease—*Continued*		
	6. Viral hepatitis (MS1 and MS2)	6. Jaundice. May be epidemic. *Chapt.* 23
	7. Yellow fever	7. Jaundice, fever, bradycardia, rapid course, often fatal. Not in U.S. Mosquito-borne
Splenomegaly	1. Brucellosis	1. Exposure to animal reservoir —cattle, sheep, goats
	2. Echinococcosis	2. Cysts—may calcify. Eosinophilia. Exposure to sheep
	3. Histoplasmosis	3. Disseminated disease, granulomas, multiple calcification. *Chapt. 17*
	4. Kala azar (leishmaniasis)	4. Large, firm spleen, marked hyperglobulinemia. Not U.S.
	5. Malaria	5. Recurrent, regular chills and fever. Parasitemia.
	6. Pyogenic abscesses (staphylococcus, salmonella, coliforms)	6. Rare. Usually septic infarcts
	7. Tuberculosis	7. Caseous granulomas, multiple calcifications. *Chapt. 16*
	8. Many viral, bacterial, and systemic mycotic infections.	
Intra-abdominal Infections		
1. Appendicitis	1. Coliforms, intestinal parasites	1. Pain right lower quadrant, vomiting, leucocytosis
2. Peritonitis-peritoneal abscess	2a. Actinomycosis	
	b. Following bowel perforation —coliforms, anaerobic streptococci, bacteroides, clostridia	
	c. Tuberculosis—associated with disseminated disease in men, pelvic infection in women	2c. *Chapt. 16*
	d. Pneumococcal	2d. Rare cause of peritonitis in children with nephrosis
Pancreatitis	1. Myxovirus parotitis	1. Complication of mumps
	2. Coxsackie B virus	2. Associated with acute febrile illness, usually respiratory
	3. Coliforms	3. Associated with duct obstruction
Cholecystitis	1. Coliforms	1. Obstructive biliary tract disease—often with cholelithiasis
	2. S. typhosa (typhoid fever)	2. Responsible for many cases of chronic carriers—particularly in women

VII. Genitourinary Tract Infections

Syndromes	Etiologic agents or disease	Clinical characteristics
Urinary tract infections	1. Ascending Infection—coliforms, Proteus, Pseudomonas, *Streptococcus fecalis*.	1. *Chapt. 24*
	2. Hemorrhagic cystitis	2. Schistosoma hematobium. Not in U.S.
	3. Metastatic infection; tuberculosis, staphylococci	3. *Chapts. 16, 19*
	4. Perinephric abscess—pyogenic bacteria, especially *Staphylococcus aureus*	4. Fever, intermittent bacteremia. Urine may be normal
	5. Urethritis—gonococcus, mimeae, mycoplasma	5. Often venereal disease in men
Venereal infection	1. Chancroid (Ducrey bacillus)	1. Painful, shallow, gray ulcer on penis in men, on vulva or vagina in women
	2. Granuloma inguinale (*Donovonia granulomatis*)	2. Phagadenic granulomatous ulcer of penis or vulva with inguinal adenopathy
	3. Lymphogranuloma venereum	3. Transient penile or vulval vesicle or small ulcer. Inguinal or perirectal adenopathy. Rectal stricture. Hyperglobulinemia
	4. Gonorrhea (*Neisseria gonorrheae*)	4. Urethritis, urethral stricture in men. Cervical-vaginal exudate in women. Tenosynovitis, arthritis
	5. Syphilis—*Treponema pallidum*	5a. Primary chancre—painless penile ulcer in men. Painless vulvo-vaginal ulcer in women b. Secondary—rash, fever, meningitis, meningovascular disease, mucous membrane lesions. c. Tertiary—late latent with positive STS. Paresis. Tabes. Aortic aneurysm. Gummata d. Congenital—fetal death. Fibrotic visceral lesions. Osteochondritis. Skin rash. Rhagades. Saddle nose. Dental deformities (Hutchinson's teeth). Eighth nerve deafness.
Endometritis	1. Gonorrhea	1. Tender, indurated salpinx, often sterility. Vaginal discharge.

VII. Genitourinary Tract Infections—*Continued*

Syndromes	Etiologic agents or disease	Clinical characteristics
Endometritis—*Continued*		
	2. Pyogenic bacteria—Streptococci, coliforms, bacteroides, mimeae, clostridia	2. Foul, purulent vaginal discharge. May occur after parturition or abortion
	3. Tuberculosis	3. May be accompanied by tuberculous peritonitis. *Chapt. 16*
Vulvovaginitis	1. *Candida albicans*	1. Exudative vaginal discharge with pruritus
	2. Herpesvirus hominis	2. Vesicular vulvar lesions, painful vaginal ulcers
	3. Trichomonas	3. Exudative vaginal discharge with pruritis
Bartholin gland abscess	1. Gonococcus	1. May be asymptomatic, perineal nodule
	2. Pyogenic bacteria	2. Tender, hot, perineal nodule
	3. Trichomonas	3. May be asymptomatic, perineal nodule
Prostatitis	1. *Streptococcus fecalis* 2. Staphylococcus 3. Trichomonas 4. Tuberculosis 5. Blastomycosis	1–5. May be acute or chronic
Orchitis	1. Coxsackie B viruses	1. Associated with acute febrile illness, usually respiratory.
	2. Myxovirus parotitis	2. Mumps
Epididymitis	1. Gonorrhea	1. Usually acute or sub-acute
	2. Tuberculosis	2. Usually chronic
Balanitis	1. Pyogenic bacteria	1. Painful penile ulcers
	2. Herpesvirus hominis	2. Painful penile ulcers

VIII. Neurological Infections

Meningitis	1. Bacterial, viral, mycotic or parasitic	1. Neutrophilic or mononuclear pleocytosis. *Chapt. 21*
Brain abscess and granuloma	1. Actinomycosis	1. Acute or chronic infection. Lung lesions
	2. Blastomycosis	2. Usually associated with granulomatous skin lesions
	3. Cryptococcosis	3. Associated with meningitis
	4. Echinococcosis	4. Rare. Exposure to infected sheep. Chronic
	5. *Entameba histolytica*	5. Complication of colonic infestation
	6. Histoplasmosis	6. *Chapt. 17*

VIII. Neurological Infections—*Continued*

Syndromes	Etiologic agents or disease	Clinical characteristics
Brain abscess and granuloma —*Continued*		
	7. Pyogenic bacteria	7. Acute infection. Direct extension from paranasal sinuses or metastatic
	8. Syphilis	8. Gumma
	9. Tuberculosis	9. *Chapt. 16*
Epidural abscess	1. Pyogenic bacteria	1. Secondary to mastoid or paranasal sinus infection. (Potts' puffy tumor)
Subdural abscess or empyema	1. Pyogenic bacteria	1. Extends from ears or sinuses. Rarely metastatic
Encephalitis—cerebritis	1. Arboviruses	1–5. *Chapt. 22*
	2. Mucormycosis	2. Orbital infection in acidosis
	3. Respiratory viruses	
	4. Syphilis	4. Paresis or meningovascular infection
	5. Trichinosis	5. Eosinophilia, orbital edema

IX. Musculoskeletal Infections

Syndromes	Etiologic agents or disease	Clinical characteristics
Myositis—severe myalgia	1. *Clostridium welchii* and other clostridia	1. Gas gangrene
	2. Coxsackie B viruses	2. Acute febrile respiratory illness
	3. Dengue (break-bone fever)	3. Mosquito-borne. Abrupt onset. Rash. Leukopenia. Epidemic
	4. Influenza viruses	4. *Chapt. 15*
	5. Leptospirosis	5. With or without jaundice. Animal disease transmitted to man
	6. Trichinosis	6. Eosinophilia, orbital edema
Tenosynovitis	1. Gonorrhea	1. Late complication
Arthritis—arthralgia	1. Many viral and bacterial infections	1. Often minor manifestation—usually sterile synovial fluid
	2. Gonorrhea	2. Polyarthritis or pyogenic monoarthritis
	3. Rat bite fevers—*Spirillum minus*, Streptobacillus moniliforms	3. Skin ulceration, lymphangitis, rash, polyarthritis
	4. Lymphogranuloma venereum	4. Hyperglobulinemia. Venereal disease
	5. Pyogenic bacteria, particularly staphylococcus and pneumococcus	5. *Chapt. 19*

IX. Musculoskeletal Infections—*Continued*

Syndromes	Etiologic agents or disease	Clinical characteristics
Arthrithis—arthralgia—*Continued*		
	6. Rheumatic fever	6. *Chapt. 20*
	7. Rubella	7. Polyarthritis with rash
	8. Syphilis	8. Charcot joint. Congenital infection usually
Osteomyelitis	1. Mycosis—systemic	1. *Chapt. 17*
	2. Salmonella	2. Particularly in patients with sickle cell disease
	3. *Staphylococcus aureus* and other pyogens	3. *Chapt. 19*
	4. Tuberculosis	4. *Chapt. 16*
Psoas abscess	1. *Staphylococcus aureus*	1–2. Loss of psoas shadow on x-ray. Pain on hip extension. *Chapt. 19*
	2. Tuberculosis	2. *Chapt. 16*
Muscle abscess	1. Pyogenic bacteria	1. Occasionally complicating intramuscular injections or foreign bodies

X. Hematological Manifestations

Leukopenia	1. Many viral diseases	
	2. Some acute bacteremias	2. *Chapt. 9*
	3. Brucellosis	3. Systemic disease, fever, splenomegaly, hepatomegaly. Cattle, goat, or sheep exposure
	4. Tuberculosis	4. *Chapt. 16*
	5. Typhoid fever	5. Ingestion of food or water contaminated by typhoid carrier
Leukemoid reaction	1. Bacteremia and severe pyogenic infection	1. *Chapt. 9*
	2. Disseminated tuberculosis	2. *Chapt. 16*
Monocytosis	1. Diphtheria	1. Membranous pharyngitis
	2. Histoplasmosis	2. *Chapt. 17*
	3. Infectious mononucleosis	3. Pharyngitis, fever, generalized lymphadenopathy, splenomegaly, positive heterophile test
	4. Rocky Mountain Spotted Fever	4. Fever, petechial rash beginning on extremities. Exposure to infected ticks
	5. Tuberculosis	5. *Chapt. 16*
Lymphocytosis	1. *Hemophilus pertussis*	1. Whooping cough. Pronounced lymphocytosis
	2. Influenza viruses	2. Relative lymphocytosis. *Chapt. 15*

X. Hematological Manifestations—*Continued*

Syndromes	Etiologic agents or disease	Clinical characteristics
Eosinophilia	1. Diffuse cutaneous infections—e.g., varicella	
	2. Many parasitic infections—e.g., intestinal, trichinosis	
	3. Coccidioidomycosis	3. Southwest U.S.
	4. Farmer's Lung	4. An allergic pneumonitis due to inhalation of moldy hay. *Chapt. 14*
	5. Group A streptococcus	5. With exfoliating scarlet fever *Chapt. 20*
Anemia	1. Common in all chronic or severe infections	1. *Chapt. 10*
Hemolysis	1. Many infections in patients with glucose-6-phosphate dehydrogenase deficiency (G-6-PD)	1–5. *Chapt. 10*
	2. *Clostridium welchii* sepsis	2. May be massive hemolysis
	3. Infectious mononucleosis	3. May be positive Coombs test
	4. Malaria	4. May be marked hemoglobinuria (blackwater fever) particularly with *Plasmodium falciparum*
	5. *Mycoplasma pneumoniae*	5. Pneumonia with cold hemagglutinins
Thrombocytopenia	1. Acute bacteremia	1. May be associated with hemorrhage. *Chapt. 9–10*
	2. Disseminated tuberculosis	2. *Chapt. 16*
	3. Infectious mononucleosis	
	4. Rickettsial infections—particularly Rocky Mountain Spotted Fever	
	5. Rubella	
Aplastic anemia	1. Disseminated tuberculosis	1. *Chapt. 16*
Coagulopathy	1. Most bacteremias	1. Related to degree of shock or hypotension. May be purpura fulminans.

Chapter 34

SELECTED REFERENCES

Viruses, Mycoplasma, Chlamydiae

Respiratory Viruses: General References

Huebner, R. J.: Viral respiratory diseases in the Americas. Ann. Rev. Resp. Dis., *88*:1, 1963.

Mufson, M. A., Webb, P. A., Kennedy, H., Gill, V. and Chanock, R. M.: Etiology of upper respiratory tract illnesses among civilian adults. JAMA, *195*:1, 1966.

Stuart-Harris, C. H.: *Influenza and Other Virus Infections of the Respiratory Tract*. Williams and Wilkins Co., Baltimore, 1965.

Tyrrell, D. A. S.: *Common Colds and Related Diseases*. Williams and Wilkins Co., Baltimore, 1965.

Adenoviruses

Beuscher, E. L.: Respiratory diseases and the adenoviruses. Med. Clin. N. Amer., *51*: 769, 1967.

Arboviruses (Dengue, Viral encephalitides, Yellow Fever)

Cassols, J., Hoogstrual, H., Johnson, K. M., Shelokov, A., Wienberg, N. H., and Work, T. H.: A current appraisal of hemorrhagic fevers in USSR. Am. J. Trop. Med., *16*:751, 1966.

Cromblett, H. G., Stegmiller, H., and Spencer, C.: California encephalitis virus infections in children. JAMA, *198*:108, 1966.

Diasio, J. S. and Richardson, F. M.: Clinical observation on dengue fever. Mil. Surg., *94*:365, 1944.

Ehrenkranz, N. J., *et al.:* The natural occurrence of V.E.E. in the United States. N. Eng. J. Med., *282*:298, 1970.

Luby, J. P., Sulkin, S. E. and Sanford, J. P.: The epidemiology of St. Louis encephalitis. A Review. Ann. Rev. Med., *20*:329, 1969.

McAllister, R. M.: Viral encephalitides. Ann. Rev. Med., *13*:389, 1962.

Miles, J. A. R.: Epidemiology of the arthropod-borne encephalitides. Bull. WHO, *22*:339, 1960.

Silver, H. K., Meiklejohn, G. and Kempe, C. H.: Colorado tick fever. Am. J. Dis. Child., *101*:30, 1961.

Work, T. H.: Serological evidence of arbovirus infection in the Seminole Indians of Southern Florida. Science, *145*:270, 1964.

Work, T. H.: Virus diseases in the tropics. In *A Manual of Tropical Medicine,* 4th ed., G. W. Hunter, W. W. Frye and J. C. Schwartzwelder (eds.), Philadelphia, W. B. Saunders Co., 1966.

Cat Scratch Disease

Spaulding, W. B. and Hennessy, J. N.: Cat-scratch disease. Am. J. Med., *28*:504, 1960.

Warwick, W. J.: The cat scratch syndrome. Prog. Med. Virol., *9*:256, 1967.

Chlamydiae (Psittacosis Group Including Trachoma)

Abrams, A. J.: Lymphogranuloma Venereum, JAMA, *205*:199, 1968.

Harding, H. B.: The epidemiology of sporadic urban *ornithosis*. Am. J. Clin. Path., *38*:230, 1962.

Jawetz, E.: Chemotherapy of Chlamydial infections. *Advances in Pharmacology and Chemotherapy,* Vol. 7, New York, Academic Press, 1969, p. 253–282.

Moulder, J. W.: The relation of the psittacosis group (Chlamydiae) to bacteria and viruses. Ann. Rev. Microbiol., *20*:107, 1966.

Schaffner, W., Drutz, D. J., Duncan, G. W. and Koenig, M. G.: The clinical spectrum of endemic psittacosis. Arch. Intern. Med., *119*:433, 1967.

Stewart, D. B.: The gynecological lesions of lymphogranuloma venereum and granuloma inguinale. Med. Clin. N. Am., *48*:773, 1964.

Thyggeson, P.: *Trachoma Manual and Atlas* (U.S. Dept. HEW, U.S.P.H.S. Publication No. 541, Revised 1960.

Cytomegalovirus

Hanshaw, J. B.: Clinical significance of cytomegalovirus infection. Postgrad. Med., *35*:472, 1964.

Enteroviruses (Coxsackie virus, echoviruses, reovirus)

Beale, A. J.: Immunization against poliomyelitis. Brit. Med. Bull., *25*:148, 1969.

El-Rai, F. M. and Evans, A. S.: Reovirus infection in children and young adults. Arch. Environ. Health, *7*:700, 1963.

Ferris, B. G., Jr., *et al.*: Life-threatening poliomyelitis: Boston, 1955. N. Eng. J. Med., *262*:371, 1960.

Huebner, R. J., Beeman, E. A., Cole, R. M., Beigelman, R. M. and Bell, J. A.: The importance of coxsackie viruses in human disease, particularly herpangina and epidemic pleurodynia. N. Eng. J. Med., *247*:249, 1952.

Kibrick, S.: Current status of coxsackie and echoviruses in human disease. Progr. Med. Virol., *6*:27, 1964.

Lepow, M. L., Coyne, N., Thompson, L. B., Carver, D. H. and Robbins, F. E.: A clinical, epidemiological, and laboratory investigation of aseptic meningitis during the four-year period 1955–1958. I. Observations concerning etiology and epidemiology. N. Eng. J. Med., *200*:1181, 1062, II. The clinical disease and its sequelae. Ibid. *266*:1188, 1962.

Lerner, M. A., Klein, J. P., Cherry, J. D., and Finland, M.: New viral exanthems. N. Eng. J. Med., *269*:678, 1963.

Ramos-Alvarez, M., Olarte, J.: Diarrheal diseases of children: The occurrence of enteropathogenic viruses and bacteria. J. Dis. Child., *107*:218, 1964.

Werner, H. A., and Low, T. Y: Virus diseases associated with cutaneous eruption. Prog. Med. Virol., *5*:219, 1963.

Chapt. 8.

Herpesvirus hominis

Brain, R. T.: The clinical vagaries of the Herpes simplex virus. Brit. Med. J., *1*:1061, 1956.

Rawls, W. E., Tompkins, W. A. F., Figueros, M. E., and Melnick, J. L.: Herpesvirus type 2: associated with carcinoma of the cervix. Science, *161*:1255, 1968.

Herpesvirus varicella-zoster

Appelbaum, E., *et al.*: Herpes zoster encephalitis. Am. J. Med., *32*:25, 1962.

Cimons, I. M., Lacher, M. J., LaMonte, C. S., Levitt, L., Cady, B. and Beattie, E. J., Jr.: Treatment of varicella pneumonia. JAMA *206*:372, 1968.

Rifkind, D.: The activation of varicella-zoster virus infections by immunosuppressive therapy. J. Lab. Clin. Med., *68*:463, 1966.

Rotern, C. E.: Complications of chickenpox. Brit. Med. J., *1*:944, 1961.

Molluscum contagiosum

Blattner, R. J., Jr.: Molluscum contagiosum; eruptive infection in atopic dermatitis. J. Pediat., *70*:997, 1967.

Mycoplasma

Chanock, R.: Mycoplasma infections of man. N. Eng. J. Med., *273*:22, 119, 1965.

Forsythe, B. R. and Chanock, R. M.: Mycoplasma pneumonia. Ann. Rev. Med., *17*:371, 1966.

Hayflick, L. (ed.): *The Mycoplasmatales and the L-phase of Bacteria*, New York, Appleton-Century-Crofts, 1969.

Chapt. 14.

Myxoviruses (Mumps, Influenza, Parainfluenza)

Chanock, R. M., Parrott, R. H., Johnson, K. M., Kapikian, A. Z. and Bell, J. A.: Myxoviruses: Parainfluenza. Amer. Rev. Resp. Dis., *88*:152, 1963.

Chanock, R. M., *et al.*: Respiratory syncytial (RS) virus. JAMA, *176*:647, 653, 657, 1961.

Hilleman, M. R.: Respiratory syncytial virus. Am. Rev. Resp. Dis., *88*:181, 1963.

Hilleman, M. R. and Stokes, J.: Live attenuated mumps virus vaccine. N. Eng. J. Med., (a) *278*:5, 227, 1968; (b) *276*:5, 243, 1967; (c) *279*:6, 300, 1968.

Russell, E. R. and Donald, J. C.: The neurologic complications of mumps. Brit. Med. J., *2*:27, 1958.

Chapt. 15.

Orf—paravaccinia

Leavell, U. W., Jr., McNamara, M. J., Meulling, R., Talbert, W. M., Rucker, R. C. and Datlon, A. J.: Orf: Report of 19 human cases. JAMA, *204*:657, 1968.

Rabies virus

Hildreth, E. A.: Rabies prevention, 1966. Ann. Int. Med., *64*:1357, 1966.

Plotkin, S. A. and Clark, H. F.: Prevention of rabies in man. J. Infect. Dis., *123*:227, 1971.

WHO Expert Committee Report on Rabies, WHO Tech. Ser. No. 321, Fifth Report, Geneva, 1966.

Rhinoviruses

Andrews, C. H.: Rhinoviruses and common colds. Ann. Rev. Med., *17*:361, 1966.

Rubella

Cooper, L. F.: Rubella: A preventable cause of birth defects. In Bergsme D. (ed.): *Birth Defects:* Original Article Series, Vol. IV, No. 7, Intrauterine Infections, The National Foundation, Dec., 1968, pp. 23–35.

Horstman, D. M.: Rubella and rubella syndrome: Problems and progress. Med. Clin. N. Amer., *51*:587, 1967.

Rubella Symposium. Am. J. Dis. Child., *110*:345–476, 1965.

Rubeola

Aznick, N. W., Shanell, S. M., and Witte, J. J.: Benefits due to immunization against measles. Public Health Rep., *84*:673, 1969.

Babbott, F. L., Jr., and Gordon, J. E.: Modern measles. Am. J. Med. Sc., *228*:334, 1954.

Weinstein, L.: Failure of chemotherapy to prevent the bacterial complications of measles. N. Eng. J. Med., *253*:679, 1953.

Variola

Dixon, C. W.: *Smallpox*. London, J & A Churchill, Ltd., 1962.

Lane, J. M.: Complications of smallpox vaccination, 1968: National surveillance of the United States. N. Eng. J. Med., *281*:1201, 1969.

Viral Hemorrhagic Fevers (Junin Virus, Machupovirus—the Tacaribe Complex of Viruses of South America)

Frame, J. D. *et al.:* Lassa fever. Am. J. Trop. Med., *19*:670, 677, 680, 692, 1970.

Johnson, K. M., Salstead, S. B. and Cohen, S. N.: Hemorrhagic fevers of Southeast Asia and South America: A comparative appraisal. In Melnick, J. L. (ed.), *Progress in Medical Virology,* Vol. 9, Boston/New York, S. Karger, 1967, pp. 105–158.

Rickettsiae

General References

Diagnostic Procedures for Viral and Rickettsial Diseases, 3rd ed., N.Y. American Public Health Assoc., 1964.

Gear, J. H. S.: Rickettsial vaccines. Brit. Med. Bull., *25*:171, 1969.

Smadel, J. E.: Status of the Rickettsioses in the U.S. Ann. Int. Med., *51*:421, 1959.

Zdrodovski, P. F. and Golinevich, H. M.: *The Rickettsial Diseases.* New York, Pergamon Press, 1960 (in English).

Zinser, H. *Rats, Lice, and History.* Boston, Little, Brown Co., 1935.

Coxiella burnetti (Q Fever)

Johnson, J. E., III, and Kadull, P. J.: Laboratory-acquired Q fever: A report of 50 cases. Am. J. Med., *41*:391, 1966.

Tigertt, W. D., and Benenson, A. S.: Studies on Q fever in man. Trans. Assoc. Am. Physicians, *69*:98, 1956.

Rickettsia akari (Rickettsial pox)

Lockman, D. B.: A review of Rickettsiae in the U. S. Clin. Pediat., *2*:206, 1963.

Rickettsia mooseri (*Endemic Typhus*)

Pratt, H. D.: The changing picture of Murine Typhus in the United States. Ann. N. Y. Acad. Sci., *70*:516, 1958.

Rickettsia prowazekii (*Epidemic Typhus*)

Moulton, F. R.: *The Rickettsial Diseases of Man.* Washington, American Association for the Advancement of Science, 1948.

Rickettsia quintana (*Trench Fever*)

Vinson, J. W., Varela, G. and Molin-Pasquel, C.: Trench fever. Am. J. Trop. Med., *18*:713, 1969.

Warren, J.: Trench fever Rickettsia. In Horsfall, F. L., Jr. and Tanner, I., (eds.) *Viral and Rickettsial Infections of Man,* 4th ed., Philadelphia, J. B. Lippincott Co., 1965.

Rickettsia rickettsi (*Rocky Mountain Spotted Fever*)

Harrell, G. T.: Rocky Mountain spotted fever. Medicine, *28*:333, 1949.

Rickettsia tsutsugamushi (*Scrub typhus*)

Traub, R. and Wisseman, C. L., Jr.: Ecological consideration in scrub typhus. Bull. WHO, *39*:209 1968.

Bacteria

Bacillus anthracis (*Anthrax*)

Brachman, P. S.: Human anthrax in the United States. In Hobby, G. L. (ed.) *Antimicrobial Agents and Chemotherapy.* Baltimore, Williams and Wilkins Co., 1965.

Gold, H.: Anthrax: Report of 117 Cases. Arch. Int. Med., *96*:387, 1955.

Bacteroides (*Gram-negative Anaerobic Bacilli*)

Bodner, S. J., Koenig, M. G. and Goodman, J. S.: Bacteremic Bacteroides infection. Ann. Int. Med., *73*:537, 1970.

Bornstein, D. L., Weinberg, A. N., Swartz, M. N. and Kung, L. J.: Anaerobic infection—review of current experience. Medicine, *43*:207, 1964.

Goldsand, G. and Braude, A. L.: Anaerobic infections. Disease-A-Month, Nov., 1966.

Bartonella bacilliformis (*bartonellosis*)

Ricketts, W. E.: Clinical manifestations of Carrion's disease. Arch. Intern. Med., *84*:751, 1949.

Weinman, D.: Bartonella group. In Dubos, R. J. and Hirsch, J. G. (eds.) *Bacterial and Mycotic Infections of Man,* 4th ed., Philadelphia, J. B. Lippincott, Co., 1965.

Brucella (*Brucellosis*)

Cluff, L. E., Trever, R. W., Peeler, R. N. Bennett, J. L., Jr., Imboden, J. B. Canter, A.: Brucellosis. *103*:381, 398, 406, 1959.

Knight, V.: Chemotherapy of brucellosis. Ann. N. Y. Acad. Sci., *53*:332, 1950.

Spink, W. W.: *The Nature of Brucellosis.* Minneapolis, University of Minn. Press, 1956.

Cholera vibrios

Carpenter, C. C. J., *et al.:* Clinical studies in Asiatic cholera. Bull. Johns Hopkins Hosp., *118:*165, 1966.

Phillips, R. A.: Asiatic cholera. Ann. Rev. Med., *19:*69, 1968.

Clostridium botulinum (Botulism)

Koenig, M. G., Spickard, A., Cardella, M. A. and Rogers, D. E.: Medicine, *43:*517, 1964.

Meyers, K. F.: Food poisoning. N. Eng. J. Med., *249:* 765, 804, 843, 1953.

Rogers, D. E.: Botulism: Vintage 1963. Editorial. Ann. Int. Med., *61:*581, 1964.

Clostridium tetani (Tetanus)

LaForce, F. M., *et al.:* Tetanus in the United States (1965–1966). N. Eng. J. Med., *280:*569, 1969.

Smith, J. W. G.: Diphtheria and tetanus toxoids. Brit. Med. Bull., *25:*177, 1969.

Corynebacterium diphtheriae (Diphtheria)

Naiditch, M. J. and Bower, A. G.: Diphtheria: A study of 1433 cases observed during a 10-year period at the Los Angeles County Hospital. Am. J. Med., *17:*229, 1954.

Smith, J. W. G.: Diphtheria and tetanus toxoids. Brit. Med. Bull., *25:*177, 1969.

Wood, W. B., Jr.: *From Miasma to Molecules.* New York, Columbia University Press, 1961.

Zalma, V. M., Older, J. and Brooks, G.: The Austin, Texas diphtheria outbreaks: Clinical and epidemiological aspects. JAMA *211:*2125, 1970.

Diplococcus pneumoniae

Chapt. 14.

Erysipelothrix rhusiopathiae (Erysipeloid)

Ewing, M.: Erisipeloid. Med. J. Aust., *1:*449, 1957.

Escherichia coli (Coliforms)

Chapts. 9, 24, 27.

Kennedy, R. P., Florde, J. J. and Petersdorf, R. G.: Studies in the epidemiology of *E. coli* infection. J. Clin. Invest., *44:*193, 1965.

Neter, E.: Enteropathogenic *E. coli,* enteritis. Pediat. Clin. N. Am., *7:*1015, 1960.

Fusobacterium fusiformis and Indigenous Oropharyngeal Spirochetes (Fusospirochetosis)

Uohara, G. I. and Knapp, M. J.: Oral Fusospirochetosis and associated lesions. Oral. Surg., Oral. Med., Oral. Pathol., *24:*113, 1967.

Granuloma Inguinale

King, A. and Nicol, C. S.: *Venereal Diseases,* 2nd ed., London, Bailliere, Tindall and Cassell, 1969.

Stewart, D. B.: The gynecological lesions of lymphogranuloma venereum and granuloma inguinale. Med. Clinics. N. Am., *48:*773, 1964.

Hemophilus (Bordetella) Pertussis (Whooping Cough)

Lapin, J. H.: *Whooping Cough.* Springfield, Ill. Charles C Thomas, 1943.

Pittman, M.: Bordetella pertussis bacteria and host factors in the pathogenesis and prevention of whooping cough. In Mudd, S. (ed.), *Infectious Agents and Host Reactions*, Philadelphia, W. B. Saunders, Co., 1970.

Hemophilus ducreyi (*Chancroid*)

Heyman, A., Beeson, P. B. and Sheldon, W. H.: Diagnosis of chancroid. JAMA, *129*:935, 1945.

Heyman, A.: The clinical and laboratory differentiation between chancroid and lymphogranuloma venereum. Am. J. Syph., *30*:279, 1946.

Hemophilus influenzae

Feingold, M. and Gellis, S. S.: Cellulitis due to *H. Influenzae* Type B, N. Eng. J. Med., *272*:788, 1965.

Holderway, M. D. and Turck, D. C.: Capsulated *H. Influenzae* and respiratory tract disease. Lancet, *1*:358, 1967.

Klebsiella—Aerobacter

Chapts. 9, 14, 24.

Listeria monocytogenes (*Listeriosis*)

Gray, M. L. and Killinger, A. H.: *Listeria monocytogenes* and Listeria infections. Bact. Rev., *30*:309, 1966.

Hoeprich, P. D.: Infections due to *Listeria monocytogenes*. Med., *37*:143, 1958.

Malleomyces mallei (*Glanders*)

Howe, C. and Miller, W. R.: Human glanders, report of six cases. Ann. Int. Med., *26*:115, 1947.

Mendelson, R. W.: Glanders. U. S. Armed Forces Med. J., *1*:781, 1950.

Malleomyces pseudomallei (*Melioidosis*)

Khaira, B. S., Korenz, W. B. and Hart, P.: Melioidosis. Brit. Med. J., *1*:959, 1959.

Spotnitz, M., Rudnitsky, J., and Rambaul, J. J.: Melioidosis pneumonitis. JAMA, *202*:950, 1967.

Weber, D. R. *et al.*: Acute varieties of melioidosis occurring in U. S. soldiers in Vietnam. Am. J. Med., *46*:234, 1969.

Mimeae (*Mima Polymorpha, Herellea*)

Reynolds, R. C. and Cluff, L. E.: Infections of man with Mimeae. Ann. Int. Med., *58*:759, 1963.

Mycobacterium leprae (*Leprosy*)

Cochrane, R. G. and Davey, T. F. (eds.): *Leprosy in Theory and Practice,* 2nd ed., Bristol, John Wright and Sons, Ltd. 1964.

Trautman, J. R.: The management of leprosy and its complications. N. Eng. J. Med., *273*:756, 1965.

Mycobacterium tuberculosis

Chapt. 16.

Neisseria gonorrheae

Dalzell-Ward, A. J.: Venereal diseases—new problems for the physician and the community. Disease-a-Month, Jan., 1971.

Keiser, H. *et al.*: Clinical forms of gonococcal arthritis. N. Eng. J. Med., *279*:234, 1968.

Trimble, C.: Gonococcal perihepatitis simulating acute cholecystitis. S. G. & O., *130*:54, 1970.

Willcox, R. R.: Some recent developments in the treatment of gonorrhea. Brit. J. Ven. Dis., *46*:141, 1970.

Neisseria meningitidis

Chapt. 21.

Pasteurella (*Franciscella*) *multocida*

Bearn, A. G., Jacobs, K. and McCarty, M.: *Pasteurella multocida* septicemia in man. Am. J. Med., *18*:167, 1955.

Olson, A. M. and Medhorn, G. M.: Pasteurella multocida in suppurative diseases of the respiratory tract. Am. J. Med. Sci., *224*:79, 1952.

Pasteurella (*Franciscella*) *pestis* (*Plague*)

Gilbert, D. N., Moore, W. L., Hedberg, L. L. and Sanford, J. P.: Potential medical problems in personnel returning from Vietnam. Ann. Int. Med., *68*:662, 1968.

Pollitzer, R.: A review of recent literature on plague. Bull. WHO No. 23, pp. 313–400, Geneva, 1960.

Pasteurella (*Franciscella*) *tularensis* (*Tularemia*)

Foshay, L.: Tularemia. Ann. Rev. Microbiol., *4*:313, 1950.

Young, L. S.: Tularemia Epidemic: Vermont, 1969. N. Eng. J. Med., *280*:1253, 1969.

Proteus Species

Chapt. 24, 27.

Tillotson, J. R. and Lerner, A. M.: Characteristics of pneumonia caused by bacillus Proteus. Ann. Int. Med., *68*:287, 1968.

Pseudomonas aeruginosa

Chapt. 9, 14, 24.

Curtin, J. A., Petersdorf, R. G. and Bennett, I. L., Jr.: Pseudomonas bacteremia. Ann. Int. Med., *54*:1077, 1961.

Tillotson, J. R. and Lerner, A. M.: Pseudomonas pneumonia. Ann. Int. Med., *68*:295, 1968.

Salmonella (*Other Types*)

Aserkoff, B. and Bennett, J. V.: Effect of antibiotic therapy in acute Salmonellosis on the fecal excretion of Salmonellae. N. Eng. J. Med., *281*:636, 1969.

Blank, P. H., Kunz, L. J. and Swartz, M. N.: Salmonellosis—A review of some unusual aspects. N. Eng. J. Med., *262*:811, 864, 921, 1960.

Robertson, R. P., *et al.*: Chloramphenicol and ampicillin in Salmonella enteric fever. N. Eng. J. Med., *278*:173, 1968.

Woodward, T. E.: Typhoid fever and other salmonelloses. Resid. Phy., 73, April, 1967.

Salmonella typhosa

Gulati, P. D., *et al.*: Changing patterns of typhoid fever. Am. J. Med., *45*:544, 1968.

Stuart, B. M. and Pullen, R. L.: Typhoid: Clinical analyses of 360 cases. Arch. Int. Med., *78*:629, 1942.

Woodward, T. E., Smadel, J. E., Parker, R. T., and Wisseman, C. L., Jr.: Treatment of typhoid fever with antibiotics. Ann. N. Y. Acad. Sci., *55*:1043, 1952.

Shigella

Barrett-Conner, E.: Shigellosis in the adult. JAMA, *198*:717, 1966.
Reller, L. B., *et al.*: Shigellosis in the United States, 1964–1968. J. Infect. Dis., *120*:393, 1969.

Staphylococcus aureus and albus

Chapt. 19.

Streptococcus (Group A and Others)

Chapt. 20.

Spirochetes

Borrelia (Relapsing Fevers)

Gefel, A., Anzarut, A. and Pruzanski, J.: Clinical picture and therapy of tickbourne relapsing fever. Israel Med. J., *23*:211, 1964.
World Health Organization. Louseborne relapsing fever. Weekly Epidem. Record, *44*:425, 1969.

Leptospira interrogans (Leptospirosis, Weil's Disease)

Edward, G. A. and Downer, B. M.: Human leptospirosis. Med., *39*:117, 1960.
Gillespie, R. W. H. and Ryno, J.: Epidemiology of leptospirosis. Am. J. Pub. Health, *53*:950, 1963.
Heath, L. W., *et al.*: Leptospirosis in the United States. N. Eng. J. Med., *273*:16, 857, 1965.
Turner, L. H.: Leptospirosis. Brit. Med. J., *1*:231, 1969.

Streptobacillus moniliformis (Rat Bite Fever)

Roughgarden, J. W.: Antimicrobial therapy of rat-bite fever. Arch. Int. Med., *116*:39, 1965.
Watkins, C. F.: Rat-bite fever. J. Ped., *28*:429, 1946.

Treponema carateum (Pinta)

Christiansen, S.: A study of pinta in Mexico. Bull. WHO, 1970.

Treponema pallidum (Syphilis)

Dalzell-Ward, A. J.: Venereal diseases—new problems for the physician and the community. Disease-a-Month, Jan., 1971.
Dunlap, E. M. C.: Problems in syphilis: A review article. Abstracts of World Med., *44*:241, 1970.
Hudson, E. H.: *Non-venereal Syphilis.* E & S Livingstone, Ltd., Edinburgh & London, 1958.

Treponema pertenue (Yaws)

Hackett, C. J. and Lowenthal, L. J. A.: Differential diagnosis of yaws. WHO, Geneva, Mon. Ser. No. 45, 1960.

Fungi

Tropical ulcer

Castellani, A.: The common ulcers of the leg, cosmopolitan and tropical. J. Trop. Med. Hygiene, *60*:55, 91, 1957.

General References

Emmons, E. W., Binford, C. H. and Utz, J. P.: *Medical Mycology,* 2nd ed., Philadelphia, Lea and Febiger, 1970.

Actinomyces israeli (*Actinomycosis in Man*)

Harvey, J. C., *et al.:* Actinomycosis, its recognition and treatment. Ann. Int. Med., *46*:868, 1957.
Peabody, J. W. and Seaburg, J.: Actinomycosis and nocardiosis. Am. J. Med., *28*:99, 1960.

Aspergillus fumigatus (*Aspergillosis*)

Ramirez, J.: Pulmonary aspergillosis. N. Eng. J. Med., *271*:1201, 1964.
Utz, J. P., *et al.:* Pulmonary aspergillosis with cavitation. N. Eng. J. Med., *260*:264, 1959.

Blastomyces brasiliensis (*South American Blastomycosis*)

Furtado, T. A., Wilson, J. W. and Plunkett, O. A.: South American blastomycosis or paracoccidioidomycosis. Arch. Derm., *70*:166, 1954.

Blastomyces dermatititis (*North American Blastomycosis*)

Abernathy, R. S. and Jansen, G. T.: Therapy with amphotericin B in North American blastomycosis. Ann. Int. Med., *53*.1190, 1960.
Harrell, E. R. and Curtis, A. C.: North American blastomycosis. Am. J. Med., *27*:750, 1959.
Palmer, P. and McFadden, S. W.: Blastomycosis. N. Eng. J. Med., *279*:18, 979, 1969.

Candida albicans (*Candidiasis, Thrush, Moniliosis*)

Ellis, C. A. and Spivak, M. L.: The significance of candidemia. Ann. Int. Med., *67*:511, 1967.
Louria, D. B. *et al.:* Disseminated moniliasis in the adult. Med. *41*:307, 1962.
Winner, H. I. and Hurley, R.: *Candida albicans.* Boston, Little-Brown and Co., 1964.

Coccidioides immitis (*Coccidioidomycosis*)

Ajello, L. (ed.): *Coccidioidomycosis.* Phoenix, University of Arizona Press, 1967.
Fiese, M. J.: *Coccidioidomycosis.* Charles C Thomas, Springfield, Ill., 1958.
Winn, W. A.: The use of amphotericin B in the treatment of coccidioidal disease. Am. J. Med., *27*:617, 1959.

Cryptococcus neoformans (*Crytococcosis*)

Bindschcr, D. O. and Bennett, J. E.: Serology of human cryptococcosis. Ann. Int. Med., *69*:1, 45, 1968.
Littman, M. L. and Walter, J. E.: Cryptococcosis. Am. J. Med., *45*:923, 1968.
Lowrin, D. B.: Deep seated mycotic infections. N. Eng. J. Med., *277*:1065, 1126, 1967.

Geotrichium candidum (Geotrichosis)

Smith, D. T.: Geotrichosis. J. Chronic Dis., *5*:532, 1957.

Histoplasma capsulatum (Histoplasmosis)

Chapt. 17.

Madurella mycetonia (Maduromycosis, Mycetoma, Madura Foot)

Mohr, J. A. and Muchmore, H. G.: Maduromycosis. JAMA, *204*:335, 1968.

Nocardia asteroides (Nocardiosis)

Murray, J. F., *et al.*: The changing spectrum of nocardiosis. Am. Rev. Resp. Dis., *83*:315, 1961.

Peabody, J. W. and Seaburg, J.: Actinomycosis and nocardiosis. Am. J. Med., *28*:99, 1960.

Weed, L. A., *et al.*: Nocardiosis: Clinical, bacteriologic, and pathologic aspects. N. Eng. J. Med., *253*:1138, 1955.

Phialophora and Cladosporium (Chromoblastomycosis)

Carrion, A. L.: Chromoblastomycosis. Ann. N. Y. Acad. Sci., *50*:1255, 1950.

Rhinosporidium seeberi (Rhinosporidiosis)

Agrawal, S., *et al.*: Generalized rhinosporidiosis with visceral involvement. Arch. Dermat., *80*:22, 1959.

Rhizopus oryzae (Mucormycosis, Phycomycosis)

Burrow, G. N., Salmon, R. B. and Nolan, J. P.: Successful treatment of mucormycosis with amphotericin B. JAMA, *183*:370, 1963.

Deal, W. B. and Johnson, J. E., III: Gastric phycomycosis: Report of a case and review of literature. Gastroenterology, *57*:579, 1969.

McBride, A., *et al.*: Mucormycosis. Am. J. Med., *28*:832, 1960.

Sporotrichum schenkii (Sporotrichosis)

Mikkelsen, W. M., Brandt, R. L. and Harrell, E. R. Sportrichosis: A report of 12 cases including two with skeletal involvement. Ann. Int. Med., *47*:435, 1957.

Wilson, D. E., Mann, J. J., Bennett, J. E. and Utz, J. P.: Clinical features of extracutaneous sporotrichosis. Med., *46*:265, 1967.

Protozoa

Ameba Histolytica (Amebiasis)

Amebiasis: Report of a WHO expert committee. WHO Technical Report Series No. *421*:1–52, 1969.

McHardy, G. and Frye, W. W.: Amebiasis. Disease-a-Month, Aug., 1957.

Balantidium coli (Balantidiasis)

Arean, V. M. and Koppisch, E.: Balantidiasis, a review. Am. J. Path., *32*:1089, 1956.

Swartzwelder, J. C.: Balantidiasis. Am. J. Diag. Dis, *17*:173, 1950

Giardia lamblia

Moore, G. T.: Epidemic Giardiasis at a ski resort. N. Eng. J. Med., *281*:402, 1969.

Hartmannella

Duma, R. J. *et al.*: Primary amebic meningoencephalitis. N. Eng. J. Med., *281*:1315, 1969.

Isospora belli (*Coccidiosis*)

Elsdon-Dew, R. and Freeman, L.: Coccidiosis in man: Experiences in Natal. Tr. Roy. Soc. Trop. Med. Hyg., *47*:209, 1953.

Leishmania braziliensis (*American Mucocutaneous Leishmaniasis*)

Shanbrom, E., *et al.*: Visceral manifestations of American mucocutaneous leishmaniasis. Am. J. Med., *20*:145, 1956.

Leishmania donovani (*Kala-azar*)

Manson-Bahr, P. E. C. and Southgate, B. A.: Recent research on kala-azar in East Africa J. Trop. Med. Hyg., *67*:79, 1964.

Leishmania tropica (*Oriental Sore or Cutaneous Leishmaniasis*)

Kozevnikor, P. V.: Two nosological forms of cutaneous leishmaniasis. Am. J. Trop. Med. Hyg. *12*:719 1963.

Malaria

Cluff, L. E.: Drugs of choice in Malaria. In *Drugs of Choice* Modell, W. E. (ed.), 1971–1972, St. Louis, C. V. Mosby Co., 1972.

Conrad, M. E.: Pathophysiology of malaria: Hematologic observations in human and animal studies. Ann. Int. Med., *70*:134, 1969.

Hunter, G. W., Frye, W. W., and Swartzwelder, J. C.: *A Manual of Tropical Medicine,* 4th Ed. Philadelphia, W. B. Saunders Company, 1966, Chapt. 35, p. 316, by Martin D. Young.

Neva, F. A.: Malaria—recent progress and problems. N. Eng. J. Med., *277*:1241, 1967.

Toxoplasma gondii (*Toxoplasmosis*)

Feldman, H. A.: Toxoplasmosis. N. Eng. J. Med., *279*:1370, 1431, 1968.

Kean, B. H.: An epidemic of acute toxoplasmosis. JAMA, *208*:1002, 1969.

Trypanosoma brucei (*African Trypanosomiasis*)

Mulligan, H. W. and Potts, W. H. (eds.): *The African Trypanosomiasis.* London, Allen and Unwin, 1970.

Trypanosoma cruzi (*Chagas' Disease*)

Chagas' Disease. WHO Tech. Report Series No. 202, 1960.

Laranja, F. S., *et al.*: Chagas' disease. A clinical epidemiologic and pathologic study. Circulation, *14*:1035, 1956.

Helminths (Metazoa)

Cestodes or Tapeworms (*Echinococcosis, Taenia, Diphyllobothrium*)

Hunter, G. W., Frye, W. W. and Swartzwelder, J. C.: *A Manual of Tropical Medicine,* 4th ed. Philadelphia, W. B. Saunders Company, 1966.

Katz, A. M. and Pan, C.: Echinococcosis disease in the United States. Am. J. Med., *25*:759, 1958.

Keeling, J. E. D.: The chemotherapy of cestode infections. In Goldin, *et al.* (eds.). *Advances in Chemotherapy.* London and New York, Academic Press, Inc. 1968, Vol, 3, pp. 109–152.

Trematodes or Flukes (Schistosomiasis, Paragonimiasis, Fasciolopsiasis)

Hunter, G. W., Frye, W. W. and Swartzwelder, J. C.: *A Manual of Tropical Medicine,* 4th ed. Philadelphia, W. B. Saunders Company, 1966. Chapt. 51, Trematodes exclusive of schistosomiasis, pp. 536–560.

Jordon, P.: Chemotherapy of schistosomiasis. Bull. N. Y. Acad. Med., *44*:245, 1968.

Wright, W. H.: Schistosomiasis as a world problem. Bull. N. Y. Acad. Med., *44*:301, 1968.

Nematodes or Round Worms

Ascariasis

Gelpi, A. P. and Mustafa, A.: Ascariasis pneumonia. Am. J. Med., *44*:377, 1968.

Ochsner, A., DeBakey, E. G. and Dixon, J. L.: Complications of ascariasis requiring surgical treatment. J. Dis. Child., *77*:389, 1949.

Cutaneous Larva Migrans

Stone, O. J.: Systemic and tropical thiabendazole for creeping eruption. Texas Rep. Biol. Med., 27 (Suppl. 2) 659, 1969.

Dirofilariasis

Beskin, C. A., Calvin, S. H., Jr., Beaver, P. C.: Pulmonary dirofilariasis. JAMA, *198*:665, 1966.

Enterobiasis

Roger, A. and Berdknikoff, K.: Pinworm infestation in children: The problem and its treatment. J. Can. Med. A., *86*:60, 1962.

Filariasis

Manson-Bahr, P.: The story of *Filaria bancrofti,* a critical review. J. Trop. Med. Hyg., *62*:53, 106, 138, 160, 1959.

Hookworm Disease

Gilles, H. M., Williams, E. J. W., and Ball, P. A. M.: Hookworm infection and anemia. Quart, J. Med., *33*:1, 1964.

Roche, H. and Layrisse, M.: Nature and causes of hookworm anemia. Am. J. Trop. Med., *15*:1031, 1966.

Onchocerciasis

Duke, B. O. L.: Onchocerciasis. Brit. Med. J., *4*:271, 1968.

Pulmonary Tropical Eosinophilia

Donohugh, D. L.: Tropical eosinophilia. N. Eng. J. Med., *269*:1357, 1963.

Strongyloidiasis

Rivers, E.: Hyperinfection syndrome with *Strongyloidiasis stercoritis*. Ann. Int. Med., *72*:199, 1970.

Stennerman, G. N.: Strongyloidiasis in migrants. Pathological and clinical consideration. Gastroenterology, *53*:49, 1967.

Trichinosis

Hall, W. J. and McCabe, W. R.: Trichinosis. Arch. Int. Med., *119*:65, 1967.
Miller, L. H.: Serologic diagnosis of parasitic infections. Ann. Int. Med., *71*:983, 1969.
Most, H.: Trichinellosis in the United States. JAMA, *193*:871, 1965.

Trichuriasis

Jung, R. C. and Jelliffe, D. B.: The clinical picture and treatment of whipworm infection. W. Afr. Med. J., *1*:11, 1952.

Visceral Larva Migrans

Beana, P. C.: The nature of visceral *Larva migrans*. J. Parasit., *55*:3, 1969.
Kerpinski, F. E., Everts-Suarez, E. A. and Sarwitz, W. G.: Larval granulomatosis (visceral *Larva migrans*). J. Dis. Child., *92*:34, 1956.

INDEX